Praise for *The 4 Habits of Healthy Families*

"There is no shortage of quick-fix diet books, but to see how well they all work, just . . . look around. What does work is a thoughtful, practical, sustainable, and family-based strategy for eating well and being active. You really CAN get there from here, but it generally requires expert coaching. Amy Hendel provides exactly that coaching in *The 4 Habits of Healthy Families*. Insightful, compassionate, and practical, this book can make your family healthier. But only if ~~ ~~ so by all means, do!"

—*David L. Katz, M.D., Medical C   nist for*
O, The Oprah Magazine

"Obesity threatens to reverse gai   ...ade in reducing mortality from heart disease and st   ...ates for obesity and type 2 diabetes are increasing and appearing at earlier ages. *The 4 Habits of Healthy Families* by Amy Hendel offers a practical plan to fight obesity by creating a useful category of food types, tips for daily eating and exercise, and many healthy recipes. Most importantly, the crucial role of the family in developing and maintaining healthy eating habits is emphasized."

—*Thomas A. Pfeffer, M.D., Chief, Department of Cardiac Surgery, Southern California Kaiser Permanente President, Board of Directors, American Heart Association, Los Angeles County*

"Amy Hendel has written an extremely helpful book for families who are ready to make the transition from overweight and unfit to healthy and fit. This guide will truly help families create healthier habits through meal planning and exercise advice and will support them every step of the way."

—*Kathie Davis, Executive Director,*
IDEA Health and Fitness Association

"This is a down-to-earth, incredibly important guide to helping families approach the epidemic of obesity. With a commonsense approach Amy Hendel combines her years of experience with patients and the media to provide a comprehensive approach to avoiding and treating unhealthy eating habits for both families and individuals. A must-read for anyone concerned about the health of their family. Excellent!"

—*Anne Peters, MD, FACP, CDE,*
Director of USC Clinical Diabetes Programs

The 4 Habits of Healthy Families

The 4 Habits of Healthy Families

··

Everything Your Family Needs
to Get Healthy and Stay Healthy for Life

··

Amy Hendel, R-PA
Family Lifestyle Therapist, iVillage Coach

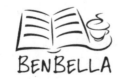

BENBELLA BOOKS, INC.
Dallas, TX

Copyright © 2008 by Amy Hendel

First BenBella Books Paperback Edition 2010

BenBella Books, Inc.
6440 N. Central Expressway, Suite 503
Dallas, TX 75206
Send feedback to feedback@benbellabooks.com
www.benbellabooks.com

Printed in the United States of America
10 9 8 7 6 5 4 3 2 1

Library of Congress Cataloging-in-Publication data is available for this title.
ISBN 978-1935251-77-4

Proofreading by Stacia Seaman
Cover design by Allison Bard
Design and composition by PerfecType, Nashville, TN
Printed by Bang Printing

Distributed by Perseus Distribution
perseusdistribution.com

To place orders through Perseus Distribution:
Tel: 800-343-4499
Fax: 800-351-5073
E-mail: orderentry@perseusbooks.com

Significant discounts for bulk sales are available. Please contact Glenn Yeffeth at glenn@benbellabooks.com or (214) 750-3628.

DEDICATION

For my dad, who I believe is one of those angels put on earth, and in memory of my mom, who so struggled with her weight and her happiness, and for my grandmother, who always made me feel like I could accomplish just about anything.

ACKNOWLEDGMENTS

There are so many people and events that shaped my life and somehow contributed to the writing of this book. I have to thank Maureen Kedes of Vertex Communications for forcing me to realize that there was a book inside of me and Boris for believing in my talents and sticking by when others would not even look my way. I also have to thank Mary for her incredible devotion, enthusiasm, warm words, and most of all for helping my written words to become a true manuscript. A huge thank you to Uwe Stender, my agent, for unbridled enthusiasm and for wanting to show "the big guys how a book deal gets done." To Glenn at BenBella Books, thanks for taking on this project and making me feel like my book was the most important book you were handling. To Leah, thanks for some fine editing and some very funny comments along the way, and to Jennifer, thank you for keeping me in the loop on how a book gets reviewed by the best. To Laura, thanks for hearing my anguish and responding. To the whole team at Krupp Kommunications, thank you for helping me spread the book's message near and far. To Paul, my lawyer and close friend, thank you for doing what most lawyers don't do: giving me more for my money. To Zahava, a special thanks for recipe inspiration and to Barbara, thanks for your cover contributions and your artistic input. To Judy, a client and friend who embraced the HFL program and never looked back, and who constantly gave me words of support, thank you. Finally, to my husband Eli and my children Melanie and Stephen, thank you for making my journey your journey as well.

TABLE OF CONTENTS

1 Facing the Facts to Save Your Family   1
2 What Kind of Food Family Are You?   29
3 Eat Like a Cow and Other Easy Ways Your Family
Can Become a "Healthy Family for Life"   51
4 The "Yes, No, Maybe So" Food Choice Plan   77
5 Focusing on "Yes" Foods: The Healthy Family
Food Superstars   129
6 Healthy Habit #1: Plan Together   157
7 Healthy Habit #2: Prepare Together   197
8 Healthy Habit #3: Portion Together   227
9 Healthy Habit #4: Play Together   253
10 The Right Way (and Wrong Way) to Support Each Other   297
11 Don't Fight the Feelings   315
12 There Are No Perfect Families: The Art of Making
Realistic Goals and Helping Your Family   335
13 Secrets for Changing Kids' and Teens' Habits   367

Yes, No, Maybe So Food Choices   405
HFL Recipes   411
Appendices   431
Useful Web Sites   465
References   467
About the Author   475

1

Facing the Facts to Save Your Family

···

Fat Habits Are Killing Families—But It Doesn't Have to Happen in *Your* Home

···

So you're brave enough to open a book that uses the "f" word, huh?

"F" as in "fat," that is.

Or maybe I should say "f" as in "family" because, in spite of all the attention being given to the obesity epidemic, family is rarely part of the story. Surprisingly little information is available today for the family who wants to develop healthy habits *as a family* to support healthy weight management.

And that's a crying shame, because fat is a family matter. We learn habits as a family, and if anything is inextricably linked to family traditions, it's food. The habits we develop in our families today can last for generations to come. The good news is that we can unlearn habits as a family, too. We can change our family food traditions, very likely saving our families in the process. And that's what this book is all about.

If you're reading this, you're probably courageous enough to start facing the truth about your family's eating habits. You are feeling symptoms of poor health at home, and are fearful of the ramifications for yourself and your family. You've probably already decided that fads don't work: you know they just mean an endless, frustrating, and self-defeating cycle of weight gain and loss. You know that extremely rigid or complicated diets are impossible to stick to—you lose weight but don't keep it off. You just want to be able to enjoy healthy, good-tasting food with your family, without spending countless hours cooking.

You want the best for your family, but somehow it's all gotten out of control—the TV watching, the loss of focus on nutrition, the everyone-for-themselves eating habits, the lack of family meals, the on-the-run eating, all the fast food and packaged food. Over and over again, you find yourself desperately asking, "How can I get a grip on this chaos?"

You may have experienced one or more of the following:

- You and/or other members of your family have tried countless diets, succeeding briefly only to return to old habits.
- You want to develop better eating habits that will benefit your whole family (especially your kids), but you can't seem to find the time or the energy to change—or you don't know where to start.
- You and/or family members have become couch potatoes who eat poorly and rarely exercise.
- Some or all of your family struggles with weight.
- You know your kids are not eating right and are at risk for a host of lifestyle-related diseases.
- You and/or family members have been diagnosed as being at risk for or already having hypertension or diabetes.

I talk to families every day who share these same challenges. I know how hard it is to climb out of that pit we call "denial" and start scaling the mountain of change. But I have helped hundreds of families do just that, and I can help yours.

You might be surprised to learn that some of the families I work with aren't overweight. That's because families can easily have unhealthy attitudes and habits that have not expressed themselves in excess weight—but you can be sure the negative consequences are there just the same.

That's because it is possible to be slim—even downright thin—and eat a high-fat, highly processed diet and/or get very little exercise. Even if it seems you are "getting away with it," inside you are setting up clogged arteries and lining them with plaque, taxing your liver with cholesterol overload, stressing your pancreas with way too much sugar, weakening your bones with no activity, and generally developing fatty organs. New research tells us that having fat deposits on internal organs like the heart, liver, or pancreas can be as dangerous, if not more so, than the symptoms of a typical over-weight person.[1] The term *TOFI* (Thin Outside Fat Inside) was created to describe this newly diagnosed subset of the population. From a behavior and health perspective, you can indeed be "fat," even if the scale isn't showing it.

Do you have a friend or someone you know who can truly take "just one bite" and be satisfied? They may not be particularly slim or thin—they may just be of average build and weight. But what they have is a "thin" attitude. Some experts describe it as a "relaxed relationship with food." They don't think about food all the time, they don't obsess about treats and desserts, they understand hunger and eat for satisfaction, they enjoy tasty food while still being able to push a half-filled plate aside when full. People with "thin" attitudes typically share these traits:

- They stop eating when they are satisfied and rarely get over-stuffed.
- They do not treat hunger like a 911 emergency.
- They don't turn to food for comfort.
- They tend to like fruits and vegetables.
- They usually follow some kind of daily, organized food schedule, with meal planning and timing as a framework.
- They exhibit restraint and self-control when it comes to eating and food sampling.

- They tend to be active—it's second nature to them.
- They have generally healthy habits, like not missing breakfast and keeping good sleep patterns.

Not surprisingly, these are the same traits shared by healthy families. Although your family may not exhibit these healthy food behaviors now, they can learn. Making that shift to a "thin" attitude and healthy habits is what this book is all about.

You Do Have the Power to Save Your Family

As a Physician Assistant who has worked with hundreds of families to achieve their nutrition, activity, and weight management goals over the past two decades, I know there is a serious disorder sweeping through homes across America. It is a *feeding disorder* and it has components that are learned, habitual, and possibly even addictive.

The obesity crisis is on the home front, and family habits are at the root of it. In many cases, busy schedules and "convenient" food choices have replaced healthier routines, and these new habits are rapidly undermining our health. For example, you may have pleasant childhood memories of home-cooked meals and family activities and gatherings. Ideally, family time, and family-meal time, should conjure up positive associations. For younger generations today, however, many of those positive feelings may be linked primarily to TV-watching and junk food.

Will your children associate happy, satisfying feelings with fat and sugar—or with nutritious meals, fun activities, and family love and support? The choice is up to you.

Those of us who are parents need to rise to the occasion, own up to our responsibility, and take charge of the situation. By monitoring our own weight, following a nutrient-rich diet (from pregnancy and even before), keeping a healthy selection of foods in the home, limiting sedentary screen-watching time, and modeling daily physical activity, we have the power to turn our families—and the future—around.

Kids don't just get fat (in their habits or in actual physical size). It happens insidiously in the home, usually because of the way parents are running the ship. Whether you realize it or not, as a parent, you are the policymaker. You are entrusted with making the decisions on everything from how recreation time is spent to how food dollars are allocated. You are responsible for the kinds and amounts of food available in the home, and the manner in which it is prepared. Your choices largely determine everything from the amount of time that is spent together as a family unit to the way your kids learn to handle their emotions (with communication or with candy bars.)

It may sound like a tall order, but if parents don't turn families around, who will? I've seen many families succeed at changing their lifestyles, so I know it can be done. Most families (like yours) just need a little practical help, and that's why I developed the Healthy Family for Life (HFL) program. It was created from more than twenty years of experience with families struggling for better control of eating habits, exercise habits, cravings, and emotional eating patterns. I've introduced this structured, easy-to-follow manual to hundreds of families, and the results have been remarkable. That's how I can tell you that this program *will work for the family who works together*.

Unlike nearly all of the healthy eating and weight loss plans available today, the HFL program is a whole-family approach. It will take you step by step through daily planning, preparation, and portioning of food for your family, as well as what you need to do to get the activity you need. This is a practical program designed by a busy parent for busy parents. You'll see how I use these ideas with my own family throughout the book.

If you are asking yourself, "Are the foods and drinks I'm serving my kids healthy and appropriately portioned?" the answer is probably no. If you are asking yourself, "Do we move enough, get enough exercise, and eat together enough?" the answer is probably no. Unfortunately, that's the answer for most families today, and most families need help with healthy lifestyle management in order to avoid the modern obesity trap and the health traps that follow. This program is about saving yourself, saving your kids, and maybe even saving their kids.

I am telling you that tomorrow is too late. If you were brave enough to pick up this book (even with its "in your face" title!), then you are ready to face the perils of your current home food and activity environment—and you're ready to take on the day-to-day changes needed to turn the situation around.

Family Wake-Up Call

In May 2005, former Arkansas governor Mike Huckabee published his book on weight loss, *Quit Digging Your Grave with a Knife and Fork.* That sober warning says a mouthful. And now our First Lady, Michelle Obama, has created her Let's Move initiative to address the alarming rising tide of childhood obesity.

Our children are expected to be the first generation of Americans who will live a shorter lifespan than their parents. We are eating ourselves to death and handing our self-destructive habits off to our kids.

It's impossible to watch the news for very long without hearing alarming updates on the escalating rates of obesity, diabetes, and metabolic syndrome, all conditions associated with how we choose to live our lives. Reality TV programs showcase their successful "losers," only many of them regain their weight after leaving the strict confines of the show's protective and secluded settings.

Obesity is one of our nation's biggest public health dangers, despite the fact that, on average, nearly two-thirds of Americans say that their doctor or health care provider has talked to them about issues like weight management and exercise. Here are some of the most startling facts, based on reports from 2005 and 2006:

- Obesity rates have not dropped in a single state in the last year (2006).[2]
- Adult obesity rates exceed 20 percent in forty-seven states and the District of Columbia; even the leanest state, Colorado, showed a 1.3 percent increase in rates of obesity among its adults from 2005 to 2006.[2]
- The rate of obesity in children more than tripled from 1980 to 2004.[2]

- There was a 167 percent spike in girls between the ages of ten and nineteen taking oral medication for type 2 diabetes, formerly known as adult-onset diabetes, in 2004.[3]
- The fastest-growing group of obese Americans consists of people who are at least 100 pounds overweight. Between 2000 and 2005, the prevalence of a BMI greater than forty (indicating clinically severe obesity) increased by 50 percent.[2]
- Almost one-third of eighteen-year-olds who applied for service in all branches of the military in 2005 were overweight, according to a recent report by the Army.[2]
- Spending in fast food restaurants grew eighteen times (from $6 billion to $110 billion) in the past three decades. In 1970, there were approximately thirty thousand fast food restaurants in the U.S.; in 2001, there were approximately two hundred and twenty-two thousand.
- A 2005 study reported in the *Archives of Neurology* concluded that obesity at midlife is associated with an increased risk of dementia and Alzheimer's disease later in life.
- Adults consumed approximately 300 more calories daily in 2002 than they did in 1985.
- Average consumption of added sugars increased 22 percent from the early 1980s to 2000.
- Obesity accounts for three hundred thousand deaths per year. (Department of HHS, 2006)

Current statistics indicate:

- Two-thirds of all American adults are obese or overweight.[2]
- Nearly one in three adults—30.6 percent—are now reported to be obese in Mississippi, the first time adult obesity rates have exceeded 30 percent in a single state.[2]
- Approximately twenty-five million children are now overweight or obese in America.
- It is estimated that 14.8 percent of youth ages ten to seventeen are overweight.[2]
- GERD (heartburn) rates are rising among kids and teens, and obesity is considered one of the possible causes. Eight of the

ten states with the highest rates of adult diabetes are also in the top fifteen states with the highest obesity rates, and nine of the ten states with the highest rates of adult hypertension are also in the top fifteen states with the highest rates of obesity.[2]

- An estimated 16 percent of active duty military personnel are currently obese and 18.9 percent of active duty soldiers under the age of twenty-one are obese.[2]

- Only one in five Americans consumes the recommended amount of fruit each day.[2]

- Sixty percent of adults are not sufficiently active to achieve health benefits.[2]

- Nearly 10 percent of high school students do not regularly participate in vigorous or moderate physical activity, only 54 percent of high school students had physical education class at least once a week, and only 33 percent had daily physical education.

- More than 20 percent of high school students played video or computer games or used a computer for something other than schoolwork for three or more hours on an average school day.

- More than 35 percent of high school students watched three or more hours of TV on an average school day.

- Obese women are more likely to have an infant with spina bifida, other neural tube defects, and heart defects as compared to normal-weight women.[4]

- The U.S. health care system spends $70 billion annually to treat obesity and related conditions.

- Obesity now rivals tobacco in terms of its impact on health risk and morbidity, with cancer deaths 50–60 percent higher in the obese.[5]

- More than 20 million adult Americans have diabetes. Approximately 176,500 individuals under the age of twenty have diabetes, 54 million Americans are pre-diabetic, and 2 million adolescents (or one in six overweight adolescents) have pre-diabetes.

- More than 75 percent of hypertension cases are reported to be directly attributable to obesity.

- Approximately 20 percent of cancer in women and 15 percent of cancer in men is attributable to obesity.

Future predictions include:

- Physical inactivity is tied to heart disease and stroke risk factors in children and adolescents. And according to studies by NIH and CDC, physical inactivity can lead to increased risk of insulin resistance and the eventual development of diabetes and heart disease in children and adolescents.
- For children born in the year 2000, the lifetime risk of developing diabetes is 30 percent for boys and 40 percent for girls, if obesity rates level off.[6]
- Currently 66 percent of U.S. adults are overweight or obese. By 2015, 75 percent of U.S. adults are expected to be overweight and 41 percent of those will be obese.

The obesity problem is not solely an American phenomenon. I recently traveled to Israel, a country where I assumed good eating habits were well entrenched. (After all, I grew up loving Israeli salad!) While working out in the hotel gym, I watched a morning news show tackle the "growing problem of obesity in Israel." I almost fell off the treadmill in shock. It seems that kids in Israel are on computers and cell phones for hours, not outdoors playing or working like previous generations. Fast food has also invaded their country.

On a trip to Italy, I saw that many Italians eat meals slowly and really savor their food. They don't serve gargantuan portions in restaurants, and there's a smart workday break in the afternoon that allows people to accomplish errands, take a long lunch, and walk. Still, thanks to the invasion of unhealthy food and more sedentary living, even Italy, along with France and Britain, is experiencing increasing rates of obesity among the adult and child populations.[7] In addition to the fast food, processed food, and high-sugar sodas available, the changing physical nature of communities and the disappearing family meal—even in these countries—all contribute to the rising tide of obesity.

Worldwide, 40 percent of men and 30 percent of women are now overweight; 24 percent of men and 27 percent of women are

THE PREGNANCY LINK

The stakes for having a healthy pregnancy are high—really high. We all know that before getting pregnant—and certainly during pregnancy—you want to stop smoking, stop drinking alcoholic beverages, take folic acid and other important vitamins, and of course, gain the right amount of weight. We also need to be aware that research is painting a disturbing picture of the interaction between women, weight, diet, blood sugar levels, pregnancy, and the health impact on children:

- Elevated blood sugars alone—not even actual diabetes—during a pregnancy can double the risk of having a child who will be overweight by age seven.[8]

- Women who are overweight *before* pregnancy are more likely to have children with higher rates of body fat by age nine, regardless of how much weight they gained *during* pregnancy.[8] Their pre-pregnancy weight directly impacted the future weight stores of their child.

- Women who ate a low-carbohydrate, high-protein diet (including a fair amount of red meat daily) had children who had an increased risk of high blood pressure and were also very sensitive to stress (had exaggerated physical responses) in middle age. [8]

Beyond genes, the environment, and the food that children eat after birth, the slogan *"You are what you eat"* is now being expanded to *"You are what your mother ate!"* David Barker, adjunct professor at Oregon Health & Sciences University, created a theory now called the Barker Hypothesis. He claims that studies have now linked adult heart disease, diabetes, stroke, high blood pressure, and even osteoporosis to low birth weight.

But the newest concern is women who are overweight, eating a poor diet, and giving birth to overly large babies. Those babies may be tomorrow's adults with diabetes and other serious health issues.

obese. Obesity has become a major clinical and public health problem in a number of countries.[9]

A rather sobering reality is that if historical obesity trends were to continue through 2020 here in the United States, without other changes in behavior or medical technology, the proportion of individuals reporting fair or poor health that directly relates to their being overweight would increase by about 12 percent for men and 14 percent for women, compared with statistics in 2000. Up to one-fifth of health care expenditures would be devoted to treating the consequences of obesity.[10]

I'm not fond of scare tactics, but in this case, the statistics are overwhelming. We need to be not just scared, but horrified, and that horror should spur us into action, for the sake of our own health, and especially for the sake of our kids.

Is It Genetics?

The first obesity gene was discovered back in 1994. Since then, almost fifty genes have been identified that may be involved in obesity.[10] Some may determine how a person lays down fat and metabolizes stored energy. Others may influence how much people want to eat, how they know when they've had enough, and how many calories they use in activities that range from fidgeting to strenuous exercise. These genes may explain why some people can gain weight from what might be considered a lower-calorie plan, because they are so efficient at storing calories.

Genetic factors may affect a variety of areas related to obesity. Many of the body's systems that regulate eating and body weight initially develop in utero during critical periods in brain development, and these may affect a child's eating and body weight—in particular, body fat—later in life.[11]

Your parents' weight directly correlates to your "weight future." A recent study found that a child is at much greater risk of being overweight by the age of seven when one parent was obese; with two obese parents, the risk was even higher.[12] When parents are obese, a child also has more than twice the risk of being obese as an adult (60 percent risk), regardless of whether he or she was obese before the

TRENDS IN THE RIGHT DIRECTION

You're not alone in taking action to turn the tide on unhealthy living. There are lots of signs that times are changing—and in a good way:

- Food companies are taking action to show that they realize the strong connection between food advertising and kids. Kraft Foods has announced that it would only advertise products that meet healthy standards to kids ages six to eleven during children's broadcast TV and radio programming, as well as in print media geared to this age group.
- *Sesame Street* has used characters to model fun ways to move and play, as well as fun and healthy snack food suggestions.
- Univision has introduced healthy lifestyle messages to its Hispanic/Latino viewing audience.
- PepsiCo has committed to reaching the goal of 50 percent of new product revenues from its healthful product line. PepsiCo has also launched a marketing program that promotes a healthier lifestyle to its consumers in print and TV ads.
- Former President Bill Clinton faced an obesity crisis and heart attack himself and resolved to change his dietary and exercise habits (once an alarming health issue was diagnosed and treated). He has joined forces with the American Heart Association to spearhead a campaign to fight childhood obesity. [13] Removing soda from school vending machines and targeting healthier snacks and lunches in school, Clinton is focusing his efforts on school food reform.
- There have been changes in national school lunch programs, vending machine policies, and even physical

> ## TRENDS IN THE RIGHT DIRECTION, *continued*
>
> education. In California, there is an ongoing movement to ensure that every child or youth participates in physical activity each day at school, that affordable fresh fruits and vegetables are available in all neighborhoods, especially low-income areas, and that junk food and soda are banned from schools.
>
> - Amish Naturals, the maker of a variety of pastas, offers whole wheat and fiber-rich pastas. They are now launching a new fiber-rich granola bar, and a campaign to promote the benefits of a fiber-rich diet and their "Amish Fiber."

age of ten. By contrast, a preschool child with parents of normal weight has only about a 25 percent chance of being overweight as an adult.[14]

New research suggests that eating is a reinforcing activity, but there appear to be significant differences, because of genetic variations, in the perceived reward that food gives to people.[15] The research suggests that *some people eat to live while others live to eat* and it adds another explanation to why some people may overeat. The study revealed that some people have lower dopamine levels (a brain neurotransmitter that helps make behaviors and substances more rewarding) so they are more likely to feel the reward of food when they stimulate those dopamine levels, so they not only eat, they overeat.

Genetically speaking, if you have more dopamine receptors, it may be easier for you to experience reward, in this case from eating food, so you will tend not to overeat. If you have fewer dopamine receptors, you may be more susceptible to the food-pleasure reward and overeat in an attempt to achieve that feeling.

Beyond genetics, other "outside" factors may play a role in fostering obesity. There is an emerging field of microorganisms and obesity called *infectobesity*. The word was coined by N. Dhurandhar, MD, head of the Biomedical Research Center in Baton Rouge, Louisiana, who sees a relationship between obesity and viruses.[16] The theory is that some intestinal microbes or viruses may be making their human hosts fat. Other theories offer the idea that since certain gut flora actually *prevent* the body from storing fat, if we could find a way to give these flora to people, perhaps we could offset a predisposition to weight gain.

Still another theory says you may actually be able to *catch a virus*—an adenovirus, to be exact—from a newly infected person who is a carrier (so he himself is not necessarily overweight) and this virus (Ad-36) can cause you either to produce more fat cells or to produce superior fat cells that can hold more fat per cell.[16] Even C-reactive protein, produced by the liver during systemic inflammation in the body and specifically implicated in heart disease and other conditions that may have an inflammatory component, may be causing a kind of chaos among fat regulation, contributing to excess fat.[16]

The Choice Is Still Yours

The reality is that genetics clearly play a role in family and individual predisposition to obesity; other factors beyond our control may do so as well. But that doesn't change the bottom line: how you choose to eat and live is up to you.

Forget the factors your family can't control because what matters are those you can: Do you choose to walk daily? Do you choose to lift weights? Do you choose to control the size of your portions? Do you choose to stock your pantry with healthy options? Do your daily life habits support weight gain or do they deter weight gain?

The healthy new habits suggested throughout this book can help minimize the impact of any negative predispositions you or your family have and give you control of your health. Regardless of your genetic heritage, you are not a helpless victim when it comes to weight or eating habits. Biology and genetics may set the stage, but it's up to you to direct the play of your life, and that includes the food and activity choices you make.

My Story

I was born into a world where food was worshipped, embraced, caressed, and enjoyed. I was born to Jewish parents.

Almost all Jewish holidays and celebrations revolve around food. There's honey and apples and sweet treats on the Jewish New Year, Hamentashen cookies on Purim, all kinds of matzo treats on Passover, not to mention the weekly challah (egg bread) and sweet wine served every Friday night. Even the Yom Kippur fast is followed by a "break the fast feast."

I was also the child of a woman who expressed her happiness, sadness, frustration, anxiety—pretty much any feeling—by eating.

My mother was not a particularly good cook. Money was tight, so she approached the week with "standards." Monday night was a fish dish (I would call that a healthy night), Tuesday was meatloaf, Wednesday was tuna noodle casserole (with three different cheeses, macaroni, and cream of mushroom soup), Thursday was lamb chops and potatoes, and Friday was always chicken or goulash (meat stew) with potatoes or kugel (a potato or noodle baked casserole). Saturday night meant pizza and Sunday night was leftovers.

You get the picture: filling comfort food, always served with a salad, though, as my mother's homage to a healthy diet. It was homemade; we didn't eat too much store-bought food during my childhood (too expensive). Except for snacks. I was from the generation of Ding Dongs® and Yodels®, apple-filled pastries and pound cake. Pop-Tarts® featured prominently, as did chips, cookies, pretzels, and licorice.

I couldn't help but notice how food seemed to calm my mother down; by association, I too began to turn to food when I received a bad grade, lost a school election, got scolded. There was always some treat available at home, ready to be hoarded and enjoyed in secret. I learned from the best, watching my mom seek solace in food secretly (or so she thought).

I knew what was going on behind the one bathroom door when she would stay in there a long time. I knew when she closed her bedroom door at night before my dad came home that she was "visiting" with food "friends," and I know a lot of eating went on while I was in school.

Over time, I developed a true hankering for sweet treats, and my palate seemed to crave these goodies. My extra weight and "thunder thighs" (a popular phrase at the time) became a serious problem around the age of sixteen, when my group of friends started dating. I was always pretty smart academically, good at sports, but I wore braces and glasses and then there was the extra weight—what an awkward stage.

One day, I had one of those true epiphanies when you just get fed up. The only options were starvation or a balanced diet. I marched myself and a friend off to a local meeting of the only structured diet program available at that time. We did the mortifying weigh-in and I settled down for my first nutrition lecture. The downside was that most of the women had forty years on me, so I didn't necessarily relate to their perspectives or feel any sort of camaraderie. The upside was that no one knew me, so I could keep my "shameful" struggle somewhat private and interact minimally.

Ultimately, that friend became my weight loss buddy and we both dropped serious pounds. By the beginning of my junior year in high school, the braces were off, contacts were in, forty-two pounds were gone—and my mother was really, really unhappy. Yup, I was no longer sharing secret binges. I now understand that my success was a real slap in the face to her, and it took me years to understand her true emotional pain.

That was the beginning of my dedication to weight management, health, and fitness. I have kept those forty pounds off ever since those teenage years, and it hasn't always been easy. I have to pay attention to what I eat and I am passionate about regular exercise to this day. And I have taken these habits into my family life. Naturally, I wanted to spare my children the struggles I experienced. Throughout this book, I'll share how I have met the nutritional health challenges of my own family, and how you can, too.

Beyond my own experience as a health-conscious wife and mother, I have worked first as a Physician Assistant and then for more than eighteen years as a Family Lifestyle Coach, focusing on family nutrition, working with clients referred from physicians.

During my training to become a Physician Assistant, my specialty was in Internal Medicine and Dependency Medicine—invaluable experience for my work today. Working with people suffering from drug and alcohol dependency enhanced my understanding of dysfunctional relationships with food. In order for addicts to have a successful rehabilitation, they needed to do many of the same things that people with food and weight problems need to do: distance themselves from their drug of choice, examine their relationship with the drug, create an ongoing plan to deal with day-to-day situations that would put them at risk for relapse, and create a support system that involves their family and others who had detoxed successfully.

As a certified personal trainer and professional member of IDEA Health and Fitness Association, my approach to family wellness integrates physical activity with nutrition education. My training and background in medicine, nutrition, and exercise have given me a strong foundation to help families transform their health habits. I have helped hundreds of families move from unhealthy eating and activity habits to healthy ones. This book is about helping your family make that move, too.

Why It Takes a Family

After working with thousands of people to help them change their eating and exercise habits, I came to the conclusion that you cannot pull off a lifestyle change in isolation. Imagine a drug addict going through rehabilitation and then coming home every day to a drug den. Do you really think an addict could avoid a relapse with that kind of temptation at his doorstep every single day?

If Mom or Dad decides to diet and starts to drink those shakes or control food portions, but they still bring home processed foods, fast foods, and temptations for the rest of the family, they'll invariably falter and fail. Kids don't fare any better when they're expected to make changes while other family members maintain old habits. Would you place a child with an allergy to grass in a room filled with a patchwork grass floor? Can you imagine this child tiptoeing around all day long trying to avoid the grass patches?

When you have one child at home who needs to lose weight and you create a set of guidelines that only he or she has to follow while other kids in the family get the extra helpings and treats, resentment and frustration inevitably emerges. It's not complicated science; it's common sense. The best way for family members to get healthy is for the family as a whole to get healthy.

That's why I believe it has to be the family way or no way, and why I chose to write a book about family rather than individual weight management. The HFL program requires—no, demands— that the entire family participate and that the participation be ongoing.

Research is mounting to support the value of a family-based approach to behavior change. A review of a range of studies found that family-based strategies in which parents and children work together are some of the most effective ways to encourage behavior change in individuals seeking to lose weight or improve their health for the long term, and that a family-based approach can "produce significant long-term sustainable results."[17]

I'm of the belief, as are many others, that the home environment will have the single most profound influence on your child's food habits, food choices, palate or taste determination, level of activity, and overall health. America on the Move did a study revealing that among 1,487 children, 71 percent said they get information on how to be healthy from their moms.

Keith Ayoob, a nationally known nutrition expert and a dietician at the Albert Einstein College of Medicine, says, "Parents are hands down the biggest influence on their kids. They need to be good role models." This speaks volumes more than genetic or family predisposition factors when it comes to kids and weight issues.

Studies have now revealed that the very choices we parents are making for our children are setting them up for obesity—and it has little to do with genetics and very much to do with exposures to certain food tastes and certain portion sizes. If you choose to feed an infant sweetened beverages and high-fat or sweet-tasting foods, it may instigate an early preference for such foods and beverages, which can then contribute in a very significant way to that child becoming overweight.[18] As a parent who has raised two children in this environment of fast food, highly processed foods, and caloric sugar-laden drinks, I have seen that kids are being given far too many of these kinds of foods, far too early in their lives and far too frequently. In fact, the Feeding Infants and Toddlers Study (FITS) found that infants as young as seven months old are being fed soft drinks (sodas and highly caloric fruit drinks) and french fries.[18]

The bottom line is that because children's preferences for high-fat, energy-dense foods are, in part, learned from their home environment and the environment in which they live, exposing children regularly to these highly caloric, very tempting, large and frequent portions of foods may reinforce their liking for them.[19]

Add to this dismal picture children who are given juice in their bottles as their significant source of hydration instead of water, kids who are kept on full-fat milk past the age of two, kids who are put in front of TVs for hours while snacking on food, and kids who are given few fruits and vegetables, and you are continuing to reinforce unhealthy habits in your home.

Experts believe family-based approaches are most effective when children are young, especially "before obesity-promoting behaviors have become well ingrained."[14] As the team leaders, parents can provide positive behavior for all family members to emulate. Research has found that a big part of this formula is to make sure the family engages in fun and productive physical activity. For example, one hugely beneficial step is to encourage kids to engage in physical activity with their peers instead of parking themselves in front of the TV or computer.[2] Because children also learn behaviors from parents, you should not be seen sitting for hours in front of the TV while telling them to go play with their friends.

So many key lifestyle patterns can be positively influenced by a family approach to behavior change from the very earliest ages. For example, one important predictor of a pudgy preschooler is a child who is still using a bottle by age three.[20] Children who are still drinking substantial calories by bottle (juice, whole milk) are probably doing so in addition to the food calories they are ingesting. Constant access to a bottle means constant consumption of calories, irrespective of hunger. Taking a bottle to bed with a liquid other than water is another bad lifestyle habit that should be discouraged; by one year, a child should be shifting over to drinking from a cup. By age two, unless a child has a health condition that warrants special caloric needs, there should also be a gradual shift to 2 percent, 1 percent, and finally, fat-free milk (this goes for all dairy products). The only way a child ends up with a nighttime bottle filled with a liquid other than water is if their mom or dad fills the bottle with something other than water. The only way a child can continue to drink high-fat milk is if their parents don't make the switch.

Another critical example of how parents can influence family health is TV watching. Studies show that eating in front of the TV can lead to overeating because: 1) you're not clued in to whether or not you're getting full, so you are just shoveling food in without any mindful awareness; 2) you might sit at the table longer to finish watching a show and keep eating just because you sit for a longer period of time, and 3) you are exposed to TV food ads, which can increase your food consumption. A study from the University of Liverpool in the United Kingdom showed that overweight and obese children increase their food intake by more than 100 percent after watching TV ads for food.[21]

Studies also confirm that the current lack of real sit-down family meals seems to be a surefire way to encourage weight gain and poor nutritional choices.[22] More often than not, several different meals are going on with no healthy food choices, parents are totally unaware of what their kids are eating, or parents are modeling poor choices. In any case, studies are clear that the loss of the traditional family meal is a definite contributor to weight and health problems on the home front.

Portion size is a unique issue because we know that until age four, no matter how much food you put on children's plates, they will only eat until they reach a comfortable fullness. They actually have a natural shut-off valve that innately controls how much they will eat.[23] Take young children and put them into an environment of food coercion or threats to "clean your plate" and, over time, they will stop listening to their natural body cues and overeat. Overfill children's plates or regularly put them among people who overeat and cajole them to eat more and you can blur their natural appetite shut-off valve and literally teach them to overeat. In older kids and adults, just the sight of extra food has been implicated in increasing their food intake, even if they're not hungry.[24]

On the other hand, overly restricting food because you struggle with weight or because you perceive your child to be overweight can backfire as well. A child who is overly controlled at meal and snack times is at risk of losing some of the inherent ability to self-regulate, to feel full, and to respond to internal cues that might otherwise guide very normal eating patterns.[25]

It is certainly true that as a society we need to work on improving our food quality, increasing opportunities for activity, developing more public health resources, and creating more responsibility in our media messages. However, as parents, we can't afford to wait for government or society to solve the problem. We have to step in and seize the right to control our home environments and change our habits and priorities.

This is the most important decision you can make as a parent. If you don't take this seriously and take action now, you and your family will join the statistics of individuals suffering with weight and health issues directly related to your lifestyle choices. You could be handing your children the punishment of a shortened or lesser quality of life, and no parent wants to do that.

The Four Habits of Healthy Families

If it seems too daunting to take care of your own individual needs and still find the energy and time to engage your whole family, that's where the HFL program steps in. It offers an organized, step-by-step approach that will maximize your weekly efforts so you minimize your planning, shopping, and preparation time.

The HFL program is organized around the four P's or four Habits of Healthy Families: 1) Planning healthy food, 2) Preparing healthy food, 3) Eating healthy Portions, and, 4) Getting enough "Play" (activity) time:

Plan

You'll be given tools and outlines to help you with everything from menus (to be discussed by all family members) to shopping lists that will cover most of your needs for a week's worth of meals and snacks. Your shopping experience will be simplified by HFL guidelines to help you select the best foods for your menus. You'll learn how to stock your fridge and pantry, plan for meals and snacks outside the home, troubleshoot challenging situations, and develop a new approach to treats.

Prepare

The core of the HFL program includes time-saving tips, habits, and techniques so that you can do most of your food preparation on one designated day each week, so you can prepare fresh, healthy meals nightly in minimal time. You will learn to keep substitute meals on hand for family members who don't participate in meal planning and don't want your main meal choice. You'll learn the easiest, healthiest ways to cook food, with strategies to involve every member of your family.

Portion

You'll learn techniques for *mindful awareness* of calories and portion sizes, so that you and your family can make responsible choices about food amounts based on your health needs and goals.

Play

You'll learn how to develop a fun, active lifestyle that matches the needs and interests of family members of all ages while it helps support healthy weight maintenance for life. You'll learn to "sneak" activity into your family life in a variety of ways.

The heart of the HFL program is the "Yes, No, Maybe So" Food Choice Plan. This is a quick and easy way for you and all the members of your family to make the healthiest food choices for you.

You'll learn to turn as often as possible to rich-in-nutrients Yes Foods that taste good, fill you up, and are good for you. You'll also learn to identify and set limits for No Foods, those personal favorites that can cause so much trouble when we either eat them with unconscious abandon or rigidly try to deprive ourselves of them. Rather than avoid them entirely, you and your family will learn how to get the most enjoyment from them while maintaining overall health and balance. Finally, you'll learn how to plan and choose the right amounts of Maybe So Foods, those calorically dense choices (with higher carbohydrate, fat, or protein content) that are part of a healthy diet *in moderation.*

A number of studies recommend that we adopt eating patterns that focus on healthier selections and limit the intake of foods with minimal nutritional value. That's the basis for the Yes, No, Maybe So approach. It's an easy to way to start recognizing that every mouthful counts. It will help you learn to shift away gradually from processed and prepared foods that are high in white flour, sugar, fat, sodium, and preservatives and toward more simple, satisfying meals you prepare yourself.

A Plan for All Budgets

Let's talk dollars and sense for real. Severely obese people are more than twice as likely as people of normal weight to be in fair or poor health and have about twice as many chronic medical conditions. That translates into higher health care costs—69 percent higher for men, 60 percent higher for women—compared with people of normal weight. It's time to realize that while we all complain about the expense of healthier food, the costs associated with NOT eating better and exercising more are substantially more dramatic and life threatening.

Clearly, poverty or very limited financial resources can make serving healthy food a challenge. But even with limited funds, kids can learn HFL guidelines, such as drinking water and 1 percent milk instead of lots of soda and juice (which shouldn't be in the home in large amounts anyway). They can learn to have healthy cereal and milk and an apple, rather than chips and dip. They can learn that dinner needs a veggie, salad, fruit, a serving of whole grain carbohydrate, and a portion of healthy protein.

In truth, we have high rates of obesity in upper socioeconomic levels, too, where kids have every electronic sit-on-your-butt device imaginable and so they aren't playing outside. They may have nannies who are making high-fat mac'n'cheese meals or they are turning to fast food takeout while their two working parents are out filling the family coffers.

I know from experience that, no matter how busy you are, you can give your family healthy choices. When I went back to work and had a nanny for a short time, I shopped and prepared food on the weekends and had a healthy food weekly menu plan for everyone to follow. One of our favorite family weekend activities was to go to a local farmer's market and taste-test with the kids.

There are lots of excuses, but regardless of your budget or your schedule, by following the HFL program, you'll discover actions you can take to become a healthier family.

You CAN Do This

Because I've been a working mom with limited time myself for more than twenty years, I know how important it is to have step-by-step weekly strategies that minimize time and maximize output in the supermarket and in the kitchen.

I know the challenges of busy families. In many cases, both of you are working long hours outside the home, the school food environment has changed, communities may no longer be safe enough for your child to play outside, more meals are being eaten outside the home or on the go, physical education is disappearing in schools, and everyone in the family brings their own unhealthy (often stress or emotion-related) habits into the picture.

Creating change is rarely easy, but it helps when you can work together as a team—a true family. You can learn to work together as you assimilate the new behaviors you need to become an HFL family. You'll find that this isn't a program of 100 percent success or failure. In my experience, families start with different challenges, move toward different goals, and progress at different rates. The same is true of family members—every individual's experience will be somewhat different, and success will not look the same for everyone.

Your family will become healthier with any and every positive change you make, and that's the simple goal. If you are increasing the number of times you eat together, improving the quality of your food choices, expanding the amount of time each member spends on physical activity, or if the overall health profiles of family members are improving through weight loss and better health screening results—you are succeeding as an HFL family.

The HFL program takes a "project view" of weight and health issues. Just as you draw up plans to build a house, the HFL program provides the planning tools you need. Just as you follow the house plan you put on paper, the HFL program walks you through the stages of implementation: shopping, stocking your fridge and cabinets, prepping food ahead of time so it's ready to be cooked later in the week with minimal effort, portioning out foods and snacks so there's no guesswork. Research has found that even small changes in diet and physical activity can yield big results in reducing people's risk for health problems ranging from diabetes to heart disease.[2] When you make small, steady changes, you are more apt to stick with them, and right now there is an absolute urgency—for the sake of your own health status and the future health of your kids—to make changes that will stick for good.

The HFL program will help you:

- Select food that tastes good and is good for your family.
- Figure out the weekly food needs of the household, learn to shop for it, and prepare it easily and quickly.
- Retrain your family's palates so they appreciate healthy and tasty food.
- Learn visual cues for portions.
- Find out how to set up your fridge and pantry with portion control in mind.
- Differentiate between true hunger and the emotional food connection.
- Work together as a family toward a worthy goal—health for all.

I won't lie to you: changing behavior takes sustained effort. Cravings do not just melt away and disappear. Complacency can be a real danger, especially after a lifestyle change has been in place for a while. We convince ourselves that we are changed people and, for the most part, we are—except that old habits and cravings and relationships with food linger for a long, long time.

With the HFL program, your family will have an arsenal of strategies and solutions for even the most daunting situations in or out of your home. Everyone in the family will learn to tackle every moment with the best possible food solutions. There will always be temptation to face and choices to make—your family just needs to have tactical solutions to draw upon. And ultimately, you will feel more in control and relaxed when you know you have time-saving solutions that make your life not just healthier but easier.

Kids tend to want to know the "why" of things, and you will be including them in the learning part of the program, in the decisions that affect their food choices, and the reasons why your family needs a serious change now. You will provide the leadership and the call to action. There may be some initial resistance, unhappiness, and even resentment, but the HFL program will take you through solutions for phases like these and other common setbacks and challenges.

As you chart a new course of action, recipes will fall flat, kids will spit food out or prefer death to tasting a new fruit or vegetable, and spouses will test the limits of your tolerance. You can expect to have low days where it just feels like it's all too much. Just like any new job, you'll have to pace yourself, allowing time for information to sink in and for new behaviors to form and then gradually feel like they're a good fit. You'll have to allow each family member to personalize the tools to their unique needs and personalities and to realize they may only be able to embrace change at their own pace—not yours. Your job will be to offer the possibilities, to set boundaries and guidelines, but also to allow some flexibility. Most rewarding of all, you will be responsible for putting an end to those unhealthy habits that, if left in place, will quite probably doom your family to so many bleak, life-threatening health consequences.

Congratulations, Let's Get Started!

Are you ready to become a Healthy Family for Life? Are you ready to move out of denial, stop listening to the food devil screaming in your ear, and start marching down the path toward better health? Well, best of all, you are taking your kids on this journey with you. Even small changes in nutrition and activity levels will produce modest gains in your health profile. Keep those changes coming in a paced, solid, organized way and the most wonderful phenomenon will occur: ongoing weight loss, health profile gains, more satisfying lives for everyone in your family. The wonderful thing about the human body is its ability to heal and often recover from disease, responding positively to lifestyle changes. It's never too late for a family to start getting healthier. The gift you are giving your kids is an early health turnaround that will keep on giving them health benefits for the rest of their lives.

Congratulations on your commitment to one of the most important family values of all: healthy living. Now let's get started!

WHAT WILL YOU AND YOUR FAMILY GAIN FROM THE HFL PROGRAM?

For your kids:
- Weight loss if needed, and a reduced chance of being overweight later in life
- A better understanding of food choices, portions, and healthy eating patterns
- Less chance of suffering from lifestyle-related diseases
- A sense of belonging to a family that operates together as a team
- A sense of support and better communication
- An understanding of the connection between lifestyle choices and long-term health
- A strong foundation for a life of healthy habits

For your spouse:
- The joy of coming home to regular, balanced, tasty meals
- More willingness to get involved, thanks to a team perspective
- A better health profile and weight loss if needed
- Lower family health costs
- Potential for more affordable life insurance with health profile changes

For you:
- Lower stress levels now that there is an organized approach to food
- More time for other things like sleep, exercise, hobbies
- Weight loss if needed and a better health profile
- Fewer arguments in the home over food
- Tools you can use to help each family member achieve individual goals
- A sense of accomplishment that your family is on the road to better health

2

What Kind of Food Family Are You?

You Can't Change Your Genes, But You
CAN Change Your Family's Food-Style

The Williams family (all names have been changed) came to my office with one very unhappy fourteen-year-old, Samantha. Samantha just scowled silently as her parents explained the situation. She was twenty-five to thirty pounds overweight, very pretty, and very embarrassed.

The mom, Anne, who had been a diabetic for ten years, was petite and needed to lose fifteen to twenty pounds to reach an ideal body weight. Mike, her husband, was a singer who wished he could drop about ten pounds. He felt better food choices could help him maintain his vocal clarity and strength. When he was younger, he had been an actor and gymnast, but he had not stayed active.

Anne's casual attitude made it clear that, although she knew her excess weight was not healthy, she was not scared enough to maintain tight control of her eating or stay on a scheduled exercise program.

She was a working professional and, like her husband, a singer. She ran her household chaotically, shopping whenever she needed to, but without much of a plan. The family rarely ate together. Most of the food was pre-packaged or fast food. Anne constantly harped on Samantha's weight, and they quarreled over typical teen issues: Samantha's choice of peer group, curfew, driver's license test, home-work, grades. The parents repeatedly felt compelled to tell me their other daughter, who was two years younger, was "fine," though the family dynamics and eating habits made it obvious to me that she was *not* fine from a health perspective. When a family has dysfunc-tional health habits, usually *every* family member is affected.

Mike reflected on his own food needs intently, but the desire to lose weight he expressed seemed motivated by his own vanity and was completely disconnected from the needs of his daughter or the rest of his family. Anne wanted to know "what [she] could do for Samantha," but she didn't make the connection between her daugh-ter's health and that of her family as a whole. I could tell that Saman-tha probably just wanted her parents to stop talking so she could go home and hide under the covers.

Anne and Mike didn't realize that their daughter wasn't the prob-lem. Instead, it was the family eating style that Samantha learned as a child that had led to her current weight problem. Anne's serious dis-ease had not provided sufficient motivation for her to change her habits. Mike was caught up in his own needs. In short, this was a typical family in food crisis.

I began by setting up appointments to meet with Samantha twice a week. When it came to the need to lose weight, Sam was old enough to "get it," but it had to be something she wanted, not some-thing her parents pushed on her.

Next, I asked Anne and Mike if they would be willing to take a crash course on food choices and start using a shopping list I would supply. I explained that families who eat together with planned menus fare much better from a health and weight perspective. Although that suggestion didn't meet with great enthusiasm, I made it clear that if they didn't try to adjust some of the habits in their home, Anne's diabetes could get worse and Samantha's weight issue would go nowhere fast.

There was a lot of work to do. If Samantha and Anne were ever going to get past the bad feelings, they would need to work together, make choices together, perhaps even shop and cook together.

It's hard to say how much of the poor relationship between mother and daughter was due to teen angst and how much was due to a mom frustrated with her own poor health and her feelings of guilt. ("I got my kid into this situation—at least partially—through my own inability to control the pantry, the fridge, and our eating patterns in a coherent, responsible way.") Parents often feel they're to blame, even when they can't articulate their guilt aloud.

Sam, on the other hand, clearly felt miserable as an overweight teen. After a couple of meetings, I could tell that the haphazard way their kitchen was run had frustrated her for some time. She knew healthier food always seemed to be available in her friends' homes, but she also knew some of the responsibility for her problem was the result of her own out-of-the-house food choices and her unwillingness to get involved in sports or physical activities.

The solution to their problem boiled down to Anne and Sam getting past their guilt and anger so they could work as partners, giving and taking on responsibilities, and finding healthy ways to verbalize frustration and encouragement, rather than nagging or criticizing. They achieved some of that with list-making (which everyone in the home contributed to), joint and shared shopping responsibilities, family conferencing, better prepping techniques, and more weekends devoted to physical activity.

Sam and her mom also became walking partners, which was a huge step toward working together for a common cause. They still had other conflicts, but they were able to join forces so both of their needs—weight loss in Sam's case, better diabetes control in her mom's case—could be met.

By now, you're probably asking the million-dollar questions: How did the family do? Did they make changes? Did Samantha lose weight? Did Anne gain better control over her diabetes? Did Mike climb on board?

This is what happened when Anne, Mike, Samantha, and Heather (the other daughter, the one who was "fine") worked together. Samantha lost twenty-three pounds and helped empower herself in the process. She learned that she needed to shop for herself when her mother's ability to stay organized and on top of menus slipped a bit. Sometimes Mike drove her to the supermarket, which brought them closer together. Mike learned to be more involved with his family. The whole family tried a lot of new recipes together, and they decided to use a delivery food option for a couple of weeks to help manage their choices and food amounts (a good learning tool for this busy family). The family began sitting down to eat together at least three times a week. They all started to exercise, albeit on their own schedules.

Samantha and Heather worked together and sometimes even shopped together to eat healthier. In the past, Heather had felt a little neglected at home, so she liked their new habit of family dinners. And she revealed to her parents that she had been afraid that she too would gain weight, and was happy the family was eating a healthier, more balanced diet.

CHRONIC HEALTH ISSUES ASSOCIATED WITH OBESITY

- Type 2 diabetes
- Heart disease
- Hypertension
- Metabolic syndrome
- Chronic respiratory diseases like asthma
- Chronic obstructive pulmonary disease (COPD)
- Asthma
- Macular degeneration
- Osteoarthritis
- Certain cancers
- Low self-esteem
- Depression
- Cavities
- Poor healing post-surgery

As the sisters gained a better understanding of their mother's diabetes, they could encourage her to cultivate better habits. Most weeks, the family made an effort to shop and prepare food on the weekend so there was plenty of healthy food in the fridge and pantry during the rest of the week. Most dinners could be prepared quickly with the nutritious ingredients on hand. The family also learned to troubleshoot their eating challenges, not to point fingers or simply give up.

They managed to change their food-style both in the home and outside it. And I felt sure that when Heather and Samantha someday became parents, they would take these new habits and behaviors into their own homes and create excellent HFL families. Are they now a family that eats perfectly? Not even close. They still eat too much fast food; sometimes they still fall back on old habits like snacking in front of the TV; they still are not consistently as active as they could be. But they have made a lot of progress by working together.

Families *Can* Change

By working together, *every* family can create healthier eating and activity habits. I know because I've seen it happen so many times. However, I also know from experience that there is no one-size-fits-all-families solution. Every family is different. Some families are constantly on the go. Others face a lot of conflict about what foods they should eat because some members want to make healthier choices than others. Sometimes one family member has developed a health or weight problem; unfortunately, all too often, this is viewed as an individual problem rather than what it really is—a family problem.

Some families make generally healthy choices, but they are hooked on big portions or they completely avoid activity. Sometimes the whole family practically lives on sugar and fat, although the weight effects may not yet be evident with every family member.

For some families, all members face similar challenges; most struggle with weight, for example. For others, there are individual considerations such as health conditions or unique lifestyle distinctions (family members who are athletes or vegetarians, who have food allergies, etc.).

For some families, serious medical consequences make it urgent to make changes promptly. For others, the consequences haven't caught up with them yet.

Your first step toward becoming a Healthy Family for Life is to assess your family's needs and take a closer look at the realities your family faces: genetics, medical indicators, and habits that could be undercutting your efforts to be healthy.

The Genetics Excuse

You can't talk about families without talking about the role of genetics, an area of research that will continue to offer new insights into family nutrition and weight management. I'm confident the emerging field of "nutritional genetics" or "nutrigenomics" will find genetic markers that predispose some individuals to store fat more easily, to be more adversely affected by high-fat or high-carbohydrate diets, and/or to burn calories less efficiently.[1,2,3,4]

Genetics contribute to body composition from birth and may influence how you process calories, both when you eat and when you exercise. Your genes can influence how much body fat you have in early life and how that fat is distributed. They can also make you more susceptible to gaining weight.

It is a genetic fact that weight management isn't a completely level playing field. Even within families, there can be considerable individual variation, which is why the Healthy Families for Life program is designed to be flexible enough to meet the unique needs of all family members. It's easy for people to point to other weight-challenged family members in current or previous generations and throw up their hands in defeat, saying, "There's nothing I can do—it runs in my family!"

However, the role of genetics is *only one factor* in the equation. As I frequently point out to patients, choosing to be a victim of real or imagined genetics is not a solution. In fact, there is plenty that you can do, regardless of genetics.

The nutritional decisions you and your family make can dramatically moderate the results of genetic predispositions. The hard truth is that *heredity doesn't destine you or your family to be fat.* The nutritional and activity choices you make greatly influence how your genes ultimately express themselves.

At the end of the day, everybody, regardless of genetics, is responsible for their own eating and activity habits. Eating poor quality food, consuming excessive quantities of food, or being inactive has the same result for all of us: poor health that puts us at risk for disease and unnecessarily diminishes the quality of our lives.

Your genetic factors should be used as motivation for you to take action, not as an excuse to give up. If your family has a history of obesity, diabetes, heart disease, strokes, high cholesterol, high blood pressure, or other conditions, understanding that history should be a wake-up call for you to make lifestyle changes.

Unfortunately, some people choose to ignore their family history, which can be just as harmful as using it to excuse poor choices. Knowledge is powerful, but only if you choose to use it.

The End of Family Denial

The whole point of this book is to put an end to family denial about health, nutrition, and weight management. If you are ignoring the truth about your family's unhealthy habits and the dangers that arise from those habits, you are contributing to a family culture of denial that your children may well take with them into their adulthoods and pass on to the next generation. And this is the kind of denial that kills. Remember how our kids could be the first generation to die sooner than their parents? We are responsible for that—but we can also work to change that outcome.

Think about where your own denial tendencies may be affecting your choices. Are you, or is one or more family members, struggling with obesity? Are you ignoring your family's history of health problems? Are your food choices irresponsible or haphazard? Do you devote inadequate time and energy to healthy meal planning and preparing? Are you conscious of portion control? Is your family inactive?

The first step out of denial is facing reality. Are you ready? Is your family ready?

The Denial Antidote: Honest Assessment

The first step to becoming a Healthy Family for Life is taking a good, hard look at where your family is now. You can use the series of assessment forms we've provided in this chapter and in the appendices at the end of the book to get a clearer picture of your family's health status. I realize that answering all these questions can seem time-consuming, but the rewards are worth it. Even small changes in your family's eating habits can create positive health results that last a lifetime. It's a sad fact that we often take better care of our car, home, or job than we do our health—but these assessment tools can help you identify where you may want to shift your priorities, and why.

The Five HFL Family Assessment Tools

1. *Family Health Tree*: a "big picture" look at health conditions and family health history (Appendix 2A)
2. *Individual Health Profile*: health status of every family member (for details, see the forms provided for Adults, Teens, and Children, Appendix 2B)
3. *Individual and Family Activity Profiles*: a look at the lifestyle and exercise habits of every family member and of the family as a whole (Appendix 2D and Appendix 2E)
4. *Family Food Intervention Stage (FFIS) Profile*: a look at factors to help you determine the level of your family's need to make lifestyle changes (later in this chapter, pages 41–43)
5. *Family Food-Style Profile*: a look at your family's current lifestyle habits (later in this chapter, pages 43–47)

How critical are these assessments? It is no exaggeration to say that these assessments could result in life-saving changes for your family, and at the very least, will significantly improve your overall health and quality of your lives for years and even generations to come.

You may be tempted to skip the assessment stage and move right to the HFL program in the chapters ahead. Certainly, any positive food, activity, or lifestyle changes that result from reading this book are valuable. However, taking the time to get an honest, realistic picture of your family's health, weight, and lifestyle will give you the strongest possible foundation for becoming a successful Healthy Family for Life.

Genetics is not the only thing you pass down to your kids when it comes to health—far from it. Teaching your children to value honest health assessment rather than to deny health problems is a wonderful legacy you can give them that will contribute to their health for the rest of their lives.

HFL Assessment Tool #1: Family Health Tree

The HFL Family Health Tree is a quick way for you to get an overall picture of your family's general medical history. You may need to call family members with questions, but think of it as a time to reconnect and get real with family members about your history. It's important to fill out as much information as you can from all the various sides of your family (or blended families).

Try to write down the major health conditions of each relative. For example, for my great-grandfather on my mother's side, I wrote: "diabetes, hypertension, died of stroke at age seventy-one." You'll end up with a typical family tree outline, but instead of just names, it will have *names and conditions* in each little box. So you'll have what I call a "comprehensive family tree." You'll also have new insight into the possible diseases that may run (or hover) in a family line. When you combine your family line and your spouse's, you'll be able to see which conditions "double dip," meaning which health issues can affect your kids from both sides of the family. (I inherited gum disease from both my mom and dad; there are stroke and cholesterol issues on my mom's side, and diabetes was prominent on my dad's side, although one great-grandparent on my mom's side had it as well.)

When you're done, you will have a better sense of the illnesses prevalent in your family that could affect you and your children's health in the future. Just remember that you aren't powerless. A disease like diabetes may be "hovering," but your health habits can greatly affect whether or not it becomes a reality for your or other members of your family.

Recently, a number of health organizations have recommended that families come together and share health information. Have your spouse and/or ex-spouses create family health trees going back to their great grandparents, if possible. Knowing that there is heart disease, diabetes, strokes, cancer, or other diseases that you may be able to fight or prevent through lifestyle changes can further spur you into action. By all means, share this information with your children when they are old enough to understand it.

HFL Assessment Tool #2: Individual Health Profile

This tool requires the help of a physician. As much as you may want to skip this step, resist the temptation. Take the opportunity to get all the information you can. Consider getting a full blood panel, urinalysis, even an EKG if you want the full health profile. These profiles will look a lot like your doctor's medical history questionnaires, and they will give you an at-home resource you can use as a reference for your HFL program.

Share your Family Health Tree with your doctor so he can guide you on which tests are appropriate for you and for your children. One of the best ways to get your family out of denial is for every member to know their "numbers."

I think of these numbers as an invaluable key to life. In fact, if there is only one lesson you take away from this book, I hope it's the importance of knowing your own health profile, so you have some objective quantification of your body's current health status.

The "numbers" are:

- *BMI*—See Appendix 2C.
- *Waist Measurement*—This tells you if you are storing dangerous excess fat in your abdominal region; see Appendix 2C.
- *Height and Weight*
- *Blood Pressure*—We now consider normal blood pressure to be 115/75 mmHg, though most people are still familiar with 120/80. Pre-hypertension would be higher than 120/80 and researchers have found that very early changes in the heart and arterial systems are already occurring when readings fall between 115/75 and 120/80.

- *Heart Rate or Pulse*—Based on your physical fitness and other health parameters, this number can vary. Your pulse will usually decrease as you condition your heart with cardiovascular exercise. My pulse rate went from 74 to 62 over a ten-year period with serious training efforts.
- *Cholesterol Levels (HDL and LDL)*—According to the American Heart Association, you want to target an HDL (good cholesterol) of greater than 40mg/dL for cardio protection. An LDL of less than 100 milligrams per deciliter is considered optimal. An LDL of 100–129 is considered near optimal, while 130–159 is borderline high. An LDL of 160–189 is high, and anything higher than 190 is very high.
- *Fasting Blood Sugar*—This should measure at or less than 100mg/dL; a reading of 100–125mg/dL is considered pre-diabetes.

You should revisit these numbers once a year, especially if there are lifestyle-related diseases in your family such as heart disease or diabetes, if you have gained or lost a significant amount of weight, or if you are on medications (in which case, check with your doctor because some number assessments may need to be done more frequently).

One of the best signs of a family evolving into a Healthy Family for Life is a slow but steady change in these numbers. Weight loss is often apparent right away from how your clothing fits, but the shift in numbers gives you a powerful guide to your success. You may even see better sleep patterns, better school performance, better energy levels, and even better concentration.

It's also important that you keep a written record of your health where you can refer to it when needed. Don't rely solely on memory. I cannot tell you how many times I've queried someone on their hospitalizations, been told he or she didn't have any, and then discovered a scar from a surgery and heard, "Oops, I forgot about that one."

That's another reason why taking the time to reconstruct your health history is crucial. If there are too many gaps in information or you haven't seen a doctor in a long time, invest in a physical exam and blood evaluation.

I know it takes time and commitment to see a physician and fill out these forms. But education is the cornerstone of any health makeover. You need to face facts. If you don't think anything is broken, you'll never be inspired to fix it.

Tips on Health Profiles for Teens and Kids

If your teen is willing to engage in this process from the beginning, great! Teens can fill out this form and even make their own appointments with a doctor to fill in the blanks. If your teen isn't willing, then fill it out to the best of your ability and consider leaving it for him or her with a personal note attached that explains why this is so important to you.

Whatever you do, don't point fingers or nag about weight or other negatives. Express your thoughts positively: "I think this could help you and all of us feel more energetic and develop healthier habits. I'm worried because I know _____ runs in our family and we can do something about it, if we're willing to make some changes. I want to start buying and preparing different foods, and become more active. I definitely want you to help make food and meal choices. Maybe we can even do some activities together or you can let me know if there are sports you want to try or a gym you'd like to join."

Obviously, the offers you make in the letter to your teen should be sincere. Don't suggest anything that time or money will prevent you from following through on, but be willing to give creative ideas, especially ones that mean you'll get to spend more time together.

For younger children, you will want to fill the form out with your pediatrician. Involve your child when age-appropriate.

HFL Assessment Tool #3: Activity Profiles

These profiles reflect the physical activity habits of your family as a whole and of each individual member. A big part of the HFL program involves getting activity and movement into your life. So often, we don't realize how little we are actually moving on a daily basis. You need to take a close look at your personal daily habits, your family's habits, and how much of your time is spent in sitting/couch potato time (and that includes TV watching, driving or riding in an

> ## DID YOU KNOW?
>
> Myeloid leukemia risk increases with a ballooning waistline. This type of cancer is the most common adult leukemia, and every extra four inches of waistline increases the risk of developing this leukemia by 37 percent.

automobile, sitting on the job, and computer time) versus exercise and physical activity time. Study upon study indicates that it's not just what you eat but how you use those calories that will partially determine weight gain. And exercise stands alone as an actual health therapy, helping to offset risk factors for disease. You can fill these forms out quickly, and they will give you a starting point for becoming more active.

HFL Assessment Tool #4: Family Food Intervention Stage (FFIS) Profile

Health care professionals organize the progression of diseases into stages to indicate the severity of the condition and how the disease will respond to possible treatment. When it comes to cancer or heart disease, for example, most of us know the value of being diagnosed in an early stage so the condition will respond to treatment more readily.

The Family Food Intervention Stage (FFIS) Profile works in the same way to help you assess the severity of your family's eating problems and the urgency needed to address them. Knowing your FFIS will help you determine which HFL tools and strategies are most suitable for your family's needs. Take a look at the four FFIS categories and determine which one best fits your family:

Stage 1: Getting Healthier Together

If you are a Stage 1 Family, you need to develop healthier habits, but you are not currently facing critical health problems. No one in your family is grossly overweight, although the adults may have shown more weight gain than is healthy and one or more of the kids may lean toward the top percentiles in weight. You have developed some unhealthy habits, such as eating on the run, making poor food choices, or not getting enough activity. Now you are ready to make some changes and get healthier together as a family.

Stage 2: Turning It Around (Facing Predisposition to Disease)

If you are a Stage 2 Family, you have concerns such as worrisome BMI, large waist size, family members with issues such as borderline high cholesterol level or blood pressure, or weight that is climbing too rapidly. Family members, however, do not yet have clear-cut, objective signs of early disease. Family members may need to lose weight to prevent full expression of diseases such as hypertension, diabetes, or heart disease.

Stage 3: Intervention Required (for Weight or Nutrition-Related Diseases)

If you are a Stage 3 Family, you and/or other family members are significantly overweight or have blood profiles or other medical tests that reveal disease. At this stage, you may be in denial due to fear, but you are also faced with the reality of health measurements that cannot be disputed.

Stage 4: Code Red (Rapid Change Required Due to Obesity or Disease)

At Stage 4, you and/or other family members have an ongoing need for a physician's care because weight and health issues require intermittent or regular healthcare. You may be in denial, and you may or may not be receiving this care.

The HFL program can help Stage 1 families integrate new, healthier habits into their lives in a reasonably paced fashion. Stage 2 families are already showing physical signs of extra weight and/or poor lab results that indicate risk factors for diseases such as diabetes, so HFL tools will specifically guide members to goals that include weight loss, a shift in HDL and LDL, and better blood glucose levels. Better quality food, portion control, and increasing activity will deliver a one-two punch on these health parameters. When it comes to Stage 3 families, who are showing early signs of disease or serious shifts in blood panels and other health measurements, the HFL program provides both assessments and a step-by-step guide to solutions that will shift poor habits and behaviors for optimal health.

The HFL program can help many Stage 4 Families stabilize health and even reduce the dosages or need for some medications, such as anti-hypertensive drugs, oral hypoglycemic medication, or medications such as Metformin (used for insulin resistance often found in pre-diabetes or early diabetes).

Note that once you or a family member has been diagnosed as a diabetic, you will always be a diabetic. But you can create a remission-type state, particularly in type 2 diabetes, in which blood sugar levels normalize and insulin resistance is diminished significantly, if not totally. Diabetes responds dramatically to weight loss and the health habits encouraged by the HFL program.

FFIS is a non-specific self-identification tool to help you increase your awareness of the medical consequences of your family's eating and activity habits. It is not intended to encourage judgments, fear, guilt or shame—only to help you consider the medical facts and take charge of your family's lifestyle choices.

Studies show that people who are suffering from serious and even life-threatening conditions can experience significant reversal of disease by committing to serious lifestyle changes. What may seem like insurmountable health hurdles may actually be conditions that can be dramatically altered by becoming a Healthy Family for Life. Whatever stage your family may be at, your goal is to intervene as early as possible to slow, stop, or prevent health deterioration.

HFL Assessment Tool #5: Family Food-Style Questionnaire

Our final assessment tool helps you identify family behaviors that sabotage your nutritional quality. Remember that these assessments are a gateway to a new way of living.

Family Food-Style Profile

Choose the eating behavior style(s) that best fits your family as a whole, as well as every individual family member. You may find that several food-styles apply both for individuals and for the family as a whole. There are many possible food-styles. We will point out some potential pros and cons for each style, but keep in mind that some of these food-styles are much healthier than others. Discuss, and see if you can identify any other patterns that have an impact on your eating habits and choices.

Q *Do you eat three square meals plus snacks in between?*

A You're a "Square" Eater. Pros: You eat regularly and don't often skip meals. You time your eating daily, never missing a meal or snack, and you never experience dramatic swings in your blood sugar levels because of your well-timed meals. You make the time to eat, realizing that skipped meals can impair your mental and physical performance. Cons: You enjoy those lunches with your coworkers at local eating haunts and those dinners out with family and friends. You always fit snacks in to their morning and afternoon slots, regardless of hunger. You don't necessarily notice the portion size or quality of food you're consuming. If your meals and/or your snacks are too big, you'll get too many calories throughout the day. Strategy: Keep your regular habits but watch portions carefully. Snacks should have between 100 and 150 calories.

Q *Do you graze throughout the day, eating few or no big "meals" but lots of mini-meals and snacks?*

A You're a Grazer. Pros: Eating more frequently discourages hunger bouts that can lead to overeating, and grazing with healthy snacks is a great way to stay energized around the clock. Grazers tend to gravitate to handheld foods like fruits, cut up veggies, energy bars, cereals and nuts. You never feel energy lows because of your approach to eating. Cons: Grazing can lead to overeating for some people because they may not realize just how much food they're actually eating, and avoiding sit-down planned and plated meals can sometimes translate into a lack of nutritional balance in the overall diet. Strategy: Portion control is the key; also pay attention to your choices, making sure you are getting adequate protein and eating from all the food groups. Healthy grazing doesn't mean eating without awareness or discernment.

Q *Do you go without food for most of the day (maybe coffee in the morning and a snack or two in the afternoon), then eat all night?*

A You're a Night Feaster. Pros: Eating a somewhat larger meal at night can be manageable if your food choices are smart and you eat a balanced meal with whole grains, lean proteins, cooked veggies, and fruit options. Cons: Eating way too much food at night, either in a large meal or in endless snacking, is unfortunately all too common—and typically results in overeating, because most people see it as an opportunity to eat through the evening hours to make up for the day's "fast." You also cannot possibly perform optimally at work or at the gym with inadequate mental and physical energy to take you through the day. Strategy: Apportion your food more evenly through the day and pay special attention to making healthier, portion-controlled choices for your evening meal and up until bedtime. Determine a cut-off time so the eating stops.

Q *Do you live on fast food, either at drive-throughs, restaurants, or by eating mostly packaged meals and pizza at home?*

A You're a Fast-Food Junkie. Pros (sort of!): Some fast food choices can be healthy and convenient. There are now a wide selection of salads with healthy proteins, fat-free dressings, low-fat yogurt and fruit parfaits, and sandwich options. Cons: Most fast food choices, however, are very unhealthy, with portions that are too large and condiments that are way too high in fat. A fast food lifestyle is one of the worst things you can do for your family's health. Strategy: Learn which fast foods are better choices, and also start to make the transition to more nutritional meals, so that fast foods become a once-in-a-while option, instead of an everyday habit.

Q *Are you always on the latest diet, from the Zone, Atkins, and South Beach to smoothies and fasts?*

A You're a Diet Junkie. Pros: It's great to stay current with new nutritional information and to stay conscious of maintaining a healthy weight. No doubt certain core elements of these eating programs have merit and one that offers a rational approach to eating could be a match made in heaven. Cons: On-and-off dieting is unhealthy and has been shown to promote weight gain, plus it encourages short-term thinking and discourages long-term lifestyle change. Dieting is the short-term solution and diets rarely help you with long-term weight maintenance. Strategy: Learn to distinguish between the unrealistic promises of radical, short-term approaches and the lasting benefits of changing the choices you make.

Q *Are you a vegetarian or close to it (you don't believe in eating meat) but still eat a fairly high-fat diet?*

A You're a High-fat Vegetarian. Healthy vegetarians make sure to eat high-grade proteins like beans and legumes, soy and tempeh, and eggs and fish (if they are only excluding animal meats and poultry). They also make sure to eat whole grains, fruits and vegetables, and only healthy oils and fats. Many people erroneously choose to shun meat, fish, and poultry in order to eat foods like pasta, pizza, and high-fat salads. Pros: Vegetarianism can be a very healthy lifestyle choice when you know how to make smart vegetarian choices. But it's not a license to simply eat everything in sight that is non-meat-based. Cons: A high-fat diet of any kind can promote weight gain and increase disease risk. You may also tend to overeat in the name of healthy eating. Strategy: Learn to make healthy vegetarian food choices and be sure to include adequate protein.

Q *Are you extremely rigid in your food choices or obsessed 24/7 with weight, calories, fat content, and/or other aspects of nutrition?*

A You're an Overly Controlled Eater. Pros: You may be well-informed about many aspects of nutrition and weight management. You may feel that due to prior dieting cycles, this is the only way to maintain control and not gain weight. You may have a strong family pattern of lifestyle-related diseases (diabetes, heart disease, stroke, hypertension) and feel that an extremely inflexible eating program emphasizing tight portion control is the way to maximize a healthy outcome. Cons: Rigidity and obsession can lead to a variety of unhealthy eating habits. You may be cutting necessary calories or food groups out of your diet in the name of health. Your obsession may also be a sign of disordered eating, or mask emotional issues that need to be addressed. Strategy: Pursue a more realistic perspective and greater flexibility in order to achieve more balance in your eating habits and your overall lifestyle approach. Vigilant eating can be a plus, but obsessive control is often detrimental to your health.

Your Family Food "Values"

Throughout the rest of the book we'll talk about strategies to change or improve your family food-style. Some patterns may need to change completely. Night Feasting, for example, almost always leads to gorging because you're hungry from starving all day. It can also lead to the "atomic bomb meal" or a very heavy, high-fat meal that can cause dangerous sudden inflammation in the arteries and even lead to a heart attack or stroke. If your family is living the "high" life of Fast Food Junkies, you're bound to be developing health problems from the poor-quality food you're eating way too regularly.

Other patterns may simply need modifying. There's nothing wrong with eating three solid meals a day with two small snacks; you may just need to downsize portions or upgrade the nutritional quality of your snacks. If your family has a Grazer food-style, you may find you need to limit high-fat and high-sugar food choices and have easy-to-grab healthy food options in the fridge and pantry.

Some extreme food-styles may require professional help. Overly rigid or obsessive dieting or uncontrollable binge eating, for example, may signal eating disorders that can be helped with professional treatment. Also, if you or a family member is having trouble managing emotional eating, professional help may be beneficial.

Taking the time to assess habits will set you on the road to becoming a healthier, happier, and even closer family. Many, many times I have seen the journey toward healthier eating result not only in better numbers (such as cholesterol, blood pressure, and weight) but in better relationships and a much more satisfying family life. Isn't that what "family values" are really all about?

CHAPTER 2 QUICK-SUMMARY

- Genetics and family history are part of the story but not "the whole enchilada."
- Involve your family's physicians, pediatrician, etc. Resist the urge to avoid the doctor. Be willing to hear the good, the bad, and the ugly. Now is the time to face your fears and take a look at the objective truth about your family's health.
- The more honest you are about where you're at, the more likely you are to make successful positive changes.

Tips for Teens

- Involve teens in health discussions: share your family health tree and talk about your own health concerns.
- Have teens list five foods they cannot live without, and discuss ways to make the choices healthier or how to substitute alternatives, smaller portions, etc.
- Have them list five new foods they'd be willing to try.
- Let them create their "fantasy menu." Talk about how it does or doesn't meet healthy, nutritious criteria.
- Have them plan one activity for the whole family to do together to "get moving." Put them in total charge of snacks, water, directions to location, picnic lunch, etc.

Tips for Kids

- Let kids make a list of foods they like, don't like, and are willing to try.
- Ask them to list differences between your kitchen routines and mealtimes and those of their friends. Ask them to rate those differences as better than, worse than, or similar to yours.
- Ask your children what they like and don't like about their meals.
- Teach them a new "Word of the Day," such as health, energy, nutrition, fats, carbohydrates, protein, exercise, treat, etc. (Make a game about using them in sentences or drawing pictures to identify their meaning.)

3

Eat Like a Cow and Other Easy Ways Your Family Can Become a "Healthy Family for Life"

....

The Basics of the Healthy Family for Life Program and the Fundamentals of Family Food

....

When clients walk into my office for the first time, they usually look like they are being marched to the guillotine (if you're less than thrilled about the idea of changing your eating habits, you can relate). My opening speech goes something like this: "Let's get one thing straight. No family eats perfectly. I haven't met one yet. And I've talked to models, celebrities, dancers, and athletes who may seem 'perfect' on the outside, but I can tell you they have habits that are very much less than perfect. So trust me, I'm not here to force you into anything unrealistic or to try and take away every eating pleasure in your life."

They usually brighten up (a bit) after that.

Fortunately, "healthy" doesn't mean "perfect." And being a Healthy Family for Life doesn't mean every family member eats perfectly every day.

I've interviewed thousands of people and I know that it is a rare person indeed who really understands nutrition completely and is able to make choices about food absent an emotional component. Just as you can be born smart and therefore need less study time than some other students, you can also be born genetically gifted when it comes to your physique.

How come we are so much less tortured by the person who aces exams without studying than the one with the unbelievable metabolism who can eat whatever they want? But, as you'll see, just because someone is at an ideal weight doesn't mean they don't have lurking health problems related to their eating.

Eating a diet high in trans fats and saturated fat can still clog arteries, even if you are slim. Eating a high-salt diet can still put you at risk for hypertension, even if you are thin. Eating a diet high in fried foods and red meats may predispose you to certain cancers, even if you are slim. Not eating enough fiber can cause elimination problems regardless of your size and weight, and not eating enough fruits and vegetables puts you at risk of nutrient deficiencies even if you are not overweight.

The Behaviors of a Healthy Family for Life

Although Healthy Families for Life (or HFL Families) are not targeting perfection, they are doing something that many families don't: paying attention to what they eat. This chapter is about surprises, and the first surprise is that making big eating improvements is probably not as hard as you may think.

In fact, even paying a *little* more attention to how your family eats could pay off in big changes. Of course, the more you work at it, the more you'll accomplish.

Let's look at some of the basic behaviors of an HFL family.

HFL Families DO:

- Organize and plan.
- Shop for food with lists and with meal plans in mind.
- Prepare healthy meal and snack options ahead of time.
- Eat meals together on a regular basis.
- Choose snacks that fuel them between meals.
- Control daily TV/video time.
- Plate food before it comes to the table.
- Factor in treats.
- Believe that exercise is important for all family members.
- Know how to celebrate without food.
- Care about their health.
- Avoid turning to food for emotional support (and turn to each other instead).
- Have breakfast every morning.
- Do not use food to reward behaviors and achievements.
- Enjoy meals slowly with attention to portion size and food quality.

HFL Families DON'T:

- Wing it when it comes to food choices and options.
- Routinely eat on the run.
- Shop for food erratically.
- Eat in different rooms of the home, while watching TV or working.
- Eat fast food and processed food meals and snacks regularly.
- Have no clue about how much time is spent watching TV/playing computer games.
- Grab food, stand and eat, eat on the run.
- Eat treats on a regular/daily basis.
- Think exercise is boring, a drag, unnecessary.
- Use food as their sole model for celebrations and holidays.
- Ignore their weight or size or risk factors.
- Use food as a comfort tool.
- Skip breakfast.

- Use food as a reward frequently.
- Eat family style, high-calorie, high-fat foods habitually.

You've already made assessments in Chapter 2; in the chapters ahead, you'll find out more about these and other healthy/unhealthy characteristics as we look at the four Habits of HFL Families:

1. Planning
2. Preparing
3. Portioning Food
4. Playing

But first, let's look at ten fundamental ideas about family and food.

1. Which Species Is Your Family? Eating Like a Cow Isn't Half Bad.

Dr. Doolittle talked to the animals. Maybe he had the right idea, because there's a lot we can learn from the animal kingdom about eating habits. Some animals eat only when they are hungry. They eat until they're full with no snacking. The snacking concept really doesn't exist among some animals. Other animals overeat during plentiful times and then go weeks or even months without eating at all. Still others graze all day long, every day.

When I work with a new family, I always take into account which "species" they are. Often, it differs from person to person even in the same family. Factors that determine eating habits include genetics, metabolic rate, and even how our day is organized or whether we engage in physical or mental labor as a profession. Someone who is on the road during the day needs a different eating approach than someone at home who can prepare food on the spot for lunch and snacks.

There is also evidence that people taste foods differently. They may have a preference for spicy or bland. Some people prefer certain textures in foods. From as far back as I can remember, I have not been able to drink plain milk. It actually causes a gag reflex. When I was a child, my mother would put a bit of chocolate syrup or a couple of teaspoons of coffee (when I was older) to get me to drink milk.

I shunned most dairy products except for American cheese and fruit-flavored yogurt. I later found out that this was a good thing because most cheeses are high in saturated fat and the calorie downfall of many an eater. Because of my taste preference, I did not introduce my kids to many cheeses, just the same two that I liked. So to some extent, how we view food and gravitate to it can have a lot to do with what our individual taste buds prefer and what we are exposed to on the home front. This may determine whether you're a vegetable eater or why you like fried foods. You may shun a certain food or food group because your palate developed without any exposures to it. At the end of the day, your kids like what they like, to a large extent, because of what you have put on the table.

You may not offer veggies if you don't like them. This is typical of parents: we tend to stock what we like. If we are stocking a lot of poor quality foods in our fridge and pantry, your kids will become accustomed to them. Whether by conditioning or genetics, some food preferences and eating habits just run in families.

Some animals are herbivores and exist solely on plants. Clearly, they can still be big animals—think giraffes or cows. Other animals are incredibly lean, with active lifestyles and animal-based diets—think lions. Others, like the polar bear, subsist on high-quality fat from blubber and oily fishes. Raccoons, opossums, and sea gulls are omnivores—they eat anything. They're like animal garbage disposals. Sound familiar?

Try to figure out if your eating pattern, body build, and preferences somehow relate to one of these animal groups and consider if that's a good thing or not. I'm a vegetarian (I do eat fish, and eggs), but I know plenty of vegetarians who eat high-fat salads and enormous quantities of pasta in the name of a healthy eating discipline. That's not quite being a giraffe. And cows do graze all day long, chewing the cud, but that is because they need enormous quantities of grass to provide the calories and nutrients necessary to support their large bodies and milk-producing efforts. If we graze high-fat foods and processed foods all day long, and remain sedentary as if we are "out to pasture," we're setting ourselves up for obesity and poor health. I also know body builders who chow down unbelievable quantities of red meat in the name of "muscle-building protein"

REAL-LIFE HFL STORIES: MAKING SLOW, STEADY CHANGE

Diane was an overweight mother of two and the wife of a man who loved fast food. He was not thrilled when she came to me for help, but he was willing not to interfere as long as her "lifestyle project" did not interfere with his passion for food. Diane struggled with her weight all her life and was eighty pounds overweight. She fed her picky kids whatever they were willing to eat, just to get food into their systems. Her ten-year-old son suffered from depression, ADHD, and possibly Tourette's syndrome. He was showing signs of rapid weight gain, and Diane blamed his medications, as well as his inability to do any team sports—he frequently got into fights with other kids. Her five-year-old daughter was age-appropriate in terms of weight.

I pointed out to Diane that if we could create good-tasting menus, her husband would probably shift some of his fast food eating—maybe not all, but it would be a start. I also pointed out that, although her son's medications might indeed have been contributing to his weight gain, she was also stocking her pantry and fridge with quick-grab processed foods. I did a pantry and fridge cleanout and evaluation, and offered her a variety of replacements and options. Any processed foods we agreed on are now in the 100-calorie packs, and after a snack like that is dispensed, if her kids want more, they have to have fruit, veggies, low-fat yogurt, or healthy cereal instead.

I also invoked the first two P's, so she began planning and preparing food on weekends. She is now buying or preparing fruit salad, healthier muffins, and entrées ahead of time. With the extra time she has during the week, she plays or read with the kids, counteracting the boredom that was leading them to ask for second or third portions of snacks.

The shift in food quality and quantity, particularly the reduced sodium, fat, and sugar, has impacted the family in a

REAL-LIFE HFL STORIES, *continued*

very positive way. Diane began to drop about a pound every one to two weeks, and the kids like being involved in menu planning and food choices. They are asking for fruit more often, and they like Mom playing with them more. Dad hasn't quite climbed on board, but he has agreed to stop taking the kids every weekend to buy fast food and is taking them for low-fat yogurt snacks instead. He eats his own fast food out of the home when he wants it and has dinner with the family more often on weeknights.

Diane decided she also needed therapy to help with ongoing issues that were leading to overeating, and she is eating less often now due to emotional stimulus. We have setbacks occasionally, especially when her son goes through a growth spurt and his meds need adjustment, but a few private sessions with him usually puts him back on track.

Like many families, Diane's may always struggle with certain food issues, but they have improved their eating patterns, added more activity, and gained a better understanding of how to organize and plan their "food life" so it doesn't rule them. Diane's most recent blood profile showed lower cholesterol and fasting blood sugar levels. Her blood pressure, which was borderline high, also came down. That's an HFL family: not perfect but making healthy progress.

but even if they're choosing lean cuts of beef, too much red meat has other health risks like certain cancers. People who love all kinds and types of food may the healthiest of all, but only if they give great regard to specific choices from each food group, portion size, and attention to exercise or calorie-burning effort.

As you consider your own personal habits, food preferences, issues and goals, you may find that they are very different from those of other family members, at minimum, because of age and gender.

Some of you may graze, some may eat square meals, and some may prefer a larger breakfast and smaller dinner. Because the HFL program helps you to organize and prepare on a weekly basis, each approach to eating can work, if you pay attention to certain core HFL principles like portion control, awareness of food choices, and awareness of physical activity.

Some of you may be at an appropriate weight, while others may need to shed pounds. However, the HFL program is flexible enough to allow diversity between families and also among family members, with core principles that apply to everyone, even if they have different goals or health needs.

2. Food Habits Die Hard: This Movie Has a Lot of Sequels!

Remember when you sucked your thumb or twirled a lock of hair or talked incessantly at school and got put in the corner a lot? You may also remember your mother threatening, cajoling, begging, bribing, and doing everything in her power to get you to stop.

Habits are really hard to break. The very nature of a habit is that it becomes physically and mentally ingrained. So it still escapes me why everyone is convinced that weight can come on slowly but disappear quickly (for good). After all, your palate grows accustomed to tastes and sensations, and when you remove those tastes and sensations all at once, you suffer.

You deny yourself.

But you only want more.

It makes sense that deprivation leads to binges and weight gain. Trying to break habits forcefully without supportive education and satisfying palate replacements will not work for most families.

Changing eating habits is a process that takes time and lots of it. You need time for your body to readjust, for your palate to create a new food history, for you to learn new, healthier habits. My own struggle with weight took years of education, many different diets, and the ability to embrace exercise before I was able to rework my relationship with food.

In short, think of this as a movie that may have a number of sequels before you've got all your new habits in place.

HEALTHY WAYS TO FEEL FULL

Fruits and veggies are low-cal/energy-dense foods, meaning they give you a big bang of energy in the form of carbohydrates with fiber. They fill you up and allow your blood sugar to rise slowly; the fiber slows your digestion so you feel full longer.

Combining a lean protein with a small amount of healthy fat and a whole grain carbohydrate will also allow you to feel full longer with less calories. Here's a good example: a whole grain wrap of white meat turkey, tomato and lettuce, plus avocado.

Choose:

- Fruit instead of gummy bears/licorice
- Sourdough/rye/100 percent whole grain/pumpernickel bread instead of white bread
- Plain non-fat yogurt plus berries instead of sweetened yogurt
- Bran or 100 percent whole grain cereals or oatmeal instead of sweetened cereals
- Baked potato with skin on instead of potato chips or fries
- Chickpeas (garbanzo beans) or brown or wild rice instead of white rice
- Plain air-popped popcorn instead of crunchy processed snacks
- Small servings of nuts instead of granola bars
- Lentils, bean dip, salsa instead of creamy processed cheeses
- Grains such as amaranth, barley, buckwheat, millet, oats, or wheat instead of refined carbohydrates
- Almond or other nut butters instead of traditional processed peanut butter

3. Palate Re-training Is the Name of the Nutrition Game

We're supposed to eat for sustenance, to supply our bodies with the fuel and nutrients that we need, right? Sure, but the palate needs pleasing, pure and simple. Research has shown that some children are actually more willing to try new tastes and new foods because they have a heightened preference and appreciation of sour-tasting foods. Studies show that if you were a child in this group, you probably were more willing to try new food tastes.[1] These "sour taste appreciators" also seemed willing to try foods with striking colors and were not put off by a strange fruit or vegetable hue.

Kids with a less developed sour taste tend to be somewhat picky with their food preferences. Most of us can probably identify whether we prefer spicy foods, bland foods, sweet or sour tastes. Our preferences may get established in childhood and persist. We fall into a taste pattern. Many of us rarely change it and we do—by the manner in which we stock our kitchens and cook—hand it off to our kids.

Although it varies from person to person, there are certain things we have in common: we want food to taste good, to feel smooth going down, and to have a crunch factor or a pleasant aroma. Based on what we have exposed our children to thus far in life, and based on what we've been trained to like, the whole family will probably need to be willing to try many new tastes with many repeated exposures over time to create new palate appreciation. Experts say it takes, at minimum, about fifteen to twenty repeated tastes in order to acclimate to a new food or taste.

Unfortunately, many of the foods our palates are drawn to just don't measure up fuel-wise. Trans fat, saturated fat, and corn syrup can make food taste really rich, turning regular foods into palate pleasers. When your palate gets used to those foods, your brain wants more, and more, and more. There is still a debate about the true nature of these fats and whether they are truly addictive.[2,3]

Experts who study food addiction offer the theory that certain foods, like a high-fat, sugary donut, may possibly offer a stronger "brain reward" than, say, a bowl of vegetable soup. Research on this is still going on in centers around the world. To use the word "addiction" accurately in association with food, we need to establish that eating is going on despite the knowledge of dire consequences, that a person is utterly preoccupied all day long with food, food preparation and meals, and that there is serious guilt about overeating without the ability to rein it in.[4,5] Until this is established or refuted by researchers, it's clear from our growing waistlines and rising diabetes rates that, once we get used to having these high-fat, sugary foods regularly, we crave these foods.

If you never introduced a child to a piece of candy and gave her a juicy, crunchy apple, do you think she'd be missing out on pleasure? If you never gave french fries to a child but instead gave him grilled slices of sweet potato, do you really think he'd be missing pleasure? But give your children candy and french fries repeatedly, and yes, over time, that will be their preference of taste and texture. No one is denying that these foods taste good, although I can tell you that once you wean yourself or your child from them, the taste will be extremely overpowering and not quite as delectable. Raise a child on high-fat, very sweet, processed foods, and that's what he will crave on a regular basis.[6] Let's call it a "corrupted palate."

Take the ever-popular birthday cake. It's usually creamy, high in fat and a real mouth pleaser, whether it's cake-based or ice cream-based. You delight in the first time your toddler celebrates her birthday and sticks her finger in the cake (or her face for that matter). That first piece of birthday cake is an American rite of passage. Now multiply the number of times that child will be exposed to that cake, thanks to thirty other pre-school friends, family parties, anniversaries, school parties, and so on. It's our own fault that our kids develop "cake palates."

To help keep your child's palate (and your own) in perspective, why not have a tiny piece of cake sometimes, and other times, sorbet or fruit dipped in dark chocolate, or a small wedge of healthier home-baked brownies or mini muffins?

Consider the state of breakfast cereals. Some of the best choices in terms of whole grain or fiber content are now adding yogurt clusters or chocolate bits. In many cases, these additions have trans or saturated fat, or simply add junk to a pretty good food.

To help retrain their palates, I suggest clients use a less healthy cereal as a two-teaspoon topping for a standard serving of a healthier one. (Or you can use chopped nuts and berries as an equally satisfying topping.) Let kids pick the "topping cereal" that accompanies their "entrée cereal." Or let them top healthy waffles or whole grain pancakes with ricotta cheese and cinnamon and a bit of light syrup. It's fun and it isn't "deprivation eating."

Maybe you can use ideas like these to help your children BEFORE they develop dominating sweet or fat palates that are harder to retrain the longer they've been entrenched. If your family is already conditioned to this kind of food, you will probably need to be slow, steady, patient and creative. Here's a surprise cooking tip: making brownies with apple butter and dark chocolate actually potentiates the flavor of chocolate, so you reduce the unhealthy fat and introduce fiber, which helps control portion size; dipping large strawberries in dark chocolate means you are now introducing a tasty treat with antioxidant benefits; using nuts and fat-free whipped cream to make a "light pound cake" more decadent means you add healthy omega-3 fatty acids, protein, and some calcium from a dairy topping. All of these can create palate pleasers with less fat and sugar, and healthier ingredients. Best of all, they can help shift palate sensitivities and ingrained taste preferences because your family will enjoy these tastes, they will not feel deprived, and you will be creating a whole new set of tasty, healthy food options. (Though they still need to be treats and not daily food habits.)

Palate shift comes slowly, however. And as I mentioned, scientifically, we know that it can take up to twenty-one exposures to a new food for a person, especially a child, to embrace a new taste. This is especially true of pungent or strangely colored fruits and vegetables. So be patient!

4. You Can Learn to Work With Your Metabolism

Some of what makes you who you are regarding food is your metabolism, no question. And as I've pointed out, some people are blessed with a faster rate of calorie burn. Some people, male and female, also carry more inherent muscle mass. We know the mitochondria or powerhouse cells of muscle tissue actually work more efficiently than those found in other cells of the body—so they are capable of utilizing calories (or specifically, the readily available glycogen stores our blood has available for energy) more efficiently. So, the more muscular you are, the more efficiently you will process and utilize calories. In the world of fitness, we encourage people to build muscle because, in addition to the sleek and toned physique you'll have, you will also usually be able to eat a bit more thanks to your muscle mass. It seems that in certain geographic locations, a metabolic gift may have actually evolved. In most cases, however, any geographic location that has had the *blessing* of American fast food move into the neighborhood has also seen an increase in weight gain and other negative health issues associated with this poor-quality food.

At Imperial College in London, researchers have been tracking 800 people of various ages and sizes and scanning them to create "fat maps" that show where people store their fat. According to the findings, people who appear thin may still be holding fat in deposits around internal organs. So, although researchers have recently gone beyond BMI to include abdominal girth or waist size in order to better predict dangerous amounts of fat and predisposition to serious diseases, an even more worrisome culprit may be the internal fat that never reveals itself clearly. As I've pointed out, thinness does not necessarily reflect good health. Even for people who seem to "magically burn what they eat," fat may be secretly stored in places not clearly evident to the naked eye.[7] Someone with a normal BMI and waist size could have dangerous stores of fat internally. There's even a new term to describe these people, as mentioned back in chapter one: TOFI, or "Thin Outside, Fat Inside."

Every time I see parents allowing "thin" kids free rein to eat all kinds of junk food and drinks, I want to shout, "Are you kidding me?" These kids' future health and quality of life will be determined to some extent by the food they're eating now. Even a great metabolism doesn't prevent plaque formation in the arteries or visceral fat deposits around vital organs. It just burns calories a bit faster.

It is possible to make friends with your metabolism. You can improve your metabolic rate by packing on some muscle mass. You can certainly burn more calories daily by exercising in general. (Different family members, due to size or gender or body make-up, may be able to eat more than others. That's life.) The key is to get the information you need, stay out of denial, and know yourself, including approximately how many calories it takes to attain and maintain your healthiest weight.

5. You Don't Have to "Open a Restaurant" to Please Everybody!

So many diet books over the decades have extolled the virtues of three square meals and two snacks, grazing throughout the day, eating five or six mini-meals, fasting one day a week, doing a fruit-only day, and on and on. How many times have you gone on a diet because a celebrity endorsed it or had success with it? Or because your friend lost amazing amounts of weight on it? Often, the plan was not quite as effective for you—or you lost the weight but quickly gained it back.

By and large, I find that many of my clients have tried numerous plans; along the way, they've gained and lost lots of pounds—mostly gained (or regained). Usually, they don't customize these plans to their own needs and preferences. So, like a dress made for another body, the plan never quite fits.

There may very well be someone in your family who does better grazing, another who needs disciplined and timed meals, and another who likes the mini-meal approach. One person may be vegetarian, another may have food allergies. But I am not for a mother being stuck in a kitchen constantly trying to meet all these different eating approaches (really, I'm not). That's why the HFL program is based on planning and prepping ahead of time. So you've got a salad cut up in the fridge, cut-up veggies for dipping, lots of fresh fruit, individual yogurts, cans of tuna, beans that are pre-rinsed, baggie-size snacks, baked crackers and peanut butter, and other foods already available for everyone, regardless of their eating style. That's how you gain control over the quality and kinds of foods your family chooses, and how you address different eating patterns and preferences without going crazy in the process.

I recently worked with a family where Dad needed to drop some pounds, Mom was slim but had a family predisposition to diabetes, the toddler was slightly overweight, and the teen son was athletic. Dad kept late hours, made even later by his efforts to get in exercise after work. The son was off to school early and then stayed after school for sports. Mom was dealing with meals on the go, meals in the home, and different needs for everyone.

With a core menu plan that involved easy-grab, pre-measured foods and snacks and healthy homemade meals that could be re-heated, the family was able to eat the same healthy core foods. Mom spent three hours each weekend creating her meal plan for the week, shopping, and preparing food. The family helped, and agreed to a minimum of three shared meals a week. Mom loved the fact that she actually saved time because she didn't need to prepare meals every day. (A quick fill-in shopping visit late in the week restocked the fridge with perishables.) The whole family had food to take with them wherever they went, and Mom had more time to play with her toddler, who benefited from the extra calorie-burn-ing activity.

With the HFL program, you will have a healthy food framework that is manageable, reasonable, enjoyable—and flexible enough to cope with lots of different tastes.

6. Hunger Can Fool You!

"I'm a big guy and there's lots of me to feed!"

"I'm an active person, so I eat for fuel and I need a lot of it!"

"I don't eat all that much, so I don't understand why I'm so big or why I'm gaining weight!"

"It's always important to clean my plate, right?"

"I'm eating healthy food, so what's the problem?"

"I'm eating for two, so I can pretty much eat anything."

Most people have lots of reasons why they're having trouble sat-isfying their hunger without eating too much or gaining weight. (I hear them every day!) In reality, hunger usually has little to do with it—and even in the best cases, hunger is a tricky indicator.

If you've ever been with people with zero food issues (yes, they do exist) at a buffet and then sat with them at a table, you will typically note:

- They observe all the offerings at the buffet—they'll scan first.
- They're selective with their choices, using measured spoonfuls.
- They don't fill their plates until they're brimming.
- Once at the table, they'll drink some water first—they don't attack their plates.
- They tend to eat slowly, putting down their fork between bites, talking leisurely.
- They usually take small bites and chew for a while.
- They leave food on their plates—there is no need to "clean their plates."
- They know how to taste dessert without gorging or they will pass on it.
- They know what fullness means, and they stop when they are comfortably full. They will push their plate away or ask that it be removed.
- They understand hunger and handle it calmly. There is no sense of desperation when you observe them eating.

Do these behaviors describe you?

For most of my clients, these are unknown behaviors and experiences. Often, they think they're listening to hunger cues, but hunger can be very misleading. There is an actual scale for determining your feeling of hunger, from one (totally satiated) to ten (ravenously hungry). Experts will often use this scale as a technique to help train someone who has not established a clear-cut sense of eating due to true physical hunger versus other food cue stimuli—in other words, someone who has no clue as to when to eat or why they are eating (see Hunger Scale on next page). I use the hunger scale to get people in touch with different levels of hunger so they can begin to associate need for fuel with hunger as opposed to eating due to emotions. I also train them to never let hunger get too strong because that is a surefire cause of overeating.

I have found that around level five to seven, when one begins feeling somewhat empty and may be beginning to have some borborygmi (gastric sounds), many people act as though they are at a level ten and will shovel in a meal so fast, they eat much larger quantities than are appropriate. Or worse, they never allow themselves to experience true hunger so never allow the tank to get really empty. Even healthy grazers, who eat on a more frequent basis, eat small enough servings so that they do feel somewhat empty and in need of another mini-meal—they're eating throughout the day but with hunger cues. I'm not a big proponent of letting your body reach the point of utter, desperate hunger, but doing so is a tool I sometimes use when retraining someone to understand hunger and the appropriate response to it.

The HFL program focuses on foods that will help keep your blood sugar stable so you don't feel sudden rushes of energy followed by plummets (typical of processed foods), which can be mistaken for hunger.

Hunger cues also get notoriously mixed up with emotions. From time to time, almost all of us suffer from some form of this scenario: "I am so . . . (sad, frustrated, anxious, upset, angry, happy, lonesome).

HUNGER SCALE

1—No sign of hunger, content and feeling very satisfied, no thought of food
2—Still very satisfied
3—Satisfied
4—Barest sense of hunger
5—Slight feeling of hunger
6—Starting to feel hungry, thinking about next meal
7—Hungry
8—Very hungry
9—Feeling low energy, empty, very seriously hungry
10—Absolutely ravenous

I know, I think I'll eat! Oh, that feels so good, oh, I'm getting calmer, oh, I'm feeling a sense of peace, oh, I know. I'll eat some more!" Food can be a powerful calming agent because of its ability to stimulate certain chemical messengers in the brain called endorphins that calm us down (see Chapters 10 and 11 for specific information on emotional eating). The more we turn to this habit of "food to calm," the more we ingrain this behavior into our eating paradigm. We can become so accustomed to this way of eating that we can actually find it odd when we encounter someone who doesn't behave this way.

When we eat to affect our emotions, whether the emotion is anxiety, boredom, stress, or happiness, a rush of satisfaction or calmness can descend over us, but it's always short-lived. When it becomes an entrenched behavior, problems arise:

- You feel ashamed or disgusted with your lack of control because you've eaten way more than you should have.
- You gain weight.
- You're led to other forms of destructive behavior, such as obsessive exercising to try to "catch up" with your eating.
- You continue to try to handle your feelings with food, rather than taking more effective action to learn to deal with your feelings, so you never get to the root of your emotional issues.

I often convince clients who really struggle with emotional eating to allow themselves a consultation with a therapist experienced with emotional eating. Although I can help you create healthy eating habits with the HFL program, you will probably need further assistance if you are in a strong, persistent cycle of emotional eating or overeating. If emotional eating is a longstanding problem, even understanding why you are eating may not be enough to help you calm those demons permanently and live harmoniously with food. Awareness that you or other family members—even kids—may be using the wrong foods for the wrong reasons is the first step to changing emotional eating habits for good. The HFL plan will help you to put structure, organization, food awareness, and other control techniques in place. But if you have serious ongoing emotional or secretive eating going on, you may need ongoing therapy as you implement this program.

7. Real Food Makes Life Easier (Really)

Back in the 1800s, convenience foods were just not part of the picture. Practically all food was "real" (not highly processed). A food was considered exotic if it wasn't readily available. It was expensive and savored when you could get your hands on it. Believe it or not, potatoes and cocoa were considered exotic back then.

Cut to the 1900s, when pasteurization and industrialization made many foods safer and more readily available. It was an amazing step toward equalizing food opportunities for different socioeconomic groups. We got better at making tasty foods that could be marketed in an eye-catching, salivation-stimulating kind of way—on TV! We started to be able to eat affordable foods that made us want to eat them more often, in larger quantities.

I remember my first Devil Dogs®: two soft hot dog bun–shaped devil's food cake halves with white cream in between. I remember the first time I had Yodels®: devil's creme–filled devil's food cakes, covered in a dark, hard chocolate glaze. I remember my first Pop-Tarts®, the same cinnamon sugar version that we have today. I still get "happy" when I think about eating these foods. They were my "friends" at a time when I was struggling with an unhappy home life. As I would eat, I would feel a physiological calm or peacefulness. Later on came the guilt from sneaking food and overeating and feeling out of control. But during the experience itself, I felt pure bliss.

I was lucky that they came on the market slowly, so they were considered unique treats. My mother was also on a tight budget, so individual boxes, rather than cartloads, were brought into our home. Still, they were immediate palate pleasers and I learned the art of hoarding them. These foods were forerunners of the now famous trans fats and high fructose corn syrup.

The idea back then was that if your mom really loved you, she would make you a Fluffernutter, a peanut butter and marshmallow fluff sandwich on white Wonder® bread. Oh my, how I envied the kids who brought those to school when I was opening my lunch bag with a hard-boiled egg, crackers, fruit, carrot sticks and a bag of chips in it. Those kids actually looked like they were on a drug trip, with kooky smiles on their faces as they plowed through those amazing sandwiches, along with their Kool-Aid®, Yodels®, and fruit shoe leather. We didn't know, then, the pitfalls of processed foods—those same kids were nodding off by 2 P.M. because their sugar rush was over and they were descending into the normal post-sugar sleepy state.

These days, we know that the so-called convenience foods aren't so convenient after all. They may be convenient in how fast they are to grab, but the time and energy required to undo the damage they cause is anything but. Today, we spend less time planning and preparing food, but much more time agonizing over weight and health problems. The HFL program is about turning that equation around to make your life easier.

Choosing the right "real" (not highly processed) foods for your breakfast, lunch, dinner, and snacks is vital to getting the best nutritional bang for your buck: high-fiber foods fill you up, slow digestion, burn up more calories during digestion, and prevent soaring blood sugar highs and lows. Often, you can even overeat these foods a little without paying a severe weight-gain price.

8. Everyone's Not Equal When It Comes to Weight Loss—But Everyone Has the Same Tools

No one really wants to accept the true secret to weight loss. It's not sexy, it's not particularly fast, it's not terribly unique, and it's not really creative. It's a relatively simple concept that seems to stress out a lot of people: don't take in more calories in a given day than you are going to use. Take in fewer calories than you need and you will burn fat stores and begin to lose weight. Eat more calories than you burn in a given day and you will gain weight.

Of course, there are factors that influence this. We've already mentioned that some people have a metabolic edge. Athletes or disciplined exercisers may be able to get away with eating more calories, although later in life, when they aren't able to be as active, they can develop serious weight issues.

There are also some newer scientific theories that bacteria in the gut may predispose some people to retain more calories from the foods they eat.[8] The results of generations of survival of the fittest are being expressed in these individuals, who may absorb more calories from certain amounts or types of food or process those calories more efficiently.

But even if the deck isn't stacked in your favor, there are great, realistic strategies that can help you reach and sustain a healthier weight for yourself.

9. You're Never Too Young to Start

The more effective you are at involving your whole family, the more success you'll enjoy. You'll want to present the changes you are going to make in a way that gets even your youngest children excited. Talk about spending more time with Mom to help pick fruits and vegetables, taste test and prepare new foods, dance or play ball, hike or bike, and become more energetic and healthy. These are the most important lessons for kids up to age ten. Offer simple sound bites of information that revolve around health, especially if weight is an issue. Kids will not feel attacked if your discussions revolve around health, encouraging better energy levels and better performance at school, and highlighting the danger of heart disease or diabetes, even if you know they need to lose weight. You want to minimize the kind of criticism that can negatively impact self-esteem and body image. Discussions that revolve *only* around weight can even instigate an eating disorder later on, so tread carefully and involve other health professionals when appropriate. After age ten, you need to decide just how mature your child is and how much more information he or she can handle regarding why they specifically may need help. The HFL program is based on four P's that even a young child can understand.

How you introduce these changes, especially to children whose palates may already be accustomed to high-fat/high-sugar processed foods or to sedentary living, will be vital to your—and their—success. It's easy to lose patience because we all want change to be swift and effective, but adding the burden of negativity will only make change more difficult. Instead, be gentle and opt for a slowly paced, positive experience for all ages (yourself included).

10. Small Choices Add Up to Big, Long-Term Success

If you could make little changes every week that positively impact your health and waistline without torturing yourself in the process, why would you seek out more challenging ones? If you could learn to modify habits slowly so that you shift the whole way you feed your body and nurture your emotions over time, why would you subject yourself to deprivation and starvation that actually impair your daily quality of life?

Don't overcomplicate things for yourself or your family. Yes, if you or a family member(s) is at FFIS Stage 3 or 4 (see Chapter 2), you will have to implement change more rapidly. Acute, serious disease commands a more rapid and dramatic change of habits, which may require the involvement of your pediatrician or other health professionals.

Ten HFL To-Dos

Even if you don't plan to do the entire HFL program, consider making just a few small changes for the health of your family. These ten "To-Dos" can make a huge difference, and the changes are not difficult to implement.

1. Eat breakfast or a more satisfying breakfast. (See Chapter 6.)
2. Plan better snacks and have them ready for every family member to take with them. (See Chapters 4 and 5.)
3. Start adding more healthy foods such as fish, beans, and nuts into your diet. (See Chapters 4 and 5.)
4. Create a list of unhealthy foods with your family and commit to limiting them—but allow occasional treats. (See Chapter 4.)
5. Teach all family members how to buy the healthier fast food options. (See Chapter 6.)
6. Create a list of foods you overeat, and make a plan for controlling the amount you eat of these foods. (See Chapter 8.)
7. Work with family members to create a plan that will include more fruits and vegetables every day. (See Chapters 4 and 5.)
8. Commit to eating together as a family three or more times a week.
9. Create and make available quick, tasty dessert options that won't pack on pounds. (See Chapter 7.)

10. Make a plan to be active as a family two to four times a week. (See Chapter 9.)

These are accessible and doable *remedies for a healthier life* and that's what the HFL program is all about. Pick several or all ten, and start working with every family member to adjust your lifestyle together. One of these changes could be your new habit of the week each week, and over the course of just a few months, you would have helped your family move into a healthier zone, all without having to make the kinds of changes that take over your life. Yes, you do have to organize and plan a bit, and that does demand a weekly time commitment, but you'll make up for it by eliminating many time-consuming last-minute grocery shopping and food preparation sessions.

CHAPTER 3 QUICK-SUMMARY

- Don't expect overnight success.
- Gradually retrain your palate so you no longer crave fat and sugar and switch to more healthy alternatives.
- Don't rely on a good metabolism to keep you healthy— even thin people suffer the consequences of bad food choices.
- Learn how to tell when you're really hungry (and not just bored or responding to emotional cues).
- So-called convenience foods aren't that convenient in the long run; learn to spend a little more time planning and preparing, so you can spend a lot less time undoing the damage.
- Yes, some family members may have a harder time losing weight, but success is never impossible if you're willing, open-minded, and patient.
- Include all family members, no matter how young (or old).
- Small changes add up. Pick a few and start today.

Tips for Kids

- Let them come shopping with you and taste test new fruits and veggies.
- Slowly teach them to read a food label so they see the difference between food in its natural or real state and processed food with all the additives and unhealthy ingredients.
- Identify whether your child is a grazer, mini-meal eater, or square-mealer and go with it within the framework of the program (refer to Chapters 5, 6, and 9).
- Limit TV/video/computer time and replace it with family activities. Instead—if you see emotional eating going on—start a dialogue with your child.
- Don't let your children skip breakfast, and let your kids be involved in food choices, which means they come shopping with you some of the time.
- Let them see you eating healthy foods because kids model their own behavior after yours.
- Let them see you exercising and weight training and explain the "muscle-metabolic" connection.
- Use water and low-cal flavored water pouches and eight-ounce cartons as instant freeze packs so they begin to drink lower calorie beverages instead of juice.
- Keep exposing them to foods, even if it takes a while to get them interested or willing to taste. Use creative presentation.
- Bake and broil healthier versions whenever possible (chicken nuggets, air fries), but realize that they are still used to the higher-fat-flavor versions.
- Don't condemn foods; do challenge portion size or frequency (applies to teens, too).
- Add puréed fruit, ground-up veggies whenever possible (applies to teens. too) and make recipe substitutions (see Chapter 7).
- Always serve a fruit salad and salad with the meal (applies to teens, too).
- Have "grab foods" in the fridge and pantry: cut-up fruit and veggies, ready-to-grab yogurts, string cheese, celery or car-

rots with bean or hummus, small containers of 1 percent or fat-free milk, small bags of cereal/nut mix, baked whole grain crackers and small peanut butter packets, grape clusters, low-fat chocolate pudding, tuna sandwich "quarters" on whole grain bread, turkey pinwheels.

• Let young kids help wash fruit, tear lettuce, add spices, fill measuring cups, grease pans with cooking spray, peel eggs, use a pizza wheel. Older kids can prepare simple recipes, use an electric can opener, use a toaster oven with mitts, or a microwave. (See more on this in Chapter 7.)

• Control TV viewing time and computer time and get them moving during TV commercials; have a short activity period about thirty minutes after dinner. It can be a short walk, freestyle dance session, or quick ball game. Do it with them so you are modeling the behavior.

• When possible, cut foods into shapes—kids love it.

• Reward exercise with a special craft, new book, or other non-food reward.

• Teach them that if it has more than eight grams of sugar (two teaspoons) per serving, it's too much.

Tips for Teens

• Involve them in taste testing healthy new food choices, and don't take it personally if they initially dislike most of the new tastes.

• Invite them into the kitchen or to shop, if they're willing.

• Try to create healthier home versions of pizza, lasagna, grilled burgers (turkey), grilled chicken, stir-fries.

• Have fruit, salad, and easy-to-grab options.

• Expose them to flavored waters.

• Review some of the healthier fast food options with them and explain why you want this program to work.

• Admit to your own poor role modeling, if applicable. Honesty appeals to teens.

• Get them involved in after-school sports or activities, and be there to cheer them on.

- Plan weekend food shopping and exercise activities, but be reasonable and patient.
- Don't condemn fast food; discuss better choices and frequency of eating.
- Stock lots of healthy condiments and spices.
- Experiment with healthy smoothie recipes. Adding protein powder is a boost for a budding athlete.
- Explore ethnic healthy home cooking recipes.
- Get your pediatrician to step in and express a perspective on health or weight and the positive implications of a lifestyle change.

4

The "Yes, No, Maybe So" Food Choice Plan

How to Live on "Yes" Foods,
Let Go of "No" Foods, and Eat the Right
Amounts of "Maybe So" Foods

With all the eating approaches and diets I tried as a teenager and a twenty-something struggling with my weight, what ultimately worked for me was learning to think about food in an entirely different way than I had been raised to do.

When I grew up, our family really had to get the most bang for our buck. My father was a schoolteacher and my mother didn't work outside the home, so money was by no means plentiful. Mom would buy the least expensive fruit-of-the-week from the grocer, usually apples. She always cut up lettuce and tomatoes for each dinner's "fill factor." White bread was the cheapest, so lunch every day was a sandwich, often peanut butter and jelly or American cheese. Potatoes were a dinner staple, and so was tuna noodle casserole (yes, the cheesy, fattening version).

I remember *so* wanting more of my favorite processed treats—Devil Dogs®, Ring Dings®, bagged chips, and Pop-Tarts®—all readily available if you could afford them, but we couldn't afford much. Like any teenager with a weight problem, I'd sneak them whenever I could save up enough money from babysitting. No doubt my mother tried to serve balanced meals, but she struggled with obesity and emotional issues with food herself. Watching her repetitive dieting only added to my body image problems and my skewed attitude about food. I saw it not only as fuel, but as a source of comfort and a friend.

My mother hoarded food and ate it secretly, although not so secretly that I didn't see it. She felt isolated because of her unhappiness about her weight—then turned to food for comfort. Her own mom, my grandmother, battled with her own weight and was rigid and controlling about food.

In my family, food was how we reacted to life. If I fell, I got food. If I got a good grade, I got food. If I was sad, I got food. Gradually, I got heavier. I learned to hate my body and thought my thighs and butt were too big. I envied my friends who were skinnier. I hated the way I looked in the short skirts and bobby socks that were popular at the time.

But I also hated the way I would hide food and then shovel it voraciously into my mouth. It felt out of control and, somehow, the way I was sneaking and eating food felt very wrong. Deep down, I knew that eating should never feel wrong. It should feel empowering. It should be savored, enjoyed, filling, and most of all, nutritious. Eating should feel like you are doing something fabulous for your health.

I had my "motivation moment" at the age of sixteen, not coincidentally just as I began to face dating. I decided that the grapefruit diet, the eat-lettuce-all-day/dinner-only diet and Carnation® liquid diet were simply not going to help me take off the weight and keep it off. I decided to try a leading commercial weight loss program of the time, which actually taught me about all the food groups, which ones tend to fill you up more or less, and how to plan daily food choices with the right amount of calories to result in weight loss.

After one year, I achieved a miracle of sorts: I lost forty pounds! I felt satisfied (not always hungry!), fabulously fit (I had also started an exercise program), and very much in control.

But that wasn't the end of the story. I continued to grapple with the fear that I could gain it all back in a moment of emotional upheaval or temptation. Part of the problem was the blandness and rigidity of the diet I was on, which worked for me during the weight loss phase but became tedious during maintenance. I struggled for years, through college and into married life, trying to maintain my weight.

Yes, No, Maybe So Is Born

Pregnancy was especially challenging for me. My appetite increased dramatically and it was hard to stick strictly with healthy foods. I wanted to eat unhealthy foods and take a long vacation from good nutrition. What helped me be more sensible was the realization that my baby's nutritional health began in the womb, and I was responsible for that.

I came up with a plan—the beginning of the Yes, No, Maybe So Food Choice Program—when I began to raise my daughter. I did not want her to struggle with weight issues like the three generations of women before her had done. I wanted her to be able to avoid the self-esteem problems and health risks. I wanted to break the cycle. I decided that each food group had a role in a daily eating program. I also decided that being as organized and aware as I could be about food choices and meal planning could actually be educational for her. I knew that having foods available in pre-portioned amounts would address calorie control. Identifying foods that should be in most of our meals and foods that were "special" would also help in a comprehensive plan. I also needed tools to help a child of two years understand the "why" of it all. These were the beginning seeds of the HFL program.

When my daughter was only a tot, I started to educate her about "Yes Foods," which have bountiful health benefits, really taste good, are easily available, and fill you up and not out. Fruits and vegetables became the staple of her diet as well as mine. As she grew older, salads became a big part of her life, with spinach for a base and fish, white meat chicken, eggs, and beans for protein.

It wasn't that there were no treats in my home; they just became "No Foods" (foods that should be eaten infrequently)—foods that were chosen with a great deal of care on food shopping day and portioned out as true treats, not daily rituals.

For "Maybe So" foods (foods that are healthy when eaten in moderation), I turned to low-fat yogurt, low-fat cottage cheese, and ricotta cheese instead of higher-fat dairy foods. Perhaps because I ate so much American cheese as a kid, I shunned hard cheeses as a teen and adult. Because most are high in fat, I felt I was doing my family a favor by not bringing too much cheese into the house.

I was never a big red-meat eater, so chicken, fish, and eggs became our protein staples. When it was age-appropriate (usually between ages four to eight, always with supervision), I introduced my daughter to nuts and seeds of all kinds, in small amounts. Our Crock-Pot® became our family's savior. Just drop in huge amounts of vegetables, liquid, seasonings, and chicken or fish, and come home to a Yes/Maybe So dinner brimming with good taste, wholesome ingredients, and healthy nutrients.

It was easy to explain to a child, "Let's get some Yes Foods," or "Time to put together some Yes and Maybe So Foods," and have her participate in the shopping, preparation, and cooking. My daughter knew exactly where to run in the supermarket for the Yes Foods and Maybe So Foods, many of which are typically in the periphery of the market—fruits, veggies, meat, fish, poultry, dairy—or down certain aisles—frozen fruits, veggies, canned beans, nuts, whole grain rice. She also knew how to recognize the healthier bread and cereals on sight and because we had ongoing "label reading lessons."

At home, fruit and veggies were always available in bowls on the table, cut up in the fridge, or in small plastic "grab bags." Some of the Maybe So foods that we enjoyed (with some measure of watchfulness) were soybeans; homemade trail mix with cereal, dried fruits, and nuts; hummus and bean dip; fat-free muffins made with applesauce and fruit; and hard-boiled eggs.

Like most people, I have struggled with food "demons" as the result of both the way my family handled food when I was growing up and from my own personality and genetics. However, since discovering my ability to handle food with the Yes, No, Maybe So principle, the desperation I used to feel about treat foods, or No Foods, has mostly passed. Now I know I can have them and that they have a place in my diet. I just can't have them all the time without consideration or limitation. Because I eat healthy Yes and Maybe So

SIX RULES OF FAMILY FOOD CHOICES

1. *Food is not the enemy.* Eating is not "bad" and starving is not "good." Food is fuel; it's how we get energy to live and do all the wonderful things we're supposed to do as human beings and as a family.

2. *Foods are not "good" or "bad."* Some foods are healthier than others and we should eat those foods more often—but nobody eats healthy 100 percent of the time, and eating an unhealthy food now and then isn't the end of the world.

3. *There is no Food Police.* As a family, we want each other to be healthy and make the best choices possible, and we help each other—but we don't make people feel guilty or ashamed about food.

4. *Food choices are individual.* No two people in the family will ever like or need or eat exactly the same things.

5. *Even a little bit better is better.* No matter how "not perfect" our food choices are, we celebrate every little improvement because they all add up.

6. *Tomorrow is another day to make good choices.* No matter what food choices we made today, it's no excuse to give up tomorrow. Making good food choices isn't a short-term (diet) thing; it's a *lifetime* thing. Some days will be better than others, but what matters is the long haul.

Foods that really satisfy my palate, I'm not emotionally or physically hungry. And when stress in my life increases, I have a fridge full of great fruits, veggies, and healthy dips to grab.

I found that the Yes, No, Maybe So system worked extremely well for me and for our growing family. It helped me tremendously when it came to shopping and meal planning for the week—and even when my kids' friends came over and clamored for treat foods. It was fun to explain that first we had to choose and prepare some Yes Foods. Soon they'd forget that they had even asked for a No Food! If they didn't, one cookie or one or two small chocolates would suffice—because they were already full from the fruits and veggies we'd had.

I learned through personal experience that Yes, No, Maybe So works. My daughter and later my son grew up with a healthy appreciation and palate for freshly prepared foods that are not necessarily time-consuming to prepare and always taste good. They understand the basics of food enjoyment such as the importance of herbs and seasonings, "tricks" such as using fruit purées instead of oils, and habits such as eating until the point of fullness—but not beyond. They are active, health-conscious adults who have broken our family's weight struggle cycle.

Your Family Can Have a Healthy Attitude Toward Food

After working with so many families over the years, I've found that the process of making food choices differs greatly between healthy families and unhealthy families. Healthy families can make food decisions virtually unhampered by emotional or physical cravings. They easily "get" eating for health. They think about how they feel after eating a certain way and are able to treat food like fuel that tastes good. They understand how to push the plate away when they're full.

Unhealthy families on the other hand, have an entirely different relationship with food. Cravings reign supreme. They habitually eat past fullness and eat whatever they want whenever they want it. They turn to food for comfort, grab food without much thought, and generally let food rule the roost.

KNOW YOUR BEANS

They're low in fat, high in protein. They also offer a variety of nutrients:

- Pinto beans have selenium.
- Kidney beans have fiber.
- White beans have iron.
- Black beans have magnesium.
- Chickpeas have folate.
- Black-eyed peas have calcium.

In my own life, I was greatly motivated to turn my own family's cycle of unhealthy eating and obesity into healthy habits. And as I worked with families in my practice, I discovered that unhealthy family habits could be transformed with education and practice.

As a mom, I wanted to do right by my family, in a way that was safe, comfortable, and practical—a way that would work with a busy family's life and, ultimately, help me raise kids who would embrace the foods that were best for them and develop healthy food attitudes along the way. The Yes, No, Maybe So approach fit the bill, and I still use it today, as do my very grown kids.

As a health professional, I found that the same principles that worked with my own family worked with clients who wanted to change their habits and become healthy families for life.

If my family can do it, so can yours!

Your Family's New Food Foundation

Healthy Families for Life make their food choices based primarily on three categories of food:

1. Yes Foods
2. No Foods
3. Maybe So Foods

Yes, No, Maybe So (YNMS) is the foundation of the HFL plan. In other words, this is where you start developing healthy family attitudes and behaviors. Once you learn the YNMS system, you'll learn to incorporate it into the four habits I call the four P's of healthy families: **P**lanning meals together, **P**reparing food together, **P**laying together and Controlling **P**ortions together. (In later chapters, you'll also learn strategies to support each other emotionally, great recipes, additional tips for succeeding, adaptations for health conditions, and much more.)

But the first—and perhaps the most important—step is to learn to look at foods using these three categories. Why is this step so important? Because *everything* starts with understanding the roles and importance of each category of food. The discussions you and your family will have and the decisions and ultimate lists you and your family members make—your choices, preferences, and your attitudes toward food—may all need to be adjusted. Before you can do any meal planning, shopping, or preparing, you need to have a foundation for making choices. If *all* you read in this book is this chapter, but you learn to make food choices based on Yes, No, Maybe So, you'll make a *huge* difference in your family's health. For life.

You are going to learn to create a family list of Yes, No, and Maybe So Foods, and also individual lists, so that each family member can create a personal plan based on their tastes, goals, and schedule. You'll also find out how to use the Yes, No, Maybe So plan when you shop, make meals or snacks, entertain, or go out.

One warning before we go any further: resist, resist, resist the urge to think of YNMS foods as "good" or "bad." This isn't about good or bad—it's just about making choices that make sense for you and your family. You are simply going to learn to say Yes more often to Yes Foods, say No more often (just not every time) to No Foods, and learn to find the right balance of Maybe So Foods for you and everyone in your family. (See the Six Rules of Family Food Choices!)

"At-a-Glance" lists of Yes, No, and Maybe So Foods appear on page 405.

HFL QUICK-TIPS FOR YES FOODS

- Your family's attitude toward Yes Foods starts with you. Let them see your enthusiasm—it may not take long for them to share it.
- If you think fruits and vegetables are boring, maybe it's because you only serve oranges, apples, lettuce, and cucumbers—get adventurous! Try new ones every week! For example, be creatively exotic with fruit: use a melon as the shell for a yogurt/nut/berry parfait; bake an apple with cinnamon and crushed nuts inside; grill pineapple.
- Challenge family members to think of new ways to add fruits and vegetables to meals and snacks.
- Have a salad and cooked vegetable with every lunch and dinner. It will greatly satisfy most appetites.
- Crunch on vegetables instead of chips and crackers for a snack.
- Get into the habit of using fruits and veggies with dips instead of traditional chips, crackers, and breads.
- Always have fruit "ready to grab" for your family.
- You can add puréed fruit even to hamburgers and meat-loaf. It will add bulk and antioxidants, plus a pleasant, subtle flavor boost.
- Change your dessert habits—have a small fruit cup with lunch and dinner.

Jazz up desserts by skewering fruit and drizzling with dark chocolate sauce, offer sweet yogurt dipping sauce with fruits, make whole-flour muffins chock-full of nuts and berries, top whole grain waffles with a variety of berries and non-fat whipped topping.

WATER ALERT

While water is the Yes beverage of choice, a study in *The Journal of Clinical Nutrition* determined that you can use other options to help you get adequate liquids during a twenty-four-hour day:[1]

- Unsweetened tea or coffee (up to forty ounces)
- Low-fat (1 percent) or non-fat milk (up to sixteen ounces)
- Diet soda/non-caloric beverages (up to thirty-two ounces—watch sodium)
- Juice (up to eight ounces)
- One alcoholic drink/day (if you already include wine, beer, or spirits regularly)
- No more than eight ounces of sweetened drinks/soda

Remember that juice and wine will replace a fruit in the HFL program. Also remember that two to three servings of wine/week is the maximum substitution and that juice will never have the same fiber content as a fruit, so it also should be used infrequently as a beverage. Finally, soda and flavored drinks are "treats" in this program.

Yeah, Yes Foods

M-m-m-m, Yes Foods. These are the foods to which you can practically always say "Yes." These are the foods you want your family to eat at every meal and as snacks, too. They're nutrient-dense, have lots of vitamins, have pleasing flavors, are often high in fiber, fill you up even though they tend to be lower in calories, and require little portion control. (I have yet to meet an individual who needed to watch fruit and vegetable intake carefully for weight loss purposes). Yes Foods are easy to remember: they're fruits and vegetables (except for starchy vegetables such as peas, corn, and potatoes of all kinds, which are treated as "bread-like" by most dieticians, nutritionists, and even Certified Diabetes Experts, who focus on carb-counting, and will go under the "Maybe So" category).

Now, wait a minute. I can almost hear some of you sighing with disappointment. Fruits and vegetables? NOT exciting, right? Well, that's where an HFL attitude adjustment comes in. If you're going to be an HFL family, you'll need to make friends with Yes Foods—and yes, that means fruits and vegetables. Ready or not, this is the "base" of your family eating from now on. Don't worry; in the next chapter we'll give you tons of ideas for getting your family to cheer for fruits and vegetables.

CALCIUM CLUES

It's a good idea to get the calcium you need from food rather than supplements. But if, for some reason, you find that calcium supplements are necessary, don't take more than 500mg at a time (you'll simply excrete it). Also, be advised that fiber can interfere with calcium absorption, so avoid taking calcium pills with high fiber ingredients such as wheat bran. (Metamucil® and oat fiber do not seem to present a problem.)

Superstar calcium sources include:

- Calcium-fortified orange juice
- Canned sardines with bones
- Non-fat milk
- Calcium-fortified soymilk
- Collard greens
- Low-fat yogurt
- Soybeans
- Turnip greens
- White beans

Let me share with you the three biggest selling points of Yes Foods:

- They're extremely satisfying (they typically leave you less hungry for other foods).
- You can eat quite a lot of them (portions are not a problem for most people).
- They're rich in fiber and bursting with antioxidants (so they're the healthiest foods you can eat).

In fact, the reason fruits and vegetables are so colorful is because of the singular or multiple antioxidant and active chemical properties they contain. These are brilliant factories of health for your family—most experts recommend eating a "bouquet of colors" because eating different colors daily ensures that you are getting the benefits of the full spectrum of vitamins and nutrients.

As far as portion control goes, yes, you could technically overeat Yes Food calories it you ate fifteen or twenty servings of fruits and vegetables on a daily basis. But honestly, what I see in my practice, and what most research shows, is that most families don't get nearly enough Yes Foods.

Family members who are eating for weight loss or have particular difficulty with overeating or portion control may need to watch caloric content of fruits and vegetables (this depends on the individual—sometimes the opposite is true, and it may be more helpful to have the freedom to fill up on Yes Foods). Fruits and vegetables have about sixty to eighty calories per serving, and you can plan on four or five servings of each group daily. Adding fruit helps to fill you up because fruit is packed with fiber, minimizes the ebb and flow of blood sugar levels because of the stabilizing fiber factor, and provides vitamin content—all with practically no fat in the mix. (You'll see that later on most meals should have a certain ratio of Yes and Maybe So foods so that you have a balanced meal.)

Non-starchy vegetables should be your primary Yes Foods; a portion is about a half-cup of cooked or chopped raw vegetables, or one cup of leafy, raw veggies such as lettuce or spinach. (Although starchy vegetables fall into the Maybe So group because they are higher in calories and require more portion control, they are still full of healthy nutrients.)

Fruits and vegetables are carbohydrates and are generally what is meant by the popular term "good carbs." That means they provide the energy your family needs to live well and perform at their best on a daily basis. Don't make the mistake of thinking all your energy needs to come from bread-like carbohydrates such as cereals, rice, pasta, and other grains.

For an At-a-Glance List of Yes Foods, see page 405, and you'll find a more extensive list on page 147 in Chapter 5.

No (Not Never) Foods

Okay, now on to No Foods. This is the most challenging issue for many of us because we instinctively don't want to give up our guilty pleasures. Before we go further, let me assure you that this list is not about banning pleasure from your life! The point of No Foods is for you and your family to understand that these foods require great caution and should not be taken lightly. No Foods should be selected as a rare treat. They need to be handled respectfully, with anticipation and pleasure, and inserted mindfully and intermittently into your family's diet.

No Foods include desserts, candy, white grains, high-fat meat and dairy products, and many processed foods, such as those that contain even small amounts of trans fat and saturated fat: baked goods, candy, granola bars, white bread, cookies, milk chocolate, whole milk and full-fat cheeses (except for children under age two or when indicated by a doctor or pediatrician in unique cases), highly sweetened cereal, red meat with marbled fat, skin on white meats, chips, full-fat dips and dressings, fried foods, deli meats (except low-sodium, fat-free ones), crackers (fried), mayonnaise, and shortening.

These foods are "occasional treats," "celebration foods," and otherwise special snack or meal foods. No does not mean never. However, these foods cannot be a regular part of your family's daily diet. Why? Because these are the foods that suck your family into the Obesity Trap. These are the foods that will kill your family if you don't pay close enough attention.

Because deprivation leads many people straight to the frustrating cycle of craving and bingeing, favorite No Foods should be thoughtfully included at a frequency of once or twice a week. But that doesn't mean each No Food gets included with that frequency! It means that you need to decide each week, based on total daily calories, which No Food you want to add . . . because you really savor it, you really miss it, or it really pleases your palate.

We often want what we are told we cannot have. But you can avoid that trap by choosing your No Foods carefully—and always with portion control and timing in mind. If there is a healthier version of something you love, say whole grain cookies, or baked (without trans fat) chips, just by cutting out some unhealthy ingredients you're making better choices. If you were eating full-fat dairy products and you switch to 1 percent or fat-free, again, that is a huge step in improving the health quality of your choices. Portion control with any treat—even dark chocolate with antioxidant benefits—is paramount. Obviously, this is a very individual area, and choices will likely be different for each family member based on taste preference and goals (health versus health and weight). For instance, a family member who is eating for weight loss will likely need to limit the frequency and quantity of No Foods as carefully as possible (always taking into account special occasions). Someone who is trying to adopt better eating habits to support health and diminish risk factors may be able to include a bit more of a Maybe So or No food.

For example, wine, as an alcoholic beverage, is in the No category. It is a caloric beverage (eighty to one hundred calories/serving) and there are a number of conflicting recommendations regarding how much wine is safe (heart protective or cancer-inducing) or beneficial to the average person. Some people look forward to its relaxing effect; some people truly enjoy the art of wine appreciation; however, because it has calories, it can't be handled irreverently. Wine also has health implications, some of which may not be beneficial. However, it has its place in health: No does not have to mean Never. I have worked with clients who choose to exclude all alcoholic beverages because they prefer to use their "treat" calories elsewhere, and other clients who have no problem integrating moderate alcohol usage into their eating and weight management plans. Your choice will depend on factors such as your age, lifestyle, and health status.

Also keep in mind that No Food strategies need to be flexible—they are likely to change often over a lifetime. Once good habits and portion control are well established, or goal weight is reached, your "treat" parameters may loosen a bit. You or a family member may find that certain new No Foods pop up as problems (you find yourself overeating them more and more often), and you may need to change your No Food strategies. (You'll find more on No Food strategies throughout the rest of the book.)

For an At-a-Glance List of No Foods, see page 407.

No with a Smile: Teaching your Family about No Foods

When you say the term "No Foods" to someone—whether adult or child—they may have one of several responses:

- Become horrified, fearful, and cease eating it entirely
- Become drawn to the "forbidden fruit" and rebelliously determined to eat it
- Crave it guiltily and fight endlessly to battle the craving for it
- Ask calmly, "Well, is it ever OK?"

Notice how three of these responses reflect emotionally extreme reactions—only the last response indicates a balanced and moderate attitude toward food. In later chapters, we will talk more extensively about emotional responses to food, but in order to use the YNMS system effectively with your family, it's critical that you understand how balance and moderation work with YNMS.

Life is about enjoyment, as is eating. An eating plan that does not acknowledge the importance of pleasure is doomed to fail. If you do not communicate this message to your family, you're unlikely to earn their cooperation for very long (if at all).

The key is balance. Enjoyment simply needs to be moderated so that we can truly treasure pleasurable experiences when they happen. This is true for kids as well as adults. Give a child a new toy daily and she'll be less likely to relish the toy's fun-giving potential fully. (Why bother? There's another one on the way!) Reward her less frequently, and she'll take more pleasure in it. We're the same way with food. If we enjoy it to excess, we lose much of the joy it can give us.

I like to think of No Foods as "No with a Smile" Foods. That means that you approach the idea of No Foods with flexibility, patience, humor, and creativity. For example, you're using the "No with a Smile" technique when you say to yourself or a family member, "You know, you already had a piece of cake on Monday, and a candy bar on Thursday, so let's wait till the weekend and maybe we'll fit in a treat then." Meanwhile, you cut up an apple and let your child (or inner child!) dip it into a tablespoon of peanut butter.

Or the "No with a Smile" approach might sound like this: "You know you don't seem to be able to have just one serving of chocolate cake, so why don't you let me split one with you at that fabulous restaurant we're going to Saturday night—and that way we'll both be in control."

No Foods and portion control may sound scary to your family at first, but the fear and anxiety will diminish as they realize they can still enjoy the pleasures of old favorite foods—just in a healthy way that will give them more "real" benefits than the taste of excess food ever could, such as getting and staying healthy, losing weight, feeling better, and looking better. Buying a small package of cookies or chips at the supermarket and deciding that your family members will have a serving of these items twice a week is not a deprivation but rather a way to stimulate true appreciation.

It may take a while to help your family get the idea. If you have been raising your family on a diet of fast foods and processed snacks, don't expect the change to occur overnight. (Patience is a virtue— and you'll need it.) But whatever you do, don't give up! You are giving your family a wonderful gift, not only in teaching them how to enjoy food with balance and moderation, but how to use those qualities to better enjoy life.

Starting Early

If you start to use the No Foods principle right from a child's birth, you are less likely to have problems with treat foods later; your child will develop a palate that appreciates and desires healthy foods. If No Foods are not commonly found in your pantry or fridge (but are

NO FOOD FOCUS: SUGAR

Sugars are simple carbohydrates found naturally in many foods such as milk, fruits, some vegetables, breads, and grains. They can be used as preservatives and thickeners and can be added to food for sweetness. From a chemical standpoint, all sugar is equal.[2] However, many sugary foods, where the sugar is added, tend to be high in calories and low in nutrients. Sugars that occur naturally in foods like fruits and vegetables are also accompanied by fiber content that helps diminish those sugars' impact on blood sugar levels. If sugar appears as one of the first four or five ingredients on a label, or appears repeatedly, the food is a No Food.

Sugar can have a number of names: watch for brown sugar, fructose, corn syrup, corn sweetener, fruit juice concentrate, raw sugar, molasses, maltose, sucrose, lactose, honey, invert sugar, and high fructose corn syrup.

Sugar substitutes, such as sorbitol, saccharin, aspartame, Sweet'N Low®, and Splenda®, do not provide significant calories, so they may be useful in your family's diet. However, food products that contain these substitutes may not be lower in calories and may not provide "fill factor." Remember—it's food with natural sweetness AND fiber like fruit that will tend to fill the "sweet, filling, low-cal" HFL dictum most of the time. Empty calories that are made low cal with sugar substitutes can't possibly rival a fruit. Some studies show that people who *consistently* rely on products with sugar substitutes may actually gain weight for a variety of reasons.[3] One reason might be a false sense of "diet benefits" that actually results in overeating. You convince yourself they are low calorie so you justify eating larger portions of these foods and you add in other foods. Another more simplistic reason is that you are ultimately not satisfied—fake food, no matter how sweet—tastes like fake food. Finally, if you are consistently turning to these foods, you've usually got other food issues going on as well. Healthy, *normal* eaters don't use these foods as a substitute or a crutch.

NO FOOD FOCUS: SODA AND JUICE

When you drink soda, you are consuming a hefty dose of caffeine plus sugar, which means lots of liquid calories without a lot of nutrients. Studies show that those who drink fair amounts of soda daily miss out on other important beverages, such as fat-free milk.[4] These individuals also miss out on the fill factor that liquid calories typically don't provide. I've seen babies with soda in their bottles and sippy cups! Introducing your child to soda should not be an American tradition.

Back in 1994, researchers noted that kids from the ages of three to five drank 15 percent less milk than their counterparts in 1977. They had, however, increased their juice consumption by 308 percent. Most parents automatically turn to juices as a bottle or cup beverage with more ounces and greater frequency of distribution than is healthy for their child.

Water is the "elixir of life" and it should be the primary hydration source after milk portions are doled out. It should be whole milk (after breastfeeding or formula has been discontinued) until age two and then low-fat or fat-free milk. Juice should be considered a treat because it really does not contain close to the vitamin, nutrient, and fiber content of whole fruit. And because many children are grazers, wouldn't you rather have an apple slice in their hand than a juice bottle hanging out of their mouth? Be aware that apple juice is not really a good source of vitamin C or folic acid, nor is unfortified grape juice. Fortified orange juice can provide vitamin C, potassium, folic acid, and even calcium, if it's added. But it should not be your or your kids' primary source of these nutrients.

not entirely forbidden either), most kids develop healthy attitudes toward eating. They learn that No Foods are simply foods that need to be treated with respect. I have learned in my practice that adults who have developed poor eating patterns suffer much more than kids raised from birth with healthy food attitudes. It is much harder to respect and portion out our treats if we've developed a "treat palate" early—and abused it for many years. So help your children now—and save them the frustrations of having to break longstanding habits in the future.

TEENS AND SODA

A growing number of studies suggest that people who drink sugary sodas consume more calories in a day than their counterparts who don't. Drinking a can of regular soda daily can add 15 pounds per year. Kids who drink three sodas daily have a 50% higher BMI than kids who drink less. Certainly we do know that soda drinkers drink less milk and have lower calcium intake as well. Soft drink consumption has also been linked to type 2 diabetes.

Consider the fact that a twenty-ounce serving of regular soda has about fifteen teaspoons of sugar. If you don't burn off those liquid calories that are being consumed right along with food calories, you're creating an easy calorie gain situation. The reality is that most teens are drinking soda daily, so it's worth targeting that habit as one of the first HFL switchouts. Emphasize water, low-calorie flavored waters, iced teas, and one or two servings of 1 percent or fat-free milk daily. I do recommend diet soda if that's the only option they'll embrace. Getting those liquid calories out of the diet should be a high priority.

NOT SO HOT FOODS

If you're bothered by hot flashes, foods high in fiber, soy, antioxidants and calcium may be your best friends. These foods are strongly emphasized in our HFL program.

What About YOUR Favorite No Foods?

I often see parents who are very good at telling their children what they should do—but not nearly so good at doing it themselves. (We can all relate to that!) It will never work to portion out single servings of "treat" crackers for your child to eat twice a week if you are munching (or sneaking) your favorite chips whenever you feel like it.

Overcoming your own unhealthy relationships with No Foods may be the greatest challenge you face in trying to turn your family's habits around. As the team leader of this family program, you have to exhibit the habits you want your whole family to embrace.

Remember that this project is a springboard for feeling better about yourself, how you look and feel, and how your kids view you, as well as their own body image and quality of life.

Creating No Food Strategies

You will need to create No Food Strategies for your family as a whole and for yourself (See sample forms, Appendix 4A and Appendix 4B), and you will need to help other family members create plans for themselves.

A No Food Strategy is simple—but not always simple to follow. It includes just two things: a list of No Foods that are a problem and the way you are going to handle each food.

Here's how a Family No Food Strategy might look:

- Pizza—Once every other week, with a salad first, light cheese and lots of vegetable toppings
- Soda—Only on special occasions, outside of home

- Sweetened cereal—only on vacation, during special events such as a slumber party, or as an occasional topping
- Chips—only with special meals
- Cookies—two each, once a week
- Cake—on birthdays and special occasions

You will want to discuss this list with everyone in the family, and get creative ideas. Also remember that you have to start somewhere—your first list may not be everything you'd like it to be ultimately. It may have too many treats or too many treats that are very

---

NO FOOD FAMILY STRATEGIES

- Don't try to rewrite your family's food habits overnight. Pick gradual strategies, such as slowly cutting down from four fast food meals to two per week—and have the kids deciding the healthy choices that will replace those meals.
- No more giant bags! Divide up individual portions of chips, cookies, or other treats and begin to limit how many times your kids have them per week, replacing them with creative fruit and veggie options such as strawberries with chocolate syrup dipping sauce, apples and peanut butter, or cut-up veggies and bean dips.
- If soda is a problem No Food, create low-cal spritzers using mostly club soda and small amounts of fruit juice.
- If white bread, pasta, and sugary cereals are family problems, alternate them with healthy breads and cereals.
- Gradually switch from full-fat dairy products by cutting in lighter, healthier versions (1 percent and fat-free).
- Use products such as flavored sprays, cinnamon, spices, and fruit to add "flavor pizzazz" that will help win family members over to healthier choices.

high in fat or calories or highly processed. Remember that unless you are dealing with very small children who have not developed ingrained habits that revolve around these treats, most kids and teens are going to fight these changes. They'll be resistant and resentful and frankly, very often your spouse will behave similarly. Make an agreement to revisit the list in a month or two or three and keep working on reducing the number of treats or substituting slightly lower fat or caloric versions of the treats.

Every family member will also want to create his or her own list. One family member may find that he or she needs to limit vending machine treats at work—or dipping into the office candy jar. Another family member's list might have to include doughnuts, milkshakes, steaks, fried chicken, tortillas, martinis or strawberry margaritas, fettuccini Alfredo, mac'n'cheese . . . the list goes on! Encourage everyone to be honest about the No Foods that they overeat, but never forget the No with a Smile philosophy. It may take time for some members to recognize or admit the foods they have problems with (and new foods can become problems at any time.) Again, set a time frame for everybody to reconsider their lists.

My Strategy for No Foods

I will often plan my snacks ahead of time to have control. There's nothing wrong with winging it sometimes or having a treat and then modifying the rest of the day's eating plan or increasing your exercise in order to accommodate it. I do believe that, especially in the early months, pre-planning helps tremendously. You'll feel more in con-

REDUCE BLOOD PRESSURE WITH SOY

Unsalted soy nuts may help to reduce blood pressure when eaten in small portion amounts (25g daily). *Source:* Archives of Internal Medicine, *May 2007;* Journal Watch Cardiology, *July 11, 2007.*

trol, and it will help your kids decide on their treats for the week. You will also be able to remind them of what they have had when they whine a bit (and they will whine for a while).

Here's a sample of how I incorporate my No Foods into a monthly plan:

Week #1:

- I plan on having two chocolate chip cookies with a cup of skim milk on Monday and do cardio and a weights workout.
- I plan on having two cups of (light) cheese puffs on Thursday and take a long run.
- I plan on sharing a piece of chocolate cake with my husband on Saturday night after we hike during the daytime.

Week #2:

- I plan on having a small frozen yogurt topped with sprinkles on Tuesday and going light on my bread servings that day.
- I plan on having two squares of dark chocolate Friday night and doing cardio and weights during the day.
- I plan on having French toast (two pieces) Sunday morning and then playing tennis and going for a walk.

Week #3:

- I plan on having five Twizzlers® on Wednesday and going for a long bike ride.
- I plan on having three pieces of California Pizza Kitchen® pizza on Saturday night after I go for a 5K run that day.

Week #4:

- I plan on having two cups of the Pirate's Booty® snack food on Monday and having a salad and protein for dinner.
- I plan on having a breakfast muffin on Wednesday morning and then doing a cardio and weights workout.
- I plan on sharing a piece of apple pie with my husband on Saturday night after running at the beach.

Food and Activity Journal

Keeping a journal of daily food intake is an enormous help for creating No Food strategies. The journal is your witness. It knows when you had the No Food last, how much you had, and the occasion. The journal doesn't lie—unless you lie. Because denial is a human trait, writing a daily accounting of your food and activity level is a way to be honest with your calories and food choices, as well as your exercise and calorie-burning activity. You may have really convinced yourself that you are a miserly eater simply because you deny or forget some of the foods you ate or the nature of those foods. You simply cannot "wing" a lifestyle change. Habits develop slowly with intentional behavior.

A journal that tracks both your food choices and your daily activities is an excellent tool for the adults and teens in the family (see sample, Appendix 4C). Even family members who are unlikely to maintain food journals for long periods of time are often able to keep one for two to three weeks to track habits and discover problem areas.

The idea is to track what you eat and how much exercise or activity you do daily/weekly (or don't do—that is, watched four hours of TV on Wednesday) and to write EVERYTHING down. You want to start noticing amounts of food, preparation methods (fried,

---

CRACKER ALERT

Crackers are notorious for hiding trans fats. They also can be devoid of nutritious ingredients unless "whole grain" is listed as the first ingredient in the label breakdown or the box is marked "100 percent whole grain." So Ritz® crackers, Wheatables®, and Multi-Grain Wheat Thins® don't make the grade. Triscuit® crackers do contain whole grain, but they have a significant fat component. Kavli® Thin Crispbread and Wasa® Fiber Rye Crispbread are better choices. So are any baked, whole grain, trans-fat-free crackers.

SUBSTITUTING FOR NO FOODS

Because most No Foods have trans fat or saturated fat (that is, are creamy, oily, fried) or are highly caloric with significant amounts of refined sugar ingredients (for example, candy or white processed food), consider finding a "healthier" or lower-calorie version that you can eat more regularly without adding too many calories.

Just remember that if you use too many No Food substitutes, you will be less likely to eat other, healthier, more beneficial foods. You'll be trying to "outsmart" the eating program. I will often ask a client, "Do you know what Webster's definition of a treat is?" I'll pause and then answer, "Well, Webster's definition is *an event or circumstance that gives pleasure*. HFL's definition is a *timed* event or circumstance or, in this case, food item that gives pleasure." Your real goal is to create a "treat mentality."

Chocolate lovers may want to substitute a small piece (instead of a whole bar or box) of decadent dark chocolate as a pleasurable treat with some added health benefits (antioxidants) and no trans fats to clog your arteries. Another alternative is to substitute a small, non-fat chocolate pudding or a cup of fat-free cocoa simply to evoke the taste of chocolate without all the calories or fat.

But be careful! I think the biggest mistake families make (other than being in denial over portion sizes and how often treats are appropriate) is peppering their diet with fat-free, low-cal, processed food versions of favorite treats. For example, a chocolate lover may decide to forgo the pleasure of their high-calorie candy pleasures and instead choose to have chocolate pudding, hot chocolate, chocolate Fudgsicle® treats, chocolate Tootsie Pops®, fat-free chocolate muffins, etc. *every day.*

I know there are diet gurus out there constantly refreshing the list of "substitute treats" that won't blow your diet. But they're missing the point—which is to retrain your palate to eat foods with high nutrient content and good taste. These treats may take the edge off your craving, but they aren't contributing positively to your health.

grilled, baked with sauces, etc.), and even emotional mood states when you eat (for example, two bags of chips when the Lakers lost) as well. If you don't measure and write everything down, journaling doesn't work. If you're eating off the dinner plates as you clear the table or grabbing candy every time you pass a receptionist's desk, you've go to "stop and jot."

Remember, your journal won't judge you. The journal may provide the key to why you are gaining weight instead of losing it, or suffering from a health condition (hypertension is directly related to salted foods, heart disease to high saturated fat/high trans fat food, weight gain to eating too many calories). It's an assessment tool that will deal you the real truth—if you're ready for it.

REAL-LIFE HFL STORIES: NO FOODS BALANCING ACT

One of my clients feels that chocolate and olives are trigger foods for her. Unfortunately, these are foods that are really hard to keep out of your life—especially when you eat out a lot, travel frequently, or entertain for business. Her strategy has been to turn to fat-free chocolate pudding and Hershey's chocolate syrup for fruit dipping—and only to book herself into hotels that have gyms.

When she feels she overeats the more caloric or fat-laden versions of these treats, she balances it out by increasing her exercise and really keeping her home pantry and fridge "pristine." Her No Foods have become part of her traveling professional life and she has basically eliminated them on the home front—or replaced them with healthier, less caloric versions. This No Foods balancing strategy has helped her create and maintain a weight loss of thirty pounds for more than two years.

LEUCINE AND PROTEIN

When choosing quality protein, leucine, an amino acid, may be the key to maintaining muscle while losing flab. Meats do have the highest concentration of leucine, but also the highest concentration of saturated fats. Better options include:

- Firm tofu, one-half cup: 1,511mg
- 1 percent cottage cheese, one cup: 1,440mg
- Reduced fat mozzarella cheese, one ounce: 670mg
- Reduced fat cheddar cheese, one ounce: 608mg
- Egg, hard-boiled: 538mg
- Couscous, one cup cooked: 464mg

When No Means No: Trigger Foods

One last thing about No Foods: although most people are successful with most No Foods by planning moderate consumption ahead of time, there are exceptions. One example is trigger (or binge) foods. A trigger food is a food that you simply cannot control, whether in quantity or frequency of consumption. Some women feel chocolate of any form is their nemesis—that it can set them off on a binge with all control lost.[5] For some guys, it's peanuts or chips.

During the weight loss phase of this process, it is particularly critical to determine whether or not you can or need to include problem foods. For example, though you may love chocolate candy bars, a small amount for you may not be enough; that small amount may trigger you to have more and more.

For those people who identify themselves as food addicts, sugar addicts, or compulsive eaters, their personal program of recovery often entails avoiding their specific trigger foods. They may exclude these foods from their diet entirely, just as an alcoholic or drug addict will remain free of their addictive substances. The medical community does not unanimously agree that food addiction exists in a pure form; they do, however, concur that a part of the population struggles with serious food control issues, and "binge eating" is a recognized medical diagnosis.

If you or a family member identifies a food that you simply can't coexist with on a reasonable No Food–frequency basis, you may have to consider just cutting it out—period. Some people find that eliminating foods permanently from their diet makes life and healthy eating much easier. Others find that after a period of time they can have small tastes or a small portion under controlled instances—only at outside dinners, perhaps, or only when sharing it with someone so they don't eat all of it themselves. And of course, many people find that working out emotional issues often translates into less use of food as "personal therapy," and a reduction of binge eating.

This is a very individual process that is often not just about willpower. Bingeing, compulsive overeating, undereating, anorexia, and bulimia are all examples of eating disorders that typically require the intervention of health professionals such as physicians, therapists, and support programs for ongoing daily management. If you or a family member suspects you may have more serious issues with food, consult a professional who can help you.

Maybe So Foods

The most important food category, by far, is the Maybe So category—foods that are healthy when eaten in appropriate amounts and in balance with the rest of your diet. Most foods fall into the Maybe So category. They require portion control and in-depth assessment to integrate them successfully into your daily eating program.

Just as with No Foods, Maybe So Food choices are very individual. For example, a child may need larger quantities of certain Maybe So Foods for growth and specifically bone support, such as dairy products. Recent studies show that it is preferable to get your calcium from foods and to only turn to supplements as a secondary back-up option.[6] Of course, there are other sources of dietary calcium, but dairy products feature prominently in most American diets. An active adult who is a serious exerciser might need more

OMEGA-3 FATTY ACIDS NEWS FLASH

The healthy fat in fish can:

- Fight pain (arthritis, inflammatory bowel disease, menstrual cramps)
- Block cancer due to its anti-inflammatory action
- Build bones
- Help to spur weight loss by improving blood flow to muscles
- Lift your mood
- May reduce the risk of sudden heart attacks and dangerous arrhythmias

protein than an older person whose metabolism is slowing down, while the older person may need more healthy omega-3 fats and calcium. Family members who are eating for weight loss will need to take that into consideration while calculating Maybe So Food choices and amounts. In short, everyone in your family will need a personalized plan for fitting Maybe So Foods into meals and snacks, in reasonable quantities, using the best options from each food group.

ANOTHER DAIRY "PLUS"

Metabolic syndrome is a condition that involves obesity, high cholesterol, high blood sugar, high blood pressure, and high triglycerides (danger signs for diabetes, coronary artery disease, and early death), and is currently being diagnosed in the adult and child population. Eating two daily servings of fat-free dairy seems to help lower the blood pressure component of this disease.[7]

MEASURING UP

Popular Maybe So Foods can be high in fat but are also very beneficial because they supply healthy fat or lean protein or calcium or other nutrients. Here are just a few examples in these measured amounts:

- Avocado, one-half cup cubed: 120 calories, 11 grams of fat
- Peanut butter (pick trans-fat-free), two level tablespoons: 188 calories, 16 grams of fat
- Olive oil, one and one-half tablespoons: 180 calories, 21 grams of fat
- Almonds, twenty-three: 164 calories, 14 grams of fat
- Very dark chocolate, one ounce: 136 calories, 9 grams of fat

Source: www.calorieking.com

MAYBE SO FOOD FOCUS: STARCHY VEGETABLES?

Although all vegetables have substantial nutrient content, peas, corn, and potatoes are actually included in the "breads/rice/pasta" food group because of their significant starch content. Treat these foods like breads when you are creating your daily food plan. Remember that sweet potatoes have far more fiber than white potatoes, which is a plus when it comes to choosing your "superstar foods." Serving size for these foods is half a cup of peas or corn or half of a small potato; you are targeting an eighty-calorie portion size.

Maybe So Foods include low-fat and fat-free dairy products, lean proteins (including the leanest cuts of red meat, skinless white meat, fish, beans and legumes, soy products, nuts, and eggs), monounsaturated and polyunsaturated fats, and high-fiber complex carbohydrates. Note that the less healthy versions of these foods—namely, the dangerous fats, which includes partially hydrogenated oils and animal-based saturated fats, fatty red meat cuts, full-fat dairy products, and processed carbohydrates—all fall into the No Food ("special treat") category.

Maybe So Food choices have nutritious elements and can be beneficial to you and your family's health, but have higher calorie counts and fat content; consider carefully how they fit into each day's worth of eating. Maybe So Foods are divided into four categories:

- Dairy
- Protein
- Bread-like carbohydrates
- Fats

REAL-LIFE HFL STORIES: CHEAT NIGHTS

I worked with a family that was addicted to junk food, and every member was overweight. The No Food solution that worked for them was a once-a-month "Anything Goes" night. Each member gets to choose three foods that they want to eat without portion control. They eat a salad at the beginning, so that they start a bit full, and then throw out any leftovers—and I mean out of the house in the outdoor garbage pail! The kids usually choose pizza and ice cream and soda, but interestingly enough, their mom reports that they still "blot the pizza" to get rid of excess oils, and actually ask for fruit on their ice cream. She has also noticed that the amount they eat on each monthly cheat night has gradually decreased because the kids know if they really want it, another cheat night is just thirty days away.

MAYBE SO: HEALTHY FATS PRIMER

Fat provides taste, consistency, stability, and a sense of fullness after eating. It also helps you absorb vitamins A, D, E, and K and carotenoids (cancer-fighting substances in vegetables). But you have to be careful which fats you choose: unsaturated fats are beneficial when consumed in small amounts; saturated and trans-fatty acids raise LDL (the bad cholesterol) and may also lower HDL (the good cholesterol).

Trans Fat: When you make liquid oils into solid fats (shortening, solid margarines, some vegetable shortenings), you get trans fat, and many processed foods have it (cookies, crackers, snack foods, french fries, doughnuts). Trans fat occurs in small amounts in butter, whole milk, cheeses, beef, and lamb. The current health recommendation is to steer clear. Americans still eat about five times more saturated fat than trans fat. Measure for measure, trans fat is more dangerous, but also be aware that too much saturated fat will dramatically increase your risk of developing heart disease, stroke, diabetes, and other ailments.

Saturated Fat: Saturated fat is the main dietary cause of high blood cholesterol. It's found mostly in foods of animal origin (meat, butter, whole milk) and in coconut oil, palm oil, and cocoa butter. Current health recommendations advise adults not to exceed 10 percent of daily calories when factoring in foods that contain saturated fat.

Monounsaturated Fat: Good fats. These are usually liquid at room temperature and are found mostly in foods of plant origin, like canola and olive oil. These fats, like polyunsaturated fats, are caloric, but they are not implicated in increasing the risk of heart disease or blood cholesterol. In fact, as

MAYBE SO: HEALTHY FATS PRIMER, *continued*

mentioned previously, they actually reduce LDL. Keep these fats to about 20 percent of your daily diet.

Polyunsaturated Fat: These fats provide omega-3 and omega-6 fatty acids. They are mostly found in vegetable oils, though some fishes, nuts, and seeds also contain polyunsaturated fats. They lower LDL (that's good), but they also lower HDL (not beneficial), so I recommend limited use of these fats.

Cholesterol: It's a naturally occurring substance (meaning our body makes all we need). The largest dietary deposits can be found in the tissues of animals, specifically liver, organ meats, egg yolks, and whole milk, which is why they are Maybe So Foods. The human body makes all the cholesterol you need, so you really don't need it in your diet. The liver does process much of the excess cholesterol we eat, but its clearinghouse function can be challenged by a high dietary intake. Some people do not process the cholesterol well, which leads to elevated cholesterol levels in their bloodstream. Eggs should be included in your diet with portion control. You can easily have one regular egg and two egg whites at a meal or just turn to a product like Egg Beaters® to control your dietary cholesterol intake.

Using these four food groups will help you plan your Maybe So choices. You'll find that Maybe So Foods give you a wide range of options, and lots to think about. For example, many Maybe So choices are nutrient-dense superstars but are also calorie-dense (for example, starchy vegetables). Proteins and dairy products are very important groups for your health, but you only need a certain number of portions daily—eat too much and you'll gain weight. Whole grains are valuable to your diet but should only be eaten in controlled amounts. Fats, too, are necessary to a healthy diet but can't be eaten indiscriminately.

Let's look at the superstars of this group—the foods that give you and your family maximum benefits in health, energy level, and performance, with minimal saturated fat. They are:

- Low-fat (1 percent) and fat-free dairy products (milk, yogurt, cheeses)
- Skinless white meats (chicken, turkey, veal)
- Whole grain, high-fiber carbohydrates (cereals/breads/rice/pasta/grains)
- "Healthy fat" foods that contain omega-3 fatty acids, monounsaturated fats (nuts and seeds, fish, avocadoes, olive and canola oil)
- Alternative sources of protein like beans and legumes
- Eggs, egg whites, and soy products (soymilks, cheeses, tempeh, tofu, soy burgers)
- Fish because it provides protein and heart-healthy omega-3 fatty acids
- Small servings of nuts and seeds (proteins with beneficial fats)
- Starchy vegetables (corn, beets, yams, potatoes, succotash, etc.)

These are the foods you'll be selecting as your Maybe So choices each day. For an At-a-Glance List of Maybe So Foods, see page 407.

A quick note on polyunsaturated fats: they lower both LDL (the bad cholesterol) and HDL (the good cholesterol) levels. They may also be implicated in contributing to the incidence of cancer. So though they are a better choice than saturated or trans fats, I don't encourage using them as a significant option for Maybe So Foods. Monounsaturated fats are a healthier choice.

Maybe So Means Portion Control

If you can remember that "Maybe So means portion control," you've got the main point about this food category. You can be much less stringent with Yes Foods, and No Foods are eaten infrequently, so

MAYBE SO FOOD FOCUS: FISH

The benefits of eating fish seem to be due to the omega-3 fatty acids it contains. This fatty acid makes up the second of two essential fatty acid groups. Omega-6 fatty acid, also called linoleic acid, is the other group and, though beneficial in small amounts, Americans get far too much of it in their diets. Omega-3 fatty acids include alpha-linolenic acid and EPA. They can be found in fresh deepwater fish (including salmon, mackerel, herring, and even sardines), fish oil, and certain vegetable oils (including flaxseed oil, walnut oil, and canola oil). Just four ounces of salmon contains 3,600mg of omega-3, mostly due to its fatty content. In comparison, four ounces of cod contains only 300mg of omega-3. Other sources include flaxseeds, flaxseed meal, hempseed oil, hempseeds, walnuts, pumpkin seeds, Brazil nuts, sesame seeds, avocados, some dark leafy green vegetables (kale, spinach, purslane, mustard greens, collards, etc.), soybean oil, wheat germ oil, anchovies, albacore tuna, and others.

While it's preferable to get most vitamins and essential nutrients primarily from their "fresh" source, if you won't eat fish (and have exhausted all methods of preparation to make it appealing to your palate) you might consider a fish oil supplement, though some experts prefer fresh sources to supplementation of this essential fatty acid. If you're a vegetarian and don't eat fish, the flaxseed family is a great source of omega-3 fatty acids in all its forms.

It would be reasonable to consider fish the new star of a healthy dietary lifestyle. Evidence continues to mount in support of the conclusion that eating fish can have a significant impact on most people and specifically on individuals at risk for or suffering from heart disease, Alzheimer's, strokes, arthritis, cancer, and other serious illnesses.

Maybe So Food amounts are the ones about which you need to be concerned. Remember, we emphasize portion control because, at the end of the day, eating healthier food is a huge step but maintaining weight has to be directly connected to calorie control. HFL *gifts* you with fruits and vegetables in abundance so you are able to be more

MAYBE SO FOOD FOCUS: HEALTHY FATS

So many diets over the years have shunned fats. But fats provide calories for energy and give food texture and taste appeal. We now know that certain fats have huge health benefits and no diet should be totally devoid of fats. Fats also help you digest certain elements better. For example, we now know that lycopene, which is found in tomatoes, is better digested and utilized by the body if it is accompanied by a small amount of healthy fat like olive oil. We also know that small amounts of healthy fats help the body process the vitamins and nutrients from vegetables. So a little olive oil helps your body to achieve the benefits a healthy raw salad has to offer. Of course, this is a Maybe So food that needs to be portion- and frequency-regulated.

Allow yourself one to two teaspoons per serving of fat, whether cooking with it or drizzling it fresh. The best fat choices include:

- Monounsaturated fats: canola, olive, peanut, other nut oils
- Polyunsaturated fats: corn oil, fish oils (omega-3 fatty acids), safflower oil, sesame oil, soybean oil, sunflower oil

The newer "healthy fat spreads," such as Benecol®, may provide health benefits but need to be portion-controlled because of their high calorie content.

conscious of the Maybe So and No Foods, which are often higher in calories.

Particularly in the early weeks of your family's lifestyle change, you should consider measuring out your portions with a weight scale or measuring cup. Why? Because you may well be used to the outsized portions that have become so common in our restaurants, supermarkets, and convenience stores. Measuring is a great way to readjust your perceptions of portions. For example, you'll find that a half-cup of rice is the size of a small scoop of ice cream—not a giant, plate-sized heap. A four-ounce serving of protein (for example, a piece of chicken or fish) is often compared to a deck of cards or the palm of a small human hand.

Maybe So for Weight Loss

If you, a family member, or your whole family wants or needs to lose weight, portion control for Maybe So Foods is even more important. Someone who is trying to lose weight needs to burn 2,500 calories more than they take in per week to shed a pound of fat successfully. You may need to be quite rigid in planning portion amounts and activity levels to achieve a one- or two-pound weight loss each week. When you achieve your goal weight, you may then be able to add on some extra servings from certain groups.

Now What? Getting Started

All right—so you and your family understand Yes, No, and Maybe So Foods. Here are some ways you will integrate YNMS into your family lifestyle:

- Create your own Family YNMS weekly shopping list and individual shopping lists for each shopping-age family member (to find out how, see Chapter 6).
- Create and post your Family No Foods Strategy, monitor your progress weekly, and consider developing a family (non-food) rewards plan. Remember you are rewarding progress, not perfection!

WHOLE GRAIN TIPS

When choosing breads for fiber content, watch for a minimum of three grams fiber/serving; cereals should have five grams/serving. Know your whole grains:

- Quinoa (one-half cup, cooked with water) has two grams fiber, 127 calories.
- Amaranth (one-quarter cup, dry) has 7 grams fiber, 180 calories.
- Barley (one cup pearled, cooked) has 6 grams fiber, 160 calories.
- Buckwheat (roasted groats, cooked) has 2.3 grams fiber, 77 calories.
- Corn (one-half cup, canned, no salt) has 2.1 grams fiber, 83 calories.
- Millet (one-half cup, cooked) has 1.1 grams fiber, 104 calories.
- Oats (twelve tablespoons, regular or instant) has 2.4 grams fiber, 108 calories.
- Brown rice (1 cup long grain, cooked) has 3.6 grams fiber, 216 calories.
- Wild rice (1 cup, cooked) has 3 grams fiber, 166 calories.
- Rye (one-quarter cup of grains) has 6 grams fiber, 140 calories.
- Sorghum (one-quarter cup) has 3 grams fiber, 160 calories.
- Spelt (one-half cup) has 7 grams fiber, 193 calories.
- Kamut (one-third cup of grains) has 4 grams fiber, 130 calories.
- Bulgur (one-half cup dry) has 12.8 grams fiber, 239 calories.
- Cracked wheat (one-quarter cup of grains) has 5 grams fiber, 140 calories.

WHOLE GRAIN TIPS, *continued*

- Wheatberries (one-half cup of grains) have 5 grams fiber, 170 calories.

You can add these to soups, salads, casseroles, and stews. After cooking whole grains, you can store them for up to five days to use in recipes. A bonus—oats and barley lower cholesterol.

- Assist family members in creating their Individual No Foods strategies, monitoring their progress weekly, and developing personalized reward plans for progress.

Planning Your Family Diet with YNMS

Food and meal planning is a highly flexible and individualized process that can be as easy or as complicated as you want to make it. Your family's lifestyle and food preferences are an important consideration. If you travel a great deal, eat out, or are constantly on the go, your plans will be quite different than if you eat most of your meals together at home. The more people there are in your family, the bigger job you have. If anyone has health conditions, weight loss objectives, or special dietary needs, you have even more factors to consider.

In Chapter 6, we will discuss in more detail how to shop and plan meals based on YNMS. Let's first look at easy ways that you can translate YNMS into healthy eating for your family.

"Quickie" HFL Meal Plan

Most families today live on the run, squeezing meals and snacks in between work, school, and other appointments. Scheduling mayhem is typically the norm. The beauty of Yes, No, Maybe So is that you can make it work for you even when there is no extra time to spare.

For example, most nutritionists feel that every meal should have a healthy, portion-controlled carbohydrate, healthy protein, and healthy fat, which facilitates a gradual increase in blood sugar levels and keeps the diet well balanced.

This simple formula, translated into the Yes, No, Maybe So philosophy, looks like the following:

Every meal:
- Two Yes Foods
- One Maybe So Protein (four to six ounces) OR low-fat or fat-free dairy (one cup)
- One Maybe So whole grain carbohydrate (optional, one to two servings)
- One healthy Maybe So fat (small portion)
- Plus No Food treat (occasional only)

A sample breakfast would be: three-quarters of a cup of high-fiber, high-protein cereal; one cup of fat-free yogurt with one-half cup of berries; half a banana; and one tablespoon crushed nuts.

A sample lunch would be: an omelet with one to two egg whites and one egg, shredded veggies, and one-quarter cup skim mozzarella cheese. Include a piece of high-fiber whole grain bread. Add in a fruit if you are still hungry.

IS BROWN BREAD BETTER?

Just because bread is brown in color or says "whole grain," it doesn't mean it's a true, significant source of whole grain. The advertised "whole grain white breads" are a good example. The wheat used to make them is a special kind that is lighter in color and sweeter, more mild-tasting than traditional whole grain. But the rest of the flour mixed in is plain old refined flour and the amount can vary. So you are really only getting a small percentage of actual whole grain.

A sample dinner would be: four ounces of grilled fish, a dinner-size salad with a drizzle of olive oil/balsamic dressing, steamed veggies, and a small scoop of whole grain rice. Add fruit if you're still hungry. If you are due for a No Food, you might choose to skip the rice and just enjoy the treat.

"Quickie" HFL Grazing Plan

Given the fact that kids (or adults) may be grazers and not sit down for a planned, balanced meal, you may want to think of your meal plan as a "grazing plan" with prepared healthy food choices ready to be eaten when needed.

Have prepared and easy-to-grab throughout the day:

- Plentiful Yes Foods
- Healthy whole grains (in measured quantities)
- Low-fat or fat-free dairy (in simple single-serve containers)
- Proteins (in measured amounts)
- Healthy fats
- Plus measured, prepared No Food servings occasionally, on a planned basis

Basic Meal Plan Options

If your family is willing and able to have planned meals and snacks for the most part, here are two Basic HFL Meal Plan templates you can try.

Snacks are factored in to prevent long periods between meals that can make you "out of control/grab hungry." You can also add snack servings to meals to make them larger or skip a snack if you are really satisfied.

Basic HFL Meal Plan Option #1

Breakfast

Two Yes Foods
One to two Maybe So Foods (protein, dairy, or bread/carb)

AM Snack

One Yes Food
One Maybe So Food (protein, dairy, or bread/carb)

Lunch

Two Yes Foods
One Maybe So (protein) Food
One Maybe So (dairy or bread/carb) Food
Plus one healthy fat serving

PM Snack

Option 1: One Yes Food plus one Maybe So Food (protein, dairy, or bread/carb)
Option 2: One to two Yes Foods

Dinner

Two Yes Foods
One Maybe So (protein) Food
One Maybe So (bread/carb) Food
One healthy fat

Plus

Occasional planned, portion-controlled No Food

Here's a sample meal plan based on this template:

- *Breakfast:* one piece of fruit, one serving of cut-up veggies, an omelet made with two egg whites
- *AM Snack:* fruit, small fat-free yogurt
- *Lunch:* medium salad, three ounces of water-packed tuna, one piece of whole grain bread, olive oil/balsamic vinegar dressing
- *PM Snack:* cut-up veggies, small serving fat-free cottage cheese
- *Dinner:* small salad, steamed veggies, grilled fish, brown rice, olive oil dressing
- Special Treat: glass of wine twice/week

Basic HFL Meal Plan Option #2

Breakfast

One Yes Food
Two Maybe So Foods (protein, dairy, or bread/carb)
One healthy fat

AM Snack

One Yes Food

Lunch

Two Yes Foods
One Maybe So (protein) Food
One Maybe So (dairy or bread/carb) Food
Plus one healthy fat serving

PM Snack

One Yes Food
One Maybe So Food (protein, dairy, or bread/carb)

Dinner

Two Yes Foods
One Maybe So Food (protein)
One Maybe So Food (bread/carb)
One healthy fat

Plus

Occasional planned, portion-controlled No Food

Here's a sample meal plan based on this template:

- *Breakfast:* fruit, whole grain cereal, skim milk, a sprinkle of nuts
- *AM Snack:* fruit
- *Lunch:* medium salad with beans, fruit salad, avocado on top of salad
- *PM Snack:* celery, string cheese

Breakfast

Two Yes Foods	One or Two Maybe So Foods
Apple and berries	Egg whites, one piece whole grain toast
	OR
	Egg whites, peanut butter (for apple slices)
	OR
	Special K® waffle, soy nut butter

AM Snack

One Yes
Fruit or veggie

OR

One Yes, One Maybe So Food
Fruit, fat-free yogurt

OR

Veggies, bean dip

OR

Baked crackers, hummus

OR

Melon and cottage cheese

Lunch

Two Yes Foods	Two Maybe So Foods (protein, bread/carb)	One Healthy Fat
Large salad	Turkey slices, one piece whole grain bread	Fat-free mayo
	OR	
Fruit salad	Cottage cheese, nuts	(Nuts)
	OR	

Salad	Chickpeas/soybeans	Olive oil
	OR	
Fruit	Tuna, baked crackers	Fat-free mayo
	OR	
Vegetables	One slice thin crust pizza (cheese)	(Cheese/oils on pizza)

PM Snack

Yes Food
Fruit or Veggie

OR

Maybe So Food (protein/dairy or protein/fat)
Yogurt

OR

Turkey slices

OR

Fat-free pudding

Dinner

Two Yes Foods	One Maybe So Food (protein)	One Maybe So Food (bread/carb)	One Healthy Fat
Salad Fruit	Grilled chicken breast	Brown rice	Olive oil
	OR		
	Grilled fish	Corn	Benecol®
	OR		
	Turkey burger *OR* Meatballs	Half a whole grain bun Whole grain spaghetti	Non-fat mayo Olive oil

- *Dinner*: fruit salad, dinner salad, grilled chicken breast, half of a sweet potato, olive oil/balsamic vinegar dressing
- *Special treat*: Dessert, one time/week

Note: One six-ounce glass of wine can be substituted for a fruit serving two or three times/week; in that case, it needs to be portion-controlled and would be a Yes Food. Otherwise, it can be a "treat or No Food."

More Meal Plan Options

Here are some more specific options you can try for a healthy meal plan (three meals plus two snacks), based on the Yes, No, Maybe So system.

Meal Planning Tips

Planning your family food choices around the Yes, No, Maybe So system can work under even the most challenging of circumstances—as long as you keep portion control and balance in mind.

Here are some additional tips:

- Yes Foods are your family's best friend—you can't be too enthusiastic a fan of them or too creative (or sneaky) in how you get them into your family's diet. If all you do is significantly increase your family's consumption of Yes Foods, you'll improve your family's health in too many ways to count.
- Mindfulness is the secret to No Foods. The more your family is able to identify No Foods and create successful strategies for handling them—whether it's planning them moderately into their food plans or cutting them out altogether—the more successful they will be at healthy eating and weight management.
- Portion control and balancing food groups are the tricks to Maybe So Foods. Everyone in the family will probably need a little education (and practice) to make smart choices.

The Practical Side of Yes, No, Maybe So

Some days are more harried than others: salad with beans or tuna accompanied by fresh fruit and a slice of multigrain bread may make more sense than grilled fish with steamed vegetables, a serving of corn, and fruit salad for dessert. Both menus marry the food groups to balance nutrients, variety, fiber needs, and taste—one meal just takes longer than the other to prepare.

You do want to consider your No Foods carefully when you are traveling so you can enjoy specialties in other countries without gaining weight and throwing caution to the wind. Maybe you will add an additional small portion or two of No Foods to the week and increase your physical activity as compensation. Obviously, if you are due a No Food, it can be dessert at either lunch or dinner or added to a smaller snack. (You decide based on your weight loss goals.)

I do recommend cutting out some calories (minimally) on the days you are going to have a No Food if you are trying to lose weight. Or conveniently plan your No Foods on exercise day so you can burn the extra calories. That way, your mindset is not "Throw caution to the wind," but rather "I'm intentionally deciding to have a No Food (or to allow my child to have it)"; all that's necessary is a conscious effort to pay back some of those calories through activity or by greater calorie awareness during the day.

Remember that calories in–calories out is tremendously important for weight control or weight loss in this program. Based on visual cues and by initially using a kitchen scale, over time you will develop an eye for portion sizes. But also remember it's easy to get blurry on measurements, so it's a good idea to revisit weighing and measuring on an intermittent basis.

YNMS Takes Time—and Common Sense

Although the Yes, No, Maybe So system is fairly simple, it can still be a BIG challenge to adjust your family's eating habits. It's important to realize that *all* eating programs have phases and transitions. You or your family may prefer a very rigid approach to begin with or a more gentle, slow-paced approach. Just don't expect it all to come together right away. Families who succeed at changing habits do so because they stick to it over the long haul, gradually integrating healthy changes despite obstacles and setbacks.

Some of the tips you find in this book may work like a charm for your family—at other times, however, you'll have to improvise to find something that works for you.

Beginning a lifestyle change is typically very exciting. You experience more control over food choices, a feeling of guiding the food rather than letting the food dictate to you. What I found personally and with many clients is that some habits require dogged (stubborn!) persistence, while other changes can be made more casually and gradually. You may find that it works to be very determined about exercising five times a week no matter what, but that you can be a little more lax about the occasional dish of ice cream. Or you may find the opposite: that desserts are too hard to control and need to be rigidly monitored, while you fluctuate your fitness program between three and four times a week, depending on your schedule.

You will also find that some weeks require different attitudes than others. There may be a week that you spend mainly dining out, partying, and entertaining. Yes Foods may not be abundantly available, despite planning ahead. Simply realize this is a week where there may be more No Foods and strategize to: 1) limit portions, 2) increase your activity level, and/or 3) ultimately learn something from the experience so you can be a bit more in control the next time.

For "unpredictable" days, I always pack some healthy meal replacement bars and small bags of nuts and dried fruit so that I can at least start the day with a healthy, balanced breakfast that includes Yes and superstar Maybe So Foods. That compensates for some choices I may have to make later in the day.

Take It Easy

Change is no small task for any family. Stress is very real, and research shows that many people use food to cope with the stress in their lives. Food is one of the most common sources of comfort for people, and that emotional connection is not easily severed.

I know from working with so many families over the years that simply understanding nutrition basics is not always enough to circumvent old tendencies to grab the foods that made you feel good or seemed to help you handle uncomfortable emotions. In later chapters, we'll discuss success strategies that can help you and your family with the deeper challenges you'll face as you change your habits. We'll also indicate when additional professional help to support this program may be necessary.

It's also important to be aware that the challenges will be different for every family member, and that you will not all move at the exact same pace through the process of learning to eat healthier for life.

It's critical that you remove the judgment factor. Simply focus slowly on achieving better choices each day and practice measuring success in new ways. Perhaps just keeping your child at his current weight so his height can catch up is all you need to do. Or consider it a success when you feel totally in control of a day's worth of menu planning. Just achieving several healthy meal plans together as a family is something you can all celebrate (just not with unhealthy food choices). Remember, every seemingly small milestone moves your family toward quality of life benefits that won't just last a lifetime—they may resonate positively for generations.

CHAPTER-4 QUICK-SUMMARY

- Remember this is a transitional process, not an overnight "quick fix."
- Really spend time learning the Yes, No, Maybe So Foods.
- Adjust portion sizes for individual needs. (Are you feeding an athlete, a growing child, someone with weight loss needs, someone who needs to address health risks, an active adult?)
- Do taste test with the family—it adds an element of fun to changing die-hard food taste preferences.
- Address the individual needs within the family needs.
- Have fun with the choosing and timing of No Foods.

Tips for Kids

- Remember that it takes repeated exposures to a new food (often as many as twenty) before kids will like it.
- Let kids choose snacks and help pack school lunches.
- Make a game out of it with red light, green light, yellow light foods to convey the same idea. Make a set of index cards and let the child use colored stickers to signify the Yes (green), No (red), and Maybe So (yellow) food categories.
- Give kids choices, taking them to the supermarket, playing taste-test games, feeling, touching, and experiencing new foods, especially fruits and veggies.
- Get your pediatrician involved in talking with your child about the purpose of this change, the need for better quality food, the implications it can have on academic performance, athletic performance, body image, long-term health consequences—whatever is age-appropriate.

- Involve kids in tracking several health parameters if appropriate (weight, cholesterol level, blood sugar level, blood pressure readings).
- Plan a physical activity with your child and during the "rest period," plot which "new foods" you'll try, which are the No Food choices for the week.
- Talk about your concessions and changes in eating, so they understand this is a family program and a family experience.
- Don't preach and lecture; be willing to have the approach fail at times, but revisit it within twenty-four to forty-eight hours so your kids know this is a change that has to happen.
- Remember that unlike many programs, the goals here are a bit more forgiving, and more in tune with the most current approaches to nutrition and better lifestyle, namely, smaller successes and achievements rather than sudden change and failure. Your attitude has to be a bit more forgiving, too.

Tips for Teens

- Remember that it will take time to readjust their palates.
- Really spend time talking about the Yes and Maybe So Foods and why No Foods need consideration.
- Engage them as often as possible in daily/weekly menu planning.
- Make sure they feel free to challenge or discuss any of the Yes, No, Maybe So Food categories but emphasize that there are no good or bad foods—each food group has its place in the eating plan.
- Remember that their friends may still be largely subsisting on fast foods, soda, and other food choices you are trying to discourage, so make sure there is balance in your approach.
- Let them know you too are struggling because teens appreciate honesty.
- Don't make it a battle of wills—appeal to their sense of health and discuss how they feel about their weight, their body image, the current food plan you've been eating.

- With dedicated athletes, larger portions and more frequent servings of HFL Yes and Maybe So Foods could be needed to sustain energy and support fitness efforts. The quantity of food (specifically portion sizes or frequency of choice of Maybe So Foods) can increase, but the quality of food should be Yes and Maybe So Foods.

5

Focusing on "Yes" Foods: The Healthy Family Food Superstars

It's Not About What Your Family Can't Eat,
It's About What They Can—and Should!

People end up at my office door for a variety of reasons. Their MD may have referred them to me because they are beginning to show signs of conditions associated with obesity. They may be feeling uncomfortably large or that their eating is out of control, or they may have a big event coming up, such as a reunion or wedding. Perhaps a life insurance evaluation revealed some worrisome findings.

Whatever the motivation, they expect to be forced into a world of *don'ts* for as long as they can take it. (And secretly, like every experienced dieter, they expect to go back to their usual habits when they can no longer stand the deprivation.) They are surprised when I tell them, "You may be having a problem with how you relate to food, but if we approach this relationship with a lot of 'No's,' you will probably give up altogether in a few weeks. Instead, what I'm going to suggest is that we agree to approach this whole process from a position of 'Yes.' In fact, the single most important change you can make in your whole relationship with nutrition is to think about what you *can* eat—not what you can't eat."

My guess is that your family will need to hear the same message. Being a Healthy Family for Life doesn't mean taking on a negative or self-sacrificing attitude toward food; instead, it's about saying yes to the right kinds of foods, and to a healthier, longer, more active and balanced life.

Why Say Yes?

Yes or Superstar Foods include most fruits and vegetables, and they are so important that I'm devoting a whole chapter to them. (Notice there's not a No Foods chapter!) What makes Yes Foods so valuable and why do I call them Superstar Foods? Well, they offer an incredible variety of benefits for their calorie count: they fill you up and sustain you with fiber, taste good thanks to their innate flavors, and offer nutrients that will keep you energized and satisfied.

Yes Foods provide a variety of benefits:

- Yes Foods satisfy your palate and hunger with the lowest penalty in calories.
- Yes Foods give you gentle ebbs and flows in your blood sugar levels, so you will be less likely to feel the swift highs and sudden plummets of a blood sugar cycle gone wild.
- Yes Foods typically have a lot of fiber and volume so your stomach stretches noticeably during digestion, allowing you to respond better to the natural feeling of fullness that normally guides eating.
- Yes Foods offer a variety of tastes, textures, and smells, so you're less likely to become bored with food choices or experience cravings because of food monotony.

Your Family Food Attitude Makeover

Every member of your family, no matter how young, has some kind of relationship with food. It may be a very healthy relationship, which means that you eat mostly for fuel, you eat to feel pleasantly full, you eat certain foods because they really appeal to you, and you eat a balanced diet because it makes you feel good mentally and physically.

In my practice of more than twenty years, I rarely see this kind of person, even in a non-professional or on a social basis. More often than not, I see kids craving junk food, even if they are eating on a regular schedule. I see people eating foods that mostly come out of boxes or containers. I see families who reward their athletic kids after a game with doughnuts, pizza, and soda. I see people whose feelings are directly reflected in the quantities and types of food that they eat. In short, the relationship we have with food is usually unhealthy. Most people I see need a Family Food Attitude Makeover. That makeover begins with shifting your focus from No Foods (and guilt) to Yes Foods (and feeling good about what you eat).

What Makes a Superstar or Yes Food

Yes Foods are:

- Low-calorie or a calorie bargain for their portion size
- Eye-pleasers, colorful and appetizing-looking
- Smell-pleasers, with a bouquet of pleasant odors
- Thirst-satisfiers (Thirst is often a component of hunger)
- Palate-pleasers, tasty, juicy, crunchy, sweet, velvety smooth, crisp, tart, spicy, salty, or succulent (These are the messages you want your brain to receive when you take a bite)
- Dense in nutrients, offering vitamins and antioxidants
- Filling, with fiber to provide a feeling of satiation when you eat reasonable quantities
- Stabilizing, causing a gentle rise and fall in blood sugar, without stimulating hunger too quickly after eating (again, because of fiber)

- Accessible; they're typically located on the supermarket's perimeter, so you don't have to delve into the aisles to get to them

While some less healthy snacks have some of these characteristics, only fruits and vegetables (again, our superstars) have *all* of them. Fruits and vegetables are natural providers of a variety of antioxidants, natural compounds that prevent cell damage caused by the effects of oxidation. The process of oxidation also releases free radicals, which are believed to contribute to causing cancer and other diseases. To understand the process of oxidation, which is caused by free radicals in the body, think of metal rusting, which means it is becoming damaged and deteriorating. The effect oxidation has on the body paves the way for a variety of diseases, including cancer and heart disease, and can also speed up the effects of aging.[1] That's why we emphasize the importance of having free radical fighters present in our daily diet and another reason fruits and vegetables are so important.

The Fiber Fullness Factor

"The Satiety Index of Common Foods" was published in the *European Journal of Clinical Nutrition*, September 1995. In this study, Dr. Suzanne Holt of the University of Sydney, Australia, designed a study in which specific portions of thirty-eight different foods were fed to test subjects, and then she recorded the subjects' perceived hunger following each feeding. The study specifically looked at the time period two hours after feeding.

The results of the study indicated that certain foods are much better than others for satisfying hunger. The researchers used white bread as their reference point, and arbitrarily assigned it a "Satiety Index" of 100. The Glycemic Index, another tool nutrition experts use to rate foods impact on blood sugar, used a similar testing procedure but reflected an absolute, namely blood sugar rise as food is digested and its carbohydrate or sugar content enters the bloodstream. Foods that did a better job of satisfying hunger were given proportionately higher values, and foods that were less satisfying were assigned lower values.[2]

Even among the most satisfying foods they tested, raw fruits stood out. Subjects that consumed the prescribed portion of these foods were less likely to feel hungry immediately afterward. It's no great surprise, based on what I've told you about processed foods, that the foods that did the poorest job of satisfying hunger included croissants, doughnuts, and candy bars.

What did surprise me is that peanuts did not fare well, even though they combine protein and healthy fat and tend to be a popular snack choice when you talk to food experts. The bottom line is that nuts do need to be eaten in small portions, though, or they become caloric bombs because of their high-fat, high-calorie content.

The Satiety Index study was a limited study, so I don't consider the food scores to be absolutes. However, the Satiety Index researchers made one very important general observation: all of the foods with the highest Satiety Index values had high weight-to-calorie ratios (I call it "low calorie for large portion"). In other words, these foods contained particularly large amounts of bulk for each calorie consumed. They help make you feel full by filling your stomach with water/fiber volume. That's why Yes Foods are salvation foods for people who are struggling to lose weight or maintain lost weight.

The following table is Holt's Satiety Index (SI), which uses foods from a number of different food groups in order to show various Satiety Index comparisons. Notice how well fruits do as foods with low-calorie/low-fat/zero-processed ingredients:

Although we are focusing on Yes Foods, it's also a good time to note that the whole grain choices like oatmeal, All-Bran®, popcorn, brown rice, and whole grain breads also achieved high ratings, but they are significantly more caloric than fruits and vegetables, which is why they get Maybe So Food status. It's also important to note that *combining* two foods like an apple with a small portion of lentils could be a good way to create a very sustaining low-cal mini-meal or snack.

Choosing Yes Foods

Some families give up before they even try when it comes to Yes Foods. They have all kinds of reasons for not stocking them: they're too expensive, too hard to get, too hard to prepare, unappetizing, or

THE SATIETY INDEX

All are compared to white bread, ranked as "100."
Each food is rated by how well it satisfied hunger.
If you want to lose weight, avoid the LOWER numbers!

Bakery Products

Croissant	47
Cake	65
Doughnuts	68
Cookies	120
Crackers	127

Snacks and Confectionary

Mars candy bar	70
Peanuts	84
Yogurt	88
Crisps	91
Ice cream	96
Jellybeans	118
Popcorn	154

Breakfast Cereals

Muesli	100
Sustain®	112
Special K®	116
Cornflakes	118
Honey Smacks®	132
All-Bran®	151
Porridge/Oatmeal	209

Carbohydrate-Rich Foods

White bread	100
French fries	116
White pasta	119
Brown rice	132
White rice	138
Grain bread	154
Whole wheat bread	157
Brown pasta	188
Potatoes	323

Protein-Rich Foods

Lentils	133
Cheese	146
Eggs	150
Baked beans	168
Beef	176
Fish	225

Fruits

Bananas	118
Grapes	162
Apples	197
Oranges	202

boring. Sometimes these attitudes are holdovers from childhood, when fresh produce actually was more difficult to get. Perhaps in your childhood you were primarily exposed only to endless apples, oranges, lettuce, and cucumbers—no wonder you got the idea produce was dull.

You're going to have to give up ideas like these if you want to do right by your family's health. Besides, old attitudes about fruits and vegetables don't hold water anymore. It's time to broaden the picture and expose your family to a whole range of amazing choices: from sweet mangos and spicy peppers to crunchy, tart berries, the sweetest of watermelons, and crunchy corn kernels. The list goes on and on: blood oranges, Satsuma tangerines, kiwis, bok choy, arugula, and yellow squash.

Although some of these fruits and vegetables are still pricey or difficult to get year-round, don't give up. With farmers' markets flourishing and the Internet making it possible to get twenty-four-hour fresh deliveries, produce is more accessible than ever before. One fabulous service that offers locally grown produce is the Community-Supported Agriculture (CSA) program—just Google it with the name of your city. Bulk-sellers like Costco® can provide great price breaks to help you keep Yes Foods stocked for your family.

Kids Can Say Yes to Fruit

A recent report (*LA Times*, May 14, 2007) suggests that a low-cost approach at schools is to offer the kids new, healthier foods by specifically asking them, "Do you want fruit or juice?" Just putting out the selections may not be enough. At a Connecticut school lunch, servers were trained to ask the question, so kids were aware that there were specific choices; 90 percent of kids took the foods offered and 80 percent actually ate them.[3] This means that kids may be more willing to try Yes Foods than we think. They just need some encouragement and enlightenment. There is a great lesson here for your Family Food Makeover, too: don't forget to give your children healthy choices verbally as well. Simply putting them out on display may not be enough to nudge them into actually trying them.

REAL-LIFE HFL STORIES: TRANSFORMING RICK, THE TEEN ATHLETE

Jennifer was the single mom of Rick, a high school student and avid baseball player. He was six feet tall and weighed 240 pounds; the majority of his weight gain had occurred in his first two years of high school when he began to subsist on fast food, smoothies, and blended coffee drinks. He ate breakfast, lunch, and snacks out of the house, a huge shift from his middle school years, when he ate breakfast before carpool at home and took brown-bagged lunches and snacks to school. Rick was initially delighted with his weight gain because he was packing on muscle mass as well. Once he passed about 200 pounds, though, much of the weight was showing up as a large belly—in his words, "not cool."

Rick realized that scouts were taking a look at prospective athletes for college teams. This motivated him. Parents can have the best intentions, but with the exception of small children, the desire has to be in the individual. Rick agreed to see me for a couple of sessions—just so we could figure out how much he needed to eat and how to balance his diet so that energy stores were maintained while he lost weight. Rick had tried a couple of fad diets that failed him, mostly because he felt tired during practice and games.

There's no doubt that Rick was eating healthfully at home (dinner and after-dinner snacks). His mom had lost thirty pounds on the HFL program and had since maintained it for two years. Rick was willing to cut back on eating out and to try healthier ways to order fast food when necessary. Dropping half of the bun, adding tomato slices, choosing white meat chicken, choosing salads with beans and lean white meat cuts, drinking water or iced tea, selecting lower-calorie smoothies and adding protein powder and more fruit, and having fat-free lattes were some of the options we discussed.

REAL-LIFE HFL STORIES, *continued*

Rick was even motivated to create daily meals and snacks that he'd prepare with his mom at home and store in a portable cooler. Frozen flavored waters became the natural ice packs in the cooler. A couple of his fellow team mates teased him at first, but not surprisingly, several began asking their moms to do the same thing. As Rick lost weight, his performance on the field, especially his base-to-base running times, improved dramatically.

Rick has shed twenty-three pounds in three and one-half months. He tells me that on weekends he'll have some extra calories, maybe one or two treats, but that thanks to his athletic involvement, it is really easy to stay motivated and to get back on track on Mondays.

Preparing Yes Foods

Yes Foods aren't hard to prepare, but you do need to give some thought to their preparation, or you'll fall prey to the Buy-It-and-Forget-It Syndrome. How many times have you bought crisper drawers full of fresh fruits and veggies, with the best of intentions, only to forget about them and throw them out weeks later? Buying Yes Foods isn't enough—you have to plan what you're going to do with them. (See more about food planning in Chapter 6 and food preparation in Chapter 7.)

Some Yes Foods preparation methods take very little time; others take more time and should be saved for special occasions. But the secret is to make Yes Foods as pleasing to the senses as possible. For example, too often we don't realize that we need to entice people visually in order to get them to welcome new foods. If you want your family to embrace this makeover with relish and enthusiasm, consider your presentation.

Don't just take it for granted that if there are some apples and oranges to grab, no additional effort is needed. You also need to have a variety of grab options cleaned, prepped, and ready to go.

Here are some tips for preparing Yes Foods:

- Follow directions and don't overcook frozen vegetables—so they can be just as tasty as fresh ones.

FRUIT THAT CAN FOOL YOU

Dried fruit, though it has fiber and nutrient content, tends to be much higher in calories per portion than fresh fruits, so even though it's tasty, you need to watch portion size. Dried fruit is sweeter, more concentrated, and easier to consume, so be wary of mindlessly munching, in larger portions. Also be aware that some manufacturers add sugar to their dried fruit products. Fruit juice, on the other hand, has sweetness and vitamins but lacks fiber; drinking liquid calories will not fill you up as much as eating an equivalent piece of fresh fruit.

One healthy option is *freeze-dried* fruit, which has all the water removed but retains the vitamins and nutrients and some of the fiber content. It also tends to be lower in calories than the same size portion of dried fruit. For comparison:

- A raw medium apple has about 70 calories and three to four grams of fiber.
- One-third cup of dried apples has 110 calories and about three grams of fiber.
- Just under an ounce of freeze-dried apples has 80 calories and one gram of fiber.
- A cup of apple juice has 115 calories and two-tenths of a gram of fiber.

As you can see, an apple gives you the most fiber and crunch factor for the least calories and will take you longer to eat.

- When you steam veggies, add fresh herbs and a bit of olive oil for great taste.
- Partially cook veggies and then finish them on the grill with a little cooking spray and some seasonings.
- Alternate fish or chicken pieces with vegetables on shish kabob spears.
- Grill pineapple to bring out the sweetness. (In fact, any sweet fruit on the grill will taste super-sweet because the grilling process caramelizes the sugar. I've even grilled papaya, watermelon, and mangos.)
- Poach pears.
- Make baked apples with cinnamon and raisins.
- Use fruit purée in turkey burgers and meatloaf made from ground chicken and turkey.

SAY DOUBLE YES TO BERRIES

The antioxidant power (as in fighting free radicals) of foods is sometimes measured with an analysis called ORAC (oxygen radical absorbance capacity).[4] Berries are among the highest-ranking Yes Foods on the ORAC scale, which is why I call them Double-Yes Foods. Fruits feature prominently on this scale. I've included a variety of highly rated fruits on this list:

- Açai: 18,500 ORAC
- Prunes: 5,770 ORAC
- Pomegranates: 3,307 ORAC
- Raisins and dark grapes: 2,830 ORAC
- Blueberries: 2,400 ORAC
- Blackberries: 2,036 ORAC
- Cranberries: 1,750 ORAC
- Strawberries: 1,540 ORAC
- Raspberries: 1,220 ORAC

- Use a Crock-Pot® to make vegetable soups and stews, including beans for protein.
- Do Chinese stir-fries with lots of veggies and tofu, cubed and marinated in a little teriyaki sauce.
- Prepare berries with dark chocolate dipping sauce.
- Get creative with fruit salads and tossed salads: different colored lettuces, spinach, mandarin orange slices, and slivered almonds are crowd-pleasers.
- Try fruit salad layered with fat-free yogurt and chopped nuts in parfait glasses.
- Take small cherry tomatoes and spear them with alternating cucumber slices to create a kid-friendly veggie dish.

Sneaking Fruit and Veggies into the Mix

You need to get creative when it comes to incorporating Yes Foods into the daily diet. Here are some great ways to sneak more Yes

---

HFL QUICK-TIP:
IN PLACE OF SPINACH . . .

Spinach is a powerhouse Yes veggie that packs in a lot of beta-carotene, vitamin B6, vitamin E, folate, potassium, magnesium, and lutein. But if you can't stomach spinach, say Yes to:

- Broccoli, carrots, sweet potatoes, and cantaloupe (beta-carotene)
- Lean meat, whole grains, nuts, and legumes (vitamin B6)
- Vegetable oils, nuts, seeds, wheat germ (vitamin E)
- Navy beans, orange juice, wheat germ (folate)
- Bananas, milk, kidney beans (potassium)
- Natural peanut butter, pecans (magnesium)
- Broccoli, brussels sprouts, kiwi (lutein)

> # HFL QUICK-TIP: SALAD BEWARE
>
> Too much fat—even healthy fat—or choices such as fried or deli meats, fried fish, whole-fat cheese, or croutons, can add a calorie and fat burden that will quickly turn a "Yes Salad" into a big No.
>
> To make the perfect Yes Salad, start with a bed of different colored lettuces, then add four or five different veggies/fruits, add some healthy fat with measured amounts of olives, nuts, or olive oil dressing, and finally, add some protein (beans, tofu, soy meats, and grilled fish are good choices) to make it a main HFL entrée.

Foods into your family's meals and snacks (chapters 6 and 7 will get more specific):

- Presentation is sometimes everything. Use toothpicks to spear melon balls or use skewers to spear a variety of fruits. Kids love a selection of different and less typical utensils when it comes to eating.
- Puréed fruit or veggies can be mixed into meatloaf. Puréed veggies can also be added to burgers and low-fat lasagna.
- Frozen berries are great in smoothies.
- Fruit soups can be refreshing in the summer.
- Add fruit to jazz up your salads.
- Always serve whole grain french toast or pancakes with fresh fruit topping.
- Always top cereal with fruit.
- Soups are a great place for both puréed and whole veggies.
- Stews including beans and veggies can be a filling meal.
- Shop the local farmers' market and get to know the vendors.
- Add healthy greens to a typical sandwich to get in a veggie serving.
- Cut-up veggies and hummus or bean dip can be a great "pick me up" snack.
- Kids love to dip—give them fruit and yogurt dipping sauce.

Patience, Patience, Patience

Most people meet their downfall by expecting change to happen too fast. You need to remember that each person in the family will move at his or her own pace, and decide when things are or are not working. Frustration, boredom with the notion of change, anger, and other feelings will often surface, sometimes repeatedly. Just be patient, and keep those Yes Foods accessible and appealing.

For the first twenty years of our marriage, the concept of "leftovers" never existed when my husband and I would go out to a restaurant. It was more like "food fest gone wild" or "the last supper." It was almost as if he needed to eat in direct opposition to the way I prepared and offered foods at home. Today (after several years!) my husband leaves restaurant food on his plate, pushes it away, and even passes on dessert for the most part, when he's full. But never fear, there are desserts and (other) ongoing treat moments. We both enjoy these foods—we just need less to be satisfied because our palates are more attuned to Yes Foods, and very rich, very sweet foods do not appeal or tempt us in the same way they once did. Our motto is "Let's share the pleasure."

Yes Foods and Weight Loss

The typical dieter is able to control food urges long enough to lose weight—that's the exciting part—but then magically expects to go back to old habits without regaining the lost weight. Unfortunately, nothing magical happens to your body in the process of dieting that allows you free rein once you get to your goal weight. You're still the same machine, and your weight is still determined by the same principle of calories in–calories out.

When it comes to losing weight and then maintaining a healthy weight (and the health benefits that go along with good eating), Yes Foods are your secret weapon. They will be the mainstay of your calorie balance. They will fill you up, providing sweetness, crunch factor, juiciness, and a bounty of nutrients. They can be a predominant component of your snack foods and add-ons to your basic meals. They can be used in a variety of creative ways to add bulk to your diet.

DO YOU KNOW YOUR MELONS?

How many melons can you name? Most people can think of honeydew and watermelon, but that's just the beginning. Different ones are in season at different times of the year. Here are some you may not be familiar with:

- Casaba
- Charantais
- Christmas melon
- Crenshaw
- Derishi, Gala
- Honeydew
- Melon-pear
- Musk melon
- Net melon
- Ogen melon
- Pepino melon
- Persian melon
- Russian/Uzbek melon
- Santa Claus melon
- Seedless watermelon
- Sweet melon
- Tree melon/Papaya
- Wax melon
- Winter melon
- Yellow watermelon
- Xigua

And that's just melons! The point is, it's time to broaden your horizons when it comes to your choices of fruits and veggies.

Fruits Plus Grains Formula for Weight Loss

If you or members of your family want to lose weight, shunning carbohydrates, even the grain selections, is really not necessary, although many of the fad diets recommend this. You will want to incorporate four to five servings each of fruits and vegetables into your daily diet, along with one to three servings of whole grain carbohydrates daily. That's one serving of grains at each of your meals, a serving of fruit and vegetable at each meal, and one fruit or vegetable as a snack. I usually recommend starting your day with one healthy grain serving because a balanced breakfast will be very filling if it includes this grain portion. If someone in the family needs to lose weight, dropping one grain serving and only having one or two grain servings of carbohydrates daily should be satisfying, and still allow for weight loss, if you are eating HFL-style and exercising. Active people or athletes may need more

---

HFL QUICK-TIP: TRY A NEW VEGGIE

You may only be only eating the "good old standards" of vegetables in your diet. Here are some new options to try and their special nutrient features:

- If you like broccoli . . . try asparagus. (It has twice the heart-healthy folate.)
- If you like carrots . . . try yellow peppers. (You'll get a nice boost of vitamin C.)
- If you like green peas . . . try edamame. (You'll get a protein boost.)
- If you like potatoes . . . try parsnips. (You'll get a fiber boost.)
- If you like romaine lettuce . . . try arugula. (You'll get a big calcium boost.)
- If you like spinach . . . try kale. (You'll get cancer-fighting sulforaphanes.)

grain servings (closer to five or six measured portions). Most people don't need to cut out the grain group entirely because it provides a variety of nutrients, as well as hunger satisfaction.

Yes Foods and Portion Control

I supply portion/calorie counts with Yes Foods merely to reflect the reality that even Yes Foods have calories. Though these foods can be eaten in relative abundance with little calorie penalty when compared to other foods, no food should be eaten without hunger and fullness awareness. That's how we get into trouble—by finding ways to justify uncontrolled eating habits. The fact that fruits and veggies are so healthy and delicious is not license to eat mindlessly. That's an attitude that the HFL program does not support. Mindful, selective eating has to be a core component of your family's new attitude about food.

Hunger vs. Thirst

Thirst and hunger signals can get confused. If you are feeling empty a short time after a well-balanced meal or snack, consider drinking a glass of water, iced tea, or calorie-free flavored water, just to see if it's your thirst that needs to be quenched.

When you eat, your blood thickens with the by-products of digestion, and the body's natural response is to want hydration. Rather than wait for this natural body reaction, drink water before and after eating. Consider including a broth-like cup of soup with the meal to fill you up and supply the necessary hydration. The high water content of the fruits and vegetables in your meals and snacks will help minimize this blood thickening effect as well.

Yes Food Success

All family members need to embrace a successful Food Attitude Makeover. If some of your kids or your spouse is reluctant or unconvinced, at least get an agreement to cooperate with the new efforts within the home. (Whatever one chooses to do outside the home may ultimately be modified by in-home changes and become healthy habits.)

WHY YES FOODS ARE BETTER THAN HIGH-PROTEIN, LOW-CARB DIETS

Satisfying your hunger with Yes Foods is preferable to high-protein, low-carb diets, which have the following disadvantages for most people:

- A low-carb diet restricts many fruits and veggies so you lose a number of important vitamins like vitamins A and C, alpha and beta-carotene, lycopene and other phytochemicals that may be instrumental in fighting disease and maintaining health. (Not to mention that these diets are very low in fiber.)
- Many low-carb diets tend to be high in fat, particularly saturated fat. It is the rare dieter who consumes only mono and unsaturated fats on these diets.
- Over time, your brain can begin to feel lethargic, blurry, and confused because it is suffering from a potentially mild form of hypoglycemia or low blood sugar. For that matter, if you are an active individual who participates in a fair amount of exercise or sports, you might also feel the negative impact on your energy level because you need to use carbohydrates and specifically the sugar they provide as an energy source to fuel your energy.
- Many people also complain of boredom or cravings on these diets. It gets a little old eating a limited range of food choices.
- The cost of the foods in the diet is often a factor as well. While it's true produce can be expensive (which is often considered to be part of why being healthy or losing weight is so challenging), the reality is that many fad diets can be even more expensive. With these types of diets, you are easily lured into buying more processed and prepared foods, supplements, and dietary aids that fit the plan but tax the wallet.

One of the easiest ways to get a reluctant family member to climb on board is to put them in charge of the weekly shopping list. Start by having them weigh in on selections, but then let them feel like they're in charge of the actual shopping. In some cases, they will have to read labels to make a decision or even compare the prices of items, so they will have the feeling of really contributing to the process and making a difference. Make it clear that only items on the list should be purchased—no personal additions that fall outside the core parameters. But do encourage them to add new Yes Food selections such as an in-season fruit that has just come out, new veggies to steam, or new ingredients for a creative fruit salad. Younger children can accompany you and help with selections. In many supermarkets now, you can ask a person in the produce section for taste tests, which can be fun and eye opening. Remember—your enthusiasm will be contagious!

HFL Program Yes Foods List

Fruits
Target: four or five servings daily.
Serving Size: as listed, approximately sixty to eighty calories
    Apple: one whole
    Banana: one small (six inches)
    Peach: one whole
    Pear: one small
    Orange: one small
    Grapefruit: one half
    Melon: one-quarter of a medium-sized one
    Strawberries: five large or seven medium
    Blackberries: one-half cup
    Blueberries: one-half cup
    Raspberries: one-half cup
    Nectarine: one medium
    Cherries: eleven large
    Grapes: twelve
    Plum: one medium
    Mango: one half
    Papaya: one half, or one cup, cubed

FRUITY TREATS

Sometimes you want your fruit to feel like a decadent treat. Try these (keeping in mind portion size and treat mentality):

- Chunky Pineapple Fruit Stix (Whole Foods)
- Dreyer's Strawberry Whole Fruit Bars (all supermarkets)
- Fruit-A-Freeze Watermelon Fruit Bars (all supermarkets)
- Palapa Azul® Cucumber Chile Frozen Fruit Bars (Whole Foods)

Pineapple: two or three (one-quarter inch) rings
Watermelon: one-sixteenth of half of a large melon, one-inch-thick slice
Kiwi: one large
Prunes: five
Tangerine: one medium
Cantaloupe: one quarter of a medium-sized one
Honeydew melon: one quarter of a medium-sized one
Kumquats: four small
Lemons: virtually unlimited (because they have negligible calories)
Limes: virtually unlimited (because they have negligible calories)
Minneola: one medium
Pummelo: one cup of sections
Tangelo: one medium
Apricot: three small
Cherries: fifteen
Pluot, plumcot: two medium
Currants: one cup
Cranberries: one and one-half cups

Vegetables
Target: five servings daily
Serving Size: one-half cup cooked or one cup chopped raw vegetables provides sixty to eighty calories; most lettuces can be measured as several cups

Asparagus: twelve spears
Arugula: unlimited
Bamboo shoots (unsalted): several cups
Bean sprouts (boiled, drained, no salt): two and one-quarter cups
Broccoli: four to five large florets
Broccoflower: five to six large florets
Brussels sprouts (boiled, drained, no salt): six to eight medium
Cabbage (raw): several cups
Chinese broccoli: two to three clusters
Onion: one medium
Artichoke: one
Jerusalem artichokes: one-half cup of slices
Jicama (raw): several cups
Cauliflower: several cups

YES FOOD COMBO TIPS

- Add vitamin C–rich peppers to iron-containing beans (such as in a pepper hummus) and you'll absorb more iron from the beans.
- Mix avocadoes and tomatoes and you'll absorb more health-enhancing lycopene from the tomatoes.
- Use turmeric on cooked cauliflower or any cruciferous veggies, and you'll get even better prostate cancer-fighting antioxidant protection.

YES FOOD TRICK: EAT BY COLORS

Pay attention to the colors of the foods you're eating because they provide big clues to the true value you're getting:

Green

Green foods contain the carotenoids, lutein and zeaxanthin, which protect eyesight and reduce your risk of developing macular degeneration. *Get Green Power by saying Yes to kiwi, broccoli, romaine lettuce, kale, spinach, Brussels sprouts, cabbage, honeydew, and avocado.* (Most "greens" also fight cancer thanks to those antioxidant components we've discussed.)

Red

Lycopene, which is found in tomatoes and watermelon, may reduce heart disease. Resveratrol, in grapes, may help treat lung disease, heart disease, and asthma. *Get Red Power from red onions, red grapes, watermelon, tomatoes, radishes, cranberries, strawberries, and red bell peppers.*

Yellow

Limonoids, found in citrus fruits, have been shown to fight cancers of the skin, lung, breast, stomach, and colon. Yellow peppers are full of vitamin C. *Foods include: yellow bell peppers, grapefruits, pineapples, lemons, and yellow squash.*

Orange

Beta-carotene may help boost immune systems, maintain healthy skin and bones, and keep eyesight healthy. Potassium in citrus fruits helps ward off heart disease. *Orange Power is*

YES FOOD TRICK: EAT BY COLORS, *continued*

found in carrots, apricots, mangos, oranges, pumpkin, cantaloupe, and sweet potatoes.

Blue

Blue foods contain antioxidants (a flavenol called kaempferol), are anti-inflammatory, and can help fight cancer. *Blueberries are the ultimate Blue Food. (Wild blueberries are the most powerful.)*

Purple

Ellagic acid, found in some purple foods, is an anti-aging compound that may protect against cancers. *Get Purple Power with plums, eggplants, blackberries, purple grapes, raisins, prunes, figs, and purple onions.*

White

Allicin, a compound in onions and garlic, may inhibit tumor growth. Flavenoids may reduce the risk of heart disease and some cancers. *Beneficial white foods include jicama, pears, bananas, cauliflower, mushrooms, onions, and garlic.*

A note on resveratrol and red and white grapes: Recent studies have shown that resveratrol is contained in the skin and flesh of both white and red grapes. When wines are made, the skin of the red grape is often included in the wine, but not in the case of white wine. It was therefore initially stipulated that the skin of grapes contained this powerful antioxidant—so white wine was assumed to be less of a source. With this new information, we now know that both white and red wine and juices have resveratrol.

Source: Produce for a Better Health Foundation.

Celery: several cups

Chicory: two to three cups

Cucumbers: unlimited

Eggplant (boiled, drained, no salt): two cups, cubed

Carrots (peeled): two medium

Escarole: several cups

Endive: several cups

Green beans, including string beans (cooked, drained, no salt): one and one-quarter cups or forty four-inch beans

Collard greens (cooked, drained, no salt): one and one-half cups

Collard greens (raw): five cups

Kale (raw): two cups

Mustard greens (raw): several cups

Turnips (boiled, drained, no salt): two cups

Lettuces: several cups

Mushrooms: one large Portabello (grilled), six shiitake (cooked), several cups small white mushrooms

Okra (boiled, drained, unsalted): one and one-half to two cups

Peppers (all colors): several cups

Parsnips (boiled, drained, no salt): one-half cup of slices

Pumpkin (boiled, drained, mashed): one and one-quarter cups

Radishes: unlimited

Radicchio: several cups

Seaweed, kelp (raw): several cups

Sprouts: several cups

Summer squash (raw): several cups

Spinach (raw): unlimited

Tomatoes: one medium or ten cherry or two small to medium Roma

Taro (cooked): three-quarters cup

Water chestnuts: eight

Watercress (raw): unlimited

Winter (butternut) squash (baked): one cup

Winter (spaghetti) squash (cooked, drained, no salt): two cups

MORE TIPS FOR STAYING FULL

Though I continuously emphasize the importance of choosing fruits because of their taste and fiber content, beans and lentils contain elements that delay their absorption as well, so you feel fuller longer. However, fruit alone will empty out of your system within two hours, which is why I recommend using it as a *component* of a meal or snack. The plus is you can include a fruit and some veggies as accompaniments to a bean or lentil dish without adding a lot of calories to the meal while enhancing that "fill factor." Also:

- Potatoes gave the highest satisfaction, seven times higher than the least-filling croissants (which actually flies in the face of the Glycemic Index, where the potato scores high, meaning it causes blood sugar to rise and fall rapidly—and we want to avoid those rapid highs and lows). Choose yams or sweet potatoes because they have the most fiber.
- Whole grain breads are 50 percent more filling than white breads.
- Cakes, doughnuts, and cookies are among the least filling.
- For fruits, oranges and apples outscore bananas and grapes when it comes to feeling full. (That's why I recommend variety and different combinations).
- Fish is more satisfying, per calorie, than lean beef or chicken.
- Popcorn is twice as filling as a candy bar or peanuts. To keep calories down, air pop it and use a flavored spray or a shake of dried herbs.

"Maybe So" Fruits and Vegetables

These fruits and veggies are considered Maybe So Foods, meaning portion control is recommended because of dense carbohydrate or some fat content. The serving size should equal about sixty to eighty calories, similar to a grain serving, which they are replacing.

Corn: one small ear or one-half cup
Peas: one-half cup
Many beans: one-quarter cup, rinsed
Potatoes (sweet, white, yams): one-half cup cubed or one small
Olives: one ounce
Beets: one and one-half cups
Avocadoes: two ounces cubed
Yucca: one-quarter cup
Succotash (corn/limas): just over one-quarter cup

For more calorie counts, see the section on starchy vegetables in Chapter 4. For other serving sizes with calorie counts, see www.calorieking.com.

CHAPTER FIVE QUICK-SUMMARY

- Yes Foods offer a big bang for the calorie count: they fill you up, sustain you, taste good, and offer nutrients that will keep you energized and satisfied.
- Your Family Food Attitude Makeover should shift your focus from No Foods (and guilt) to Yes Foods (and feeling good about what you eat).
- Give up your old stereotypes about Yes Foods and your excuses for avoiding them (too expensive, too hard to get, too hard to prepare, unappetizing, or boring).
- Make Yes Foods as pleasing to the senses as possible. Don't just take it for granted that if there are some apples and oranges to grab, no additional effort is needed.
- Be patient, and keep those Yes Foods accessible and appealing.

Tips for Kids

- Ask kids to try one bite. Be willing to do this with the same food for a while.
- Put out the foods you want them to eat at every meal so they get used to seeing them daily, and make sure they see you eating them.
- Offer choices, preferably two or three on a small platter.
- Don't get too caught up in the "healthy message" featured on many boxed products—those labels can be very misleading and there are no strict guidelines governing many of the claims.
- Make the foods readily available—in the fridge, on the kitchen counter, at the dinner table—so kids can grab them when they want them.
- Let them make faces on a plate with cherry tomato eyes, pepper eyebrows, a celery nose, a strawberry mouth.
- Offer crunchy snacks and side dishes and offer healthy dips: kids love to dip.
- Try exotic fruits and veggies: it's like a fun science experiment when it's new to you, too.
- Let them help to clean, prep, and prepare. Kids love to eat the things they help to prepare.
- Add fruits and veggies to foods they already love to add volume and sweetness.
- Get some age-appropriate kid cookbooks; invest in a kid cooking class series.
- Let them help pick out table settings from placemats to color-themed napkins and tablecloths to glass size so they are really a part of the whole meal experience.
- Remember that dried, raw, cooked, canned, and frozen all count from a nutrient perspective, so you don't need to offer only fresh fruits and veggies.

Tips for Teens

- Don't nag.
- Be creative and appeal to their athletic sense, body image, energy needs, and even intellectual needs.
- Create tasty smoothies with fruit and egg wraps with veggies. Offer a variety of healthy cereals along with a bowl of fruit for topping.
- Add veggies to sandwiches.
- Make cooler foods teens can take with them: frozen flavored water, a wrap, sides of fruits and veggies, some healthy dips, a small bag of nuts, hard-boiled eggs, English muffin halves with peanut butter, healthy trail mix.
- Teens love fajitas, baked potatoes (add healthy toppings), air fries (french fries baked at a high temperature), chunky soups, and salads with grilled chicken.
- Do a weeknight home salad bar and a weekend breakfast bar with egg, healthy cereal and grains, and fruit selections.

6

Healthy Habit #1:
Plan Together

Remember the old adage, "Fail to plan and you plan to fail"? I can almost guarantee that your family will not succeed at healthy eating unless you plan for it. This is a hard reality for many of us because we prefer to go on "automatic pilot" when it comes to food, and make choices based on whim or opportunity—whatever happens to be on the menu or around at the time.

Some of my patients associate food planning with dreaded "diets," and I have to explain that planning is not about restricting, depriving, or losing flexibility or freedom. However, having a plan does give you a sense of structure, some control, and some boundaries for your food choices. Deciding in advance on menus, how much food you need, and the best options to save you time and money can help you avoid last-minute anxiety and confusion, as well as sudden or impulsive food decisions that you might later regret. Believe it or not, you will see that having a plan is about giving yourself and your family *more* flexibility and freedom, and more and better choices.

Planning is the #1 tool of eating with awareness, or mindfulness, and probably the most important part of the HFL program. My clients often expect that planning food for the week is going to be an unpleasant, time-consuming, tedious chore. What they usually find is that it's much easier than they thought it would be, especially once they've got the routine down. In reality, when you have a plan, shopping is usually less time-consuming, not more. And shopping with a good plan probably will also take less time than you now spend panicking about what to eat/make and scrambling for last-minute meal solutions.

My clients are also often surprised to discover that planning is one of the easiest secrets around for losing excess weight and keeping it off. Once you've made sure that you've got great (healthy AND tasty) food choices around whenever you need them, the need to nosh on empty calories diminishes greatly.

Healthy Families Are (Somewhat) Organized

Even the most creative, wild, wacky, free-spirited, or artistic family needs some organization in order to succeed. If you don't believe me, think about finances. Financially successful people and families tend to budget. They decide on a goal (buy a house, replace an expensive appliance, get a new car, take a vacation, invest in college, etc.) and plan how they will meet it, either by fitting regular payments into their budget or by saving up. Once they make the purchase, they also *care* for the purchase. The house is maintained, the car is taken in for checkups, and appliances are serviced. Careful and planned steps are taken to maximize the purchase's value and keep it in good condition for as long as possible. So planning is crucial to any goal being achieved and maintained.

I find that healthy families in general tend to approach most of their tasks in an organized fashion. Just like in finances, success in eating doesn't just happen—it's planned. Successful eating includes strategies to help you make the best choices possible, and cope if anything goes awry. If you have a plan or specific strategies to cope with most situations, you are less likely to be "thrown" by unexpected situations (which you can always expect to happen).

Planning food and meals means less wasted time, less stress, less arguing, and more feeling in control, all which help to prevent "grab and overeat." This is a common behavior for people who don't think ahead and who respond to emotional upheaval by grabbing the first food available to make them "feel better." You're establishing a routine that will help your whole family develop healthy habits. If your small child is raised expecting to be involved in choosing, preparing, and organizing meals, he or she will be more likely to develop an appreciation of foods and how to enjoy them properly. If you *plan* treats judiciously and *plan* the development of a palate that appreciates the natural sweetness and tartness of fruits and vegetables, chances are you and your family will be less likely to overeat processed foods and much more likely to develop a healthier attitude toward foods in general.

Planning menus, and figuring out the ingredients you need for meals, snacks, and "emergencies," is crucial in coping with time issues, weight issues, and health issues. It will also help you develop some necessary parameters, especially with kids. Kids do need to know that eating between meals is *healthy* snack time, that only one dinner will be served, that water is the beverage of choice, that certain treats need to be special, not daily, options. Does everyone have to eat the planned meal 100 percent of the time? No. Being organized is good; being inflexible is not. Smart planning allows for flexibility. But flexibility does not mean anything goes. I know too many families where four different meals are taking place on any given evening, and there's endless snack grabbing.

The rule in my home has always been that the kids weigh in on the weekly meal plan, and if a meal is made that they don't like or aren't in the mood to have, they can have a planned alternative, such as:

- A salad topped with whatever protein is on hand—turkey, tuna, or beans
- Fruit salad or fruit topped with fat-free yogurt, cereal, and nuts

- A peanut butter and banana sandwich on whole grain bread, plus fruit

However, I do NOT prepare a separate, labor-intensive meal.

There are also ways to work alternative meals into the basic meal plan. If I make a stir-fry with chicken and veggies, I always prepare an extra chicken breast that can be broiled separately. So when you prepare your family's shopping list, you'll all agree on certain staples that will appear on the list every week for back-up "no fuss" meals.

Planning will also help you decide on items you can buy in bulk to save money; it also means less spoiled food as you become better at calculating your family's needs.

Planning to Shop with YNMS

So, how do you come up with a shopping plan that works for your family? The answer is easy (at least on the surface): you just use your Yes, No, Maybe So food lists—the Family and Individual food lists you created in Chapters 4 and 5 (or use the samples provided), along with the Meal Plan formulas provided in Chapter 4 (see pages 117–121).

Creating and combining your YNMS lists and meal plans may well be the most challenging part of the HFL plan for you and your family. Just remember that it will all become second nature after a while. Think of it as an investment in your future.

Planning your meals and shopping lists does not give you license to throw caution to the wind in other ways. You will need to pay attention to your budgets (both financial and caloric) and your food choices and quantities.

Especially when you're getting started, your planning should include every dietary aspect you can think of, from anticipating portion sizes to making sure you incorporate adequate amounts of Yes Foods into your daily meal plans, from selecting cooking techniques to having main course alternatives available (I call them standbys) in case any planned meals fall flat. Your planning should also include scheduling dinners so that everyone can sit down together as often as possible.

When to Make Your Family List and Shop

What has worked for me, and a lot of my clients, is designating the morning or afternoon of one Saturday or Sunday each weekend to do the food shopping for the week. If you can get into a steady routine, you may only have to make one quick "fill-in" shopping trip during

HEALTHIER SWEET SNACKS

- Pineapple and fat-free cottage cheese
- Frozen grapes and blueberries
- Mixed dry fruit and raw nuts in small quantities
- Sweet potato half with a little maple syrup
- Sweet potato half with cottage cheese and cinnamon
- Unsweetened applesauce, yogurt, with four ginger snaps
- Fat-free yogurt with fresh strawberries
- Angel food cake with All-Fruit® preserves spread thinly on top and a sprinkle of nuts
- Gelatin with fresh sliced peaches
- Non-fat pudding with sliced bananas
- Cereal sprinkled on apple slices
- Hot cocoa made with unsweetened cocoa powder, skim milk, sweetener
- Yogurt and fruit
- Special K® waffle and one teaspoon peanut butter
- Homemade bran/fruit/nut muffin
- Baked apple with cinnamon and nut topping
- Dried plums/slivered almonds/semi-sweet chocolate chips (healthy trail mix)
- Skim latte and a ping-pong-ball-sized homemade fruit, nut, or whole grain muffin

the week. (Kids do bring friends home, food can spoil in certain seasons, etc.) You can either grab each family member individually ahead of time to have them weigh in on choices and share their schedule issues (especially older kids, so that you know when they'll be able to share a family meal and when they need transportable food or a late meal), or you can designate a family "powwow time." Encourage everybody to make individual food lists that can be handed off to you for integration into the master list. This way, someone who can't meet at the designated time can still provide input.

Oh, yes, there may be resistance, surprise, skepticism, unhappiness, defiance—you name it! Just be patient (another very important

HEALTHIER SALTY SNACKS

- Raw veggies and fat-free bean dip or hummus
- Hard-boiled egg with seasoning dip and baked crackers
- Baked whole grain crackers, reduced fat cheese, and diced tomato
- Shrimp cocktail
- Cup of homemade veggie and bean soup
- Small handful of mixed raw nuts
- Fat-free popcorn
- Rice cakes with mango chutney
- Matzo, fat-free cottage cheese, and Old Bay® seasoning
- Tomatoes and fat-free cottage cheese
- Celery and peanut butter
- Small can water-packed tuna and baked whole grain crackers
- White meat, low-salt turkey slices and pickle relish
- Fat-free refried beans and mini rice cakes
- A wedge of Laughing Cow® light cheese and baked crackers

P word that will get a huge workout in the early weeks and months). Realize that little children initially will have difficulty getting used to new eating habits because they may be somewhat conditioned to a higher fat meal with lots of processed sugars and to snacks that clearly taste really good but are not good for them. Help them make choices, be patient and creative, and take special care to let them feel that their input is important.

Make sure that all family members give you their top ten fruits and veggies as well as new ones they are willing to try, which will help to create your initial shopping list of Yes Foods. No (With a Smile) Foods should be easy—get everyone's two or three favorite snacks and treats that can be timed and portioned out; try to come up with some group favorites, too. Maybe So Foods (the meat dishes, fish dishes, bean dishes, pasta dishes, egg dishes, dairy foods, etc.) will determine the main course of many meals, so get a sense of how many Maybe So preferences are shared by family members (maybe everyone likes turkey meatballs, grilled chicken breast, or vegetable chili, for example). Then agree on the two standby meals (maybe tuna salad and sliced turkey breast and hard-boiled eggs) that family members can substitute for a Maybe So entrée that isn't to their liking.

My Sample Shopping Lists

It may help for you to see some sample lists I've used for my family of four, based on the menu plans that we typically create. These menu plans follow the shopping list.

Amy's Maybe So Foods Sample Weekly Shopping List

Eight Light 'n Fit™ fat-free yogurts
Four Yoplait® low-fat yogurts
One package fat-free American cheese
One gallon 1 percent milk
One gallon skim milk
Shredded part-skim mozzarella cheese
One gallon of orange juice (calcium-fortified, low sugar)

One box Corn Bran cereal

One box Cheerios®

One box Bran Buds®

One box Cocoa Puffs®

One package 100 percent whole grain bread

One box frozen 100 percent whole grain waffles

Medium-sized fat-free tortillas (100 percent whole wheat)

One box Barilla® high-protein pasta

One jar natural fresh ground peanut butter

Twelve four-ounce chicken breasts (skinless and boneless)

One pound of ground white meat chicken

Four four-ounce pieces of salmon fillet

Four small sweet potatoes

One bag frozen corn

One bag brown rice (eight portions)

Two large cans of tuna in water

Four four-ounce packs of low-sodium, fat-free turkey (deli-style)

One box of fat-free vegetable broth

Tomato sauce (no oil)

One can of evaporated skim milk

Two cans of beans (garbanzo and black beans)

One avocado

Two dozen brown, omega-3 enriched eggs

One container Benecol®

One bag of almonds

One bag of cashews

One box of soybeans

One box of whole grain baked crackers

One container of fat-free frozen yogurt

One container of protein powder

One container of low-fat vanilla soymilk

Container of hummus dip, salsas

If needed:

- Olive oil
- Low-sodium soy sauce
- Low-sugar teriyaki sauce

Amy's Yes Foods Sample Weekly Shopping List

Vegetables

Enough salad fixings for four large family-size salads (you may need to do one midweek fill-in), including:

Carrots
Celery
Cherry tomatoes
Peppers, onions
Scallions
Radishes
Stir-fry vegetables (buy pre-packs)
Five bags of frozen assorted vegetables
Five large cucumbers
Three large tomatoes
Extra spinach and arugula

Plus: vinegar, fresh and powdered spices

Fruits (changes seasonally; this is a summer sample)

Four containers of mixed, pre-cut fruit
Ten plums
Ten peaches
Large watermelon
Bunch of bananas
Two or three different melons
Tangerines
Apricots
Blueberries
Strawberries
Bag of apples
Grapes
Lemons and limes
Several bags of frozen fruit and berries

Plus: flavored waters, regular water, unsweetened teas, flavored seltzers

HEALTHY LUNCHBOX PLANNING TIPS

- First, you need the right stuff: an insulated lunch bag, lunchbox, or mini-cooler; an insulated drink cup (or you can freeze water bottles or cartons); cold packs; plastic utensils; durable containers; and foil or plastic wrap. Nobody likes a warm, mushy lunch.

- A tip to keep stews, soups, or noodles warm: pour hot water into a thermos bottle and let it stand for five to seven minutes. Pour out the water and replace it with hot food. Obviously, if a microwave is available at school or work, you can reheat.

- Kids like many little choices. Pack lots of them: a hard-boiled egg, a small sandwich bag of baked crackers, a small box of raisins, a small bag of cut-up apples, a small bag of cherry tomatoes or carrots, pudding, a small bag of cereal, dried fruit, nuts (make sure school allows nuts; some don't due to allergies). Then see what comes home, so you'll know what to leave out next time. Ask them what their friends are bringing that they like. If they want chips, buy baked and send a small bag. The same goes for most treats: sometimes find the healthier version and sometimes send "the real deal" in very small quantities.

- Other great options: mini rice cakes with small cubes of low-fat cheese, pinwheel sandwiches with fat-free cream cheese and veggies, baked chicken nuggets, cubed fruit and yogurt, pita wedges with salsa and beans, tomato soup and half a sandwich, peanut butter or apple butter sandwiches shaped with a cookie cutter, melon balls. Add hummus or bean dip.

- Teens love wraps, yogurt parfaits, pita sandwiches, smoothies, and "breakfast for lunch" (waffles and fruit

---

HEALTHY LUNCHBOX PLANNING TIPS, *continued*

or peanut butter, cereal and dried fruit in a container with milk on the side), pudding, cut-up veggies and hummus dip, nutrition bars (lean toward high-protein bars and watch trans and saturated fat as well as high fructose corn syrup (HFCS). They may also want to buy their lunches; home discussions can help to guide them on best choice options.

Amy's No with a Smile Foods Sample Weekly Shopping List

Skinny Cow® fat-free ice cream sandwiches
Fudgsicle® frozen treats
Jell-O® Devil's Food 100-calorie puddings
Pringles® 100-calorie baked chips packs
Kraft® Lorna Doone® cookies 100-calorie packs
One bag dark chocolate chips
Five Balance® bars
One box South Beach Diet® 100-calorie bars

Easy Meals to Go with the Lists

Not too enthralled with the idea of coming up with family meal plans? Don't worry, you can borrow mine! They're fairly fast and easy, and they work for most families. Just keep these guidelines in mind:

- Always be conservative about the number (and portion size) of grain servings. This is a Maybe So Food that does require strict portion control.
- Try to include salad and fruit at every meal: start lunch or dinner with a veggie broth or dinner salad to help you cut down on calories if you are targeting weight loss.

HEALTHIER FROZEN DELIGHTS

If ice cream snacks or frozen treats are your passion, you can simply buy light or fat-free frozen yogurt or ice cream and top it with fruit and nuts or turn to these low-cal, low-fat treats. They average from sixty to one hundred calories) and don't skimp on flavor:

- Fudgsicle® (usually low-cal and satisfying)
- Frozen fruit bars that are pure fruit only
- Healthy Choice® mocha fudge swirl (2.5 ounces)
- WholeFruit® frozen yogurt and sorbet swirl
- Breyers® double-churned 100-calorie ice cream cups
- Yoplait® double fruit smoothie
- Häagen-Dazs® fat-free sorbet and yogurt (two and one-half ounces)
- Weight Watchers® sherbet and ice cream, or sorbet swirl (two to four ounces)
- Klondike Slim-a-Bear® 100-calorie ice cream sandwich
- Creamsicle®
- Palapa Azul® mango fruit bar
- Tropicana®, Edy's®, and Breyers fruit bars and cups (many have 20–60 calories)

- In the winter, a hearty soup with puréed vegetables, beans, and white meat chicken can offer cold weather comfort and fill you up.
- In the summer, consider lightening up your meals; an omelet with veggies or yogurt and fruit with nuts may be ideal.

In general, meal and ingredient portion sizes will depend on whether you are serving kids or adults, trying to lose weight vs. just get healthier, serving an athletic teen or adult, or dealing with a specific disease such as diabetes, but the quality of food and menu options work for everyone.

Also, keep in mind that breakfast foods typically work for lunches as well.

Breakfast Foods

Hard-boiled eggs
Yogurt/fruit and cereal
Cereal (or oatmeal) with fruit and milk
Waffles and fruit (with yogurt or milk)
Smoothies with protein powder

DIPPING DOS

Salsas are great dips for veggies and are usually low in calories and bursting with flavor. Bean dips and hummus are also great protein/healthy fat dips. Guacamole is great; it's high in fat, but it's healthy fat. Fat-free dressings are also fine as dips in small amounts, but remember that a little bit of healthy fat allows you to absorb certain vitamins more readily from vegetables; I usually dress a salad with an olive oil vinaigrette. You can also create dips with fat-free plain yogurt or fat-free sour cream and chives, seasonings, or purées of veggies or fruit.

Dipping can become mindless instead of mindful, so always portion out some dip on a plate and move away from the area.

Here are some prepared dips and spreads that offer a low-cal/low-fat option (just watch serving sizes; see page 212):

- Grande® grilled and roasted salsa
- Ortega® black bean and corn salsa
- Marina® cocktail sauce
- Wegmans® tzatziki dip
- Fresh Food Concepts five-layer party dip with guacamole
- Fritos® bean dip

Frozen berries, nuts and frozen fat-free yogurt
Peanut butter on whole wheat toast with fruit and milk

Lunch Foods

Bean and veggie wraps
Bean salads
Yogurt and fruit "parfaits"
Tuna salad
Hard-boiled eggs
Grilled cheese sandwiches
Tuna, turkey, and peanut butter sandwiches or wraps

Dinner Foods

Grilled fish
Chicken stir-fry with brown rice
Ground white meat turkey and veal meatballs and spaghetti
Tofu stir-fry
Bean and veggie stew in the Crock-Pot®
Omelets with veggies
Homemade tortilla pizzas
Grilled chicken

Lunch and Dinner Sides

Mixed salad
Fruit salad
Fresh fruit
Corn
Rice/pasta (wild and brown rice, couscous, high-protein pasta)
Sweet potatoes
Occasional "bread food," such as whole grain wraps, tortillas, or
sandwich bread

Snacks

Cut-up veggies with hummus, salsa, or bean dip
Fresh fruit
Fat-free pudding, yogurt
Homemade trail mix
"No Foods" (treats for each person three times a week)

Sample HFL Breakfast Meals

- Whole grain English muffin with poached egg, sliced tomato, spray of butter-flavored Pam®, and a piece of fruit
- Fat-free yogurt in half of a cantaloupe, topped with whole grain cereal and a sprinkle of nuts
- A smoothie blended from silken tofu, frozen berries, a splash of orange juice, a scoop of frozen yogurt, and ice
- High-protein cereal on top of oatmeal made with skim milk, berries
- Whole grain french toast made with Egg Beaters®, low-sugar maple syrup, and a piece of fruit
- Veggie omelet with a piece of whole grain toast, tomato slices, fruit
- Toasted whole grain English muffin topped with cottage cheese, apple butter, and a sprinkle of nuts
- Bran cereal mixed with protein cereal, skim milk, berries
- Whole grain waffle with apple butter, peanut butter, and a skim milk latte
- Whole grain toast with ricotta cheese, bananas, cinnamon
- Wrap with scrambled eggs, veggies, tomato slices
- Two hard-boiled eggs, cup of oatmeal, berries, skim milk
- Half an English muffin, scrambled egg, turkey or soy bacon, tomato slices, a piece of fruit
- Whole grain toast, cottage cheese, diced apple, cinnamon

Sample HFL Lunch Meals

- Open-face, low-fat cheese and veggie sandwich with basil, berries, and a fat-free pudding
- A whole grain wrap with hummus, veggies, and fat-free turkey, a piece of fruit
- A scoop of cottage cheese topped with fresh fruit and nuts, baked crackers
- Half a whole grain pita stuffed with beans and shredded salad and a fruit cup
- A large salad topped with three or four ounces of grilled fish or grilled chicken *or* one-half cup of beans *or* two or three ounces of grilled tofu *or* three or four ounces of soy/deli slices with four baked crackers and a cup of fresh fruit salad
- A yogurt parfait made with fresh fruit, nuts, and whole grain cereal
- Steamed veggies and brown rice (one-half cup) topped with grilled fish (three or four ounces) *or* grilled chicken (three or four ounces) or grilled tofu (two or three ounces)
- Tuna or chicken salad (made with relish/fat-free mayo) in a whole grain wrap with veggies, with fruit on the side
- A grilled Portabello mushroom with melted low-fat cheese (one-quarter cup), diced tomatoes, and rosemary on half of a whole grain bun, plus fruit
- A black bean burrito (whole grain tortilla) with shredded or grilled veggies, and a side of fruit
- Homemade Chinese chicken salad (four ounces) with rice vinegar and four baked crackers and one piece of fruit
- A homemade Waldorf salad with fat-free sour cream, one-quarter cup of nuts and a side dinner salad topped with a one-quarter cup of beans
- Vegetable and bean soup (made with fat-free chicken stock) with four baked crackers and fruit
- Six pieces of brown rice sushi, with a side salad and fruit
- Whole grain or high-protein pasta salad (one-half cup), cold, with tuna (three ounces) *or* grilled chicken (three ounces) and veggies added, and fruit

- Whole grain pita or tortilla pizza with cooked veggies, crushed tomatoes, part-skim shredded mozzarella cheese (one-quarter cup) and a piece of fruit
- A stuffed pepper or tomato with tuna (three ounces) or chicken salad (three ounces), dinner salad and fruit
- A stuffed pepper or tomato with ricotta cheese, dinner salad, and fruit
- Turkey or soy bacon (three ounces) and fat-free cheese (one-eighth cup) with tomato, grilled open-face on one slice of whole grain bread
- Fajitas with whole grain tortillas (one or two, depending on calories), grilled veggies and chicken (three ounces) and a piece of fruit
- Egg salad (two eggs) with fat-free mayo, shredded veggies in a whole grain wrap with fruit
- Whole grain tortilla, no-fat refried beans (three ounces), shredded part-skim mozzarella (one-eighth cup), diced tomatoes and peppers
- Veggie burger on an open whole grain bun, salad, steamed veggies

Sample HFL Dinner Meals

- Tofu stir-fry, dinner salad, fruit
- Crock-Pot® chicken or bean stew, fruit, salad
- Grilled fish, corn, steamed veggies, fruit
- Small baked sweet potato with two to four ounces of protein, steamed veggies, fruit
- High-protein spaghetti with veggies, dinner salad, fruit
- Eggplant parmigiana with low-fat cheese and fat-free ricotta, dinner salad, fruit
- BBQ chicken, chopped salad, half a sweet potato, fruit
- Chicken or shrimp shish kabob, couscous, dinner salad, fruit
- Rice, beans, and grilled veggies, dinner salad, fruit

MAKING TO-GO FOOD PLANS FOR TRAVEL

Hotels

- Most hotels will provide a refrigerator (if you call ahead) and directions to a local supermarket where you can stock up on cereal, milk, juice, fruit, and yogurt, as well as nuts, mini carrot bags, and nutrition bars.
- Bring along sandwich bags to make cereal/nut trail mix and to transport fruit. Also pack healthy beverages. You'll save money that way and have some food to turn to for snacks.
- You can also see hotel menus online so you know if on-site restaurants or in-room dining offer healthy choices.
- Local Chinese food can always be delivered; order it steamed with sauces on the side.
- Take advantage of large buffet breakfasts and refrigerate fruit and hard-boiled eggs for later use.
- Scout out hotels that have gym facilities (or a gym nearby).

Car Travel

- Use a cooler to pre-pack food and snacks, as well as frozen water bottles to keep everything cool while defrosting. Home-packed trail mix and wraps travel well.
- Map out healthy fast-food options before you travel with the kids if you are going to eat out.

International Travel

- The hotel manager and concierge can be invaluable in helping you navigate food menus, local restaurant

MAKING TO-GO FOOD PLANS FOR TRAVEL, *continued*

options, and hotel food. In many cases, you'll be able to make arrangements for a fridge in the room, know where a local food mart is, know restaurant accessibility, or at least be forewarned so you can plan ahead.

- Keeping your daytime calories a bit lower allows you to splurge at dinnertime; in most countries, you can enjoy a nice post-dinner walk to help burn off some of those evening calories.

- When we travel as a family, we often eat a hearty American-style breakfast (cereal, fruit, egg whites, lattes) at the hotel and take fruit and nuts on the road for a light lunch, buy yogurt or smoothies along the way, and then enjoy a well-balanced dinner.

More Meal Plan Guidelines

In Chapter 7 we'll talk about the many different marinades, cooking techniques, seasonings, and strategies to "jazz up" healthy food so that it not only is good for you, but tastes good, too. You'll notice many of my menu suggestions are made from simple, accessible ingredients and prep time is pretty quick. That's the whole idea. As long as you plan menus so you have ingredients on hand, you'll have no problem offering your family fabulous-tasting and constantly changing menu plans.

To visualize correct portion size, think of an airline meal: it's actually a good guide. The standard trays used in most frozen meals are as well (though the meal itself may be high in fat or sodium). We'll talk more about specific portions in Chapter 8. Note that most of your breakfast selections should weigh in at about 300–400 calories; lunch and dinner come in at around 400–600. Or you can flip this and make breakfast your big meal of the day, with lunch and dinner a bit lighter. Depending on your weight and health goals, one or two daily snacks (if you have them) should run around 100–150 calories each. Remember that large or athletic people may need to eat larger portions to meet their higher daily calorie needs, but they should still follow the basic HFL outline and food and menu choices and suggestions.

Most health professionals agree that your daily calorie count should *not fall* to less than 1,200 or 1,300 calories. You can always increase activity to burn off extra calories, but ingesting too few calories can actually slow your metabolic rate in response to what it perceives as starvation.

Seriously obese people or Stage 4 individuals (see the chart on page 42) should be under the care of a physician and/or nutritionist. In most cases, these professionals will concur with the HFL food and menu choices, although they may add very strict calorie guidance and other supportive suggestions. A current dietary approach for diabetics, who need to be very aware of their blood sugar levels and the impact of different foods on those levels, is to count carbs. In the HFL program, we monitor carbs (Maybe So Foods) by controlling daily servings and portion sizes.

Shopping the HFL Way

Consider approaching the supermarket experience with a "MapQuest® mentality." Before you go in, know your floor plan and target zones for Yes Foods, No Foods, and Maybe So Foods. I'm all for exploration, but that should mostly happen in the Yes aisles and the aisles that provide main course Maybe So Foods. If you find yourself browsing too intently in the No Foods section, red alert! You're putting yourself through needless temptation. Don't give the marketers the time they need to hook you. You don't need to know about every new cereal and snack. In fact, the processed food aisles should be "run through" aisles. Don't linger on foods that are high in fat, sodium, high fructose corn syrup, or other poor quality ingredients. You should know which foods are on your No list; don't linger—just grab them and GO.

Take a trip with me through the HFL Supermarket Strategic Shopping map.

Yes Zones

The fresh fruits and veggies section is usually a long wall on one of the four sides that make up the supermarket perimeter; this is a safe place to linger as you fill up your cart and do some taste testing. Remember, though, that corn, peas, and potatoes are dense and more like bread foods, so buy small with portion size in mind. Cleaning products, paper goods, and toiletries are also safe aisles.

No Zone (or Special Treat Areas)

Think of the pastry aisles, candy and soda aisles, cookies, chips, creamy foods, crackers, chips, and all aisles with heavily processed food as unfriendly territory. You may need to pick up a few items here to meet your family's entitlement to some weekly treats, but don't make a practice of hanging out in these bad food neighborhoods! Come with specific requests and then clear out.

Selective Frozen Zone (Yes, No, and Maybe So Are All Here)

The frozen food section is great for frozen fruits and veggies, frozen healthy waffles, fat-free ice cream, frozen soy foods and lean meats, emergency frozen entrées (acceptable as an occasional back-up to home cooking). But make sure to read labels so you understand each selection's serving size, calories per serving, sodium, fat, and protein content. Also review individual ingredients and always go trans-fat-free with no more than two to three grams of other fat for every 100 calories of serving (i.e., a 300-calorie serving size could have between seven and nine grams of fat). You'll notice how difficult these numbers are to find, another reason preparing food at home usually means not only fresher, but healthier, too.

Hydration (Beverage) Zone

Certainly explore the beverage aisle—choose calorie-free flavored waters, and new kinds of unsweetened tea beverages (or make your own with a twist of lemon or lime or a splash of orange juice). But beware: liquid calories can add up. Also note that many caloric beverages contain *more than one serving* per small bottle.

Oil Slick Zone (Slide Through with Caution)

We all need some healthy fat in our diets, but this aisle needs careful selectivity. The best oils include extra virgin olive oil, olive oil, nut oils, canola oil, and soybean oil. Vegetable oils are not quite as healthy, so limit these as a choice. And don't forget to buy vinegars: they are great on their own or mixed in to reduce the amount of fat in salad dressings and marinades. Oil does enhance the absorption of certain vitamins, so we do not want to live "oil free."

Deli Zone (Can Be Fun but Beware of Salt and Fat)

Products from the deli and cheese area need careful evaluation for saturated fat, sodium, and calories per portion. Deli meats should be purchased in two- and four-ounce packages; I always buy in four-ounce packages, and choose low-sodium versions whenever possible. When buying fish and meat, consider having it pre-cut into portions for easier prep at home.

Salad Bar Zone

Yes, they're great—as long as you avoid the creamy and high-fat dressings and the marinated and prepared offerings! Choose a bounty of cut-up vegetables and fruits that are fresh and try some selections new to you.

Ready-Made Zone

Many supermarkets have a prepared foods section and often list ingredients so, though you may not have exact calorie counts, you can tell which types of fats and sweeteners were used, and make healthier choices accordingly. A cutting board with fresh white meat turkey, slim slaw made with vinegar, steamed veggie salad, and prepared baked sweet potatoes can help you pull off a healthy meal when prep time is limited.

Cereal Zone

Your cereal choices should fall into the *high-fiber, low-sugar* category (unless you decide to buy one sweet version for topping) or be *high-protein and whole grain cereals*; bran cereals are great as mix-ins to add fiber. Spend a bit of time reading labels and get a clear-cut idea of which choices fall into your regular daily selections and which need to be categorized as a "treat topping" or "mix-in treat."

Canned Goodies Zone

This is another aisle where you do need to spend time and read labels. Anything from the canned goods aisle needs to be assessed for sodium. Remember, beans (even canned) always need to be rinsed. Breads, wraps, tortillas, and pastas should be whole grain, as should rice. Condiments like mayo can now be purchased in fat-free versions, ketchup comes in less sugar versions, and mustards, which come in a large flavor variety, are naturally low-cal marinade ingredients or sandwich condiments. I sometimes buy some Balance® and Genisoy® bars and fat-free pudding. When combined with fresh fruit, these make quick-grab pre- or post-exercise snacks.

Dairy Zone

Healthy dairy options include 1 percent or fat-free milk, yogurts, cheeses (I tend to buy organic so that no hormones are present), omega-3 infused eggs, or Egg Beaters®. I often buy a small fresh-squeezed orange juice (with pulp) or calcium-fortified orange juice to add to smoothies and other recipes.

How Healthy Is Your Pantry?

Your pantry can either be a safe haven where family members feel relatively secure in finding healthy, tasty ingredients for meals and snacks . . . or it can be "temptation island," a constant, nagging reminder of processed foods, sweet and creamy flavors, artificial colorings, and artery-clogging, caloric treats.

If there is order to your pantry (remember that healthy families are organized), you are less likely to waste money buying items that you already have or replacing items that have gotten buried in the back and passed their expiration date. You'll also feel that you have control of the space, which is so important when it comes to developing habits that save you both time and money. An orderly pantry means you can notice what is running out or missing, and having specific locations for different food groups makes it easy to assemble ingredients for meals.

Here's a plan for your cabinet that works, regardless of size. You can use separate shelves or cabinets if it's a small space, or separate areas within a larger space or pantry closet. Group your food into these categories:

- Cereals
- Rice/pasta/grains
- Beverages
- Crackers
- Treats (keep higher up)
- Nutrition bars
- Condiments/spices
- Oils/sprays/dressings/marinades/vinegars/broth
- Nuts and nut butters
- Dried fruits
- Teas/coffee/sweeteners
- Canned goods (separate out categories—soups/beans/ sauces/fish)
- Onions/potatoes (though I personally keep these in the fridge)
- A specific area for homemade, pre-portioned trail mix bags and 100-calorie snack bags
- Non-perishable milks (evaporated skim, small boxes of 1 percent, soy)

How Healthy Is Your Fridge?

Successful professionals rely on tidy and organized offices to help save precious time and energy. Why not approach your fridge and freezer with the same clerical skills? Creating *food files* with corresponding refrigerator locations—categorizing your food and filing it in certain places—is a great way to keep on track and in control of your family's daily diet.

TEN SHOPPING DOS AND DON'TS

1. Do realize that the process truly gets easier with time.
2. Do use a list every time: try to manage impulse shopping.
3. Don't shop hungry.
4. Do buy in bulk to save bucks, but create portions immediately when you get home.
5. Do spend some time reading labels so you get better at eyeing and evaluating processed food products.
6. Do create a Top Ten List of foods that always get incorporated into your weekly menus: mine is veggie broth, fresh herbs, evaporated skim milk, Bran Buds®, frozen broccoli, high-protein pasta, whole grain tortillas, tuna, tomato sauce, slivered almonds. Varying the list will help you come up with new recipes.
7. Do come up with menu categories like stews, soups, stir-fries, pasta dishes, egg dishes, grilling, wrap night, or salad bar night. These will help your family focus more easily on options. You can then create menu plans for a dish from each group and more easily list shopping needs.
8. Do buy ingredients that allow for multi-tasking recipes. Chicken can be grilled, stir-fried, and baked with tomato sauce or incorporated into a healthy chicken salad. Tuna can be made into a wrap or served on a salad. Grilled fish can be made into a stew or added to a thick vegetable soup.
9. Do invest in a well-equipped kitchen, which should have a scale, blender, Crock-Pot® (which allows you to cook with little or no fat), food processor, and measuring cups.
10. Do create exchange lists: substitute veggie broth for higher-fat sauce ingredients, evaporated skim milk instead of half-and-half, fresh fruit instead of dried fruit, cooking sprays instead of oils, egg whites instead of eggs, apple butter instead of oils, etc.

Fridge Food File: Fruits and Vegetables
Location: Lower bins (for fresh produce and snack bags of pre-cut fruits and veggies) and upper refrigerator shelf (for a large tossed salad and fruit salad)
Filing Tips:

- Shop for enough variety to fill both refrigerator drawers.
- Once home, take the time to cut up and bag some of the carrots and celery in snack-size amounts. Cut up three days' worth of fruit salad and tossed salad and store in airtight plastic containers.
- Create containers of grated carrots and chopped onions, peppers, celery, and squash to add to high-protein pasta and omelets.
- Pack a small container with salad and another with fruit salad to take to work the next day. You can keep it in a mini-cooler if there's no fridge.
- Make sure to buy quick-grab apples, tangerines, and other seasonal fruit. Consider buying bags of frozen berries (great for smoothies and healthy muffins) and always have bags of frozen vegetables on hand.

Fridge Food File: Dairy Products, Juice, Eggs
Location: Upper shelf for large containers of milk and juice; second shelf of fridge for yogurt, cheese, and a bowl of hard-boiled eggs.
Filing Tips:

- Buy single-serve containers of fat-free yogurt and cottage cheese so you can toss one in your lunch bag daily.
- Buy half-gallon containers of fat-free milk, 1 percent milk, and soymilk.
- A bag of shredded, part-skim mozzarella cheese and a package of low-fat American cheese can round out your dairy choices.
- Low-fat puddings are a great snack.

- If you do buy orange juice, take advantage of the kind that comes "calcium-fortified." New juices like mangosteen and açai offer antioxidants as well in a four-ounce gulp.
- Eggs can now be purchased DHA/omega-3 fortified, and Egg Beaters® and liquid egg whites in individual ready-to–microwave cups offer portability.
- Have four to six hard-boiled eggs already made for lunches on the go or to add to salads.

Fridge Food File: Whole Grain/High-Fiber Bread, Waffles, Muffins (a small folder)
Location: Lower shelf of fridge, right-hand side.
Filing Tips:

- Reading bread labels and choosing 100 percent whole grains and high-fiber brands allow you to make healthy open-face sandwiches and breakfasts. Consider buying low-fat tortillas and whole wheat pita and mini-bagels: many brands now offer fortified, whole grain options.
- Whole grain English muffins and wraps are also good portion-controlled choices.

PANTRY ITEMS TO KEEP IN STOCK

- Canned evaporated skim milk
- Non-fat sweetened condensed milk
- Veggie broth
- Cooking spray
- Applesauce (unsweetened)
- Apple butter
- Butter sprinkles (Molly McButter®) or butter-flavored cooking spray
- Mustard
- Rice wine and flavored vinegars

Fridge Food File: Fish, Meats, Proteins
Location: Lower shelf of fridge, left side.
Filing Tips:

- This is an important folder because it really does need to be pre-determined weekly. Buy your raw fish and meats in four-ounce (for women and kids) and six-ounce (men and athletes) portions, and marinate and/or pre-cook some of them so you have less daily after-work prep stress.
- Buy fresh low-sodium/low-fat deli meats in four-ounce portion packs. Try some of the soy alternative deli "meats."
- Keep a box or two of edamame (soybeans) so you can grab a quick protein snack or sprinkle on salad.
- Mix tuna with fat-free mayonnaise or with pickle relish in small containers to have on hand for lunches. You can have healthy egg salad and rinsed beans ready as well.

Fridge Food File: Condiments, etc.
Location: Fridge door.
Filing Tips:

- These items are purchased on a less-frequent basis and include mustards, salsa, relish, balsamic vinegar, all-fruit jam, lemon and lime juice, spray salad dressings, mashed garlic, hummus (which you can now buy in individual 70-calorie squeeze packs), cholesterol-lowering spreads, and fat-free mayonnaise, mustards, and ketchup.
- Set aside one shelf in the door specifically for bottled and flavored waters, club soda, and unsweetened teas.

More Quick Food Filing Tips

- Label and date containers, especially leftovers.
- Always separate newly purchased foods from those you still need to finish up.
- Get in the habit of doing a clean-out/evaluation once a week.
- Keep a magnetic pad on the door of the refrigerator so you can jot down items you need to buy or replace.

- Keep your refrigerator tidy and always use the same storage areas: it helps give you visual cues on what's running out and what's available to be grabbed.

Planning to Eat Out

This section should really be called "dodging the dangers of eating out" or maybe, on a more positive note, "delighting in eating out." The truth is that if you are not careful, dining out can be a true weight and health challenge.

Plates have gotten larger, there is no clear calorie, fat, or sodium information, and we often pile the unhealthy choices one on top of another: wine or alcoholic beverage, appetizer, main dish, dessert, and coffee with creamer. And in many cases, when food is served "family style," we take more than one portion without realizing it.

Dim lights can make you underestimate calories and the size of portions. The adjectives that describe appetizers and entrées on menus are designed to stimulate you and make you engage with the food. Background music and chatter can help you throw caution to the wind and eat too much and too quickly because you're just not focused on the food itself. Wine or liquor can blur your portion perspective.

It's a real rat race out there in restaurants, but you can make it through the maze. It's usually best not to respond to the challenge by going to extremes. If you just have a salad to be virtuous, you're much more likely to go back to work or home and pig out in frustration from hunger. (Always add the healthiest protein choice to a salad and have dressing on the side). I once read an article that compared the battle with food to the one between the angel and devil within. The angel says, "Be virtuous all the time." The devil says, "Eat whatever the heck you want—all the time." I think when most people contemplate eating out, they see it as an opportunity to forget caution and have a good time. "After all, eating out is special so I should be able to choose anything and everything I want because these food excursions are occasional." But that's not the reality anymore.

We eat out an awful lot these days. But at the same time, we see each birthday celebration, each social gathering, as a separate and unique experience rather than as one in an ongoing string of overindulgences. So the calories and the weight creep up on us.

What we really need to do is invoke the "Moderator Within" who urges us to remember how often we eat out and to designate which moments are truly special treat or entrée or appetizer moments. (That's why keeping a food journal or food calendar is so important: it keeps us honest and in touch with reality.)

If you're following the HFL program, you should only be eating out a couple of times a week at most, and you should have already made the decision to be more active or tack on some exercise on those days, especially if they are days on which you are planning to indulge. And don't forget that happy hour should only be a rare indulgence, not a daily event!

Eating Ethnic (and Healthy)

It can be particularly difficult to stay healthy when we eat out at ethnic restaurants, which are becoming more common dining choices. Here are some guidelines that can help you reduce the calories, fat, and sodium.

Mexican: Your best choices are fajitas with vegetables and lean beef, chicken, or shrimp; quesadillas with chicken or shrimp and cheese on the side (so you can add just a bit); a burrito or enchilada with lean protein and cheese on the side. Avoid sour cream, lots of cheese, refried beans, chips, and large amounts of guacamole (a little bit goes a long way).

Japanese: Your best choices are sushi with brown rice, sashimi, teppanyaki dishes (dishes cooked on an iron griddle), sukiyaki dishes, teriyaki dishes (with teriyaki sauce on the side so you can control it), or sunumono salad. Avoid tempura, yakitori, and regular sushi (six pieces is a meal).

Chinese: Your best choices are steamed vegetables and sauces on the side for dipping, low-oil, stir-fried dishes (you can ask), brown rice, steamed wontons, and vegetable soup. Avoid fried egg rolls and spring rolls, pancakes and thickly battered fish and meat, sweet and sour dishes, lo mein dishes, spare ribs, and Kung Pao chicken.

Italian: Your best choices are vegetable antipasto, pasta and bean soup, minestrone soup, grilled fish, chicken or lean cuts of meat, and thin-crust vegetable pizza with light cheese. Avoid creamy white pasta dishes, deep-fried foods, carbonera dishes, calzone and cannelloni dishes, lasagna, eggplant parmigiano, and Caesar salad.

HFL QUICK-TIPS FOR EATING OUT

- Have a light snack about an hour before going out.
- Start with a salad or broth soup.
- Don't be afraid to customize your meal: ask for dressing and sauces on the side, no bread basket, no rice, extra veggies, and fruit or sorbet for dessert.
- Limit alcohol to one drink.
- Practice portion control: take half your entrée home or share it.
- Eat slowly and ask the waiter to put in your main order after you finish your salad.
- Remember that even though it sounds healthy on the menu, it still may be very calorie-heavy.
- Beware of the word "light" in descriptions: ask for information on calories, fat, and sodium, or at a minimum, find out the ingredients so you can assess the dish.
- Pick the best and leanest protein.
- Double your steamed veggie side dish.
- If you are due for dessert, truly enjoy it!

French: Best choices include ratatouille, fish dishes with sauces on the side, and root vegetables. Avoid creamy sauces, pâté, mousses, hollandaise, beurre blanc, béarnaise, and pommes frites.

Indian: Best choices are tandoori and tikka white meat chicken and shrimp, saag dishes, and biryani rice. Avoid creamy yogurt sauces, deep-fried dishes, samosas, and korma dishes.

Fast Food, Good Food?

When it comes to fast food, it's good to have emergency options, but as a rule it's best to avoid fast food altogether. The following choices are better than most, but are still too high for regular HFL consumption. If you turn to this food option for one of your meals, you need to be very vigilant with the rest of your food choices that day.

Burger King®: Best bets include a veggie burger with half a bun, hold the mayo; fire-grilled shrimp garden salad with fat-free dressing; chicken Whopper® sandwich on a small bun, hold the mayo, plus dinner salad.

Wendy's®: Best bets include Mandarin Chicken® salad (add baked potato if you want a carbohydrate), Ultimate Chicken Grill sandwich and side salad, and large chili (with crackers).

McDonald's®: Best bets include Chicken McGrill (open) sandwich, hold the mayo, and apple dippers. For the Southwest grilled chicken salad, only drizzle on the creamy dressing lightly.

Kentucky Fried Chicken®: Best bets include Honey BBQ KFC Snacker™, mashed potatoes without gravy, Tender Roast® sandwich without sauce, baked beans, three-inch corn on cob.

Pizza Hut®: Best bets include tomato, mushroom & jalapeno, Fit 'N Delicious fourteen-inch large (slice); ham, pineapple & diced red tomato, Fit 'N Delicious fourteen-inch large (slice); Veggie Lover's® six-inch personal pan pizza; diced chicken, red onion & green pepper, Fit 'N Delicious fourteen-inch large (slice).

Taco Bell®: Best bets include Fresco-style bean burrito, Fresco-style Ranchero chicken soft taco.

Chili's®: Best bets include Guiltless Grill® Salmon (hold the cheese for the veggies), Guiltless Grill® Pita (ranch dressing on the side), Guiltless Tomato Basil Pasta (share and ask for light cheese or cheese on the side).

Applebee's®: Best bets include teriyaki steak and shrimp skewers, grilled tilapia with mango salsa, sizzling chicken skillet.

Chick-fil-A®: Best bets include chargrilled chicken sandwich, chargrilled chicken garden salad (hold the cheese and use light dressing), wheat bagel with fruit cup (add some protein), Spicy Chicken Cool Wrap®.

Denny's®: Best bets include veggie omelet (ask them to make it with a bit of oil instead of butter), grilled tilapia dinner (ask them to use only a bit of oil in the cooking process), grilled chicken breast salad (hold the cheese and use fat-free dressing), Boca® burger (hold the cheese and go open bun), vegetable beef soup with side garden salad.

Sbarro®: Best bets include side sautéed mixed veggies and garlic roll (add a protein).

Panera®: Best bets include low-fat vegetarian black bean soup and baked potato, grilled salmon salad with dressing on the side and fruit cup, classic café salad with dressing on the side.

Jamba Juice®: Best bets include light smoothies (add protein powder).

Baskin-Robbins®: Best bets include non-fat soft serve yogurt (chocolate, vanilla), Nonfat Capuccino Blast®.

Cold Stone Creamery®: Best bets include Sinless Very Berry Good, Berry Trinity™ Smoothie, Sinless Sweet Cream Ice Cream, sorbet.

Subway®: Best bets include Fresh Fit® combo meals.

Starbucks®: Best bets include skim or fat-free lattes (grande if iced, tall if hot), Frappuccino® light (grande), coffee with skim milk and a low-fat blueberry muffin.

Planning For Parties

The HFL Plan is obviously not meant to be dull—you and your family should have fun with your food! Parties and entertaining are definitely encouraged—you just need to do it mindfully, with as much advance planning as possible.

My friends call me the "salad gal." They know I will always contribute a tossed salad bursting with veggies, a crudités (fancy name for cut-up veggies) platter with healthy dip, or an exotic fruit salad or fruit dessert. I love thinking up new presentations and recipes to wow their palates. I will often also supply a separate container of rinsed beans or nuts to top salads and add some protein. This also means that I never have to worry about what I will eat. It especially helps during weeks of holiday partying or summer barbecues when we are eating out a lot and I want some control over my core menu choices. It means I can have my salad, and then pick and choose what I want to accompany it.

When I entertain at home, I try to find out ahead of time if guests prefer fish or chicken or are vegetarian. My menus often include a grain salad, a tossed salad, a fruit salad, a main protein, some kind of steamed or cooked veggies, and a sweet potato, rice, or hot grain dish. I always have frozen yogurts or sorbets to add to the fruit, or angel food cake and a fat-free whipped topping or chocolate sauce for dipping. That's how I cook for my family, and that's how I entertain. I get really creative with my poultry and fish rubs and marinades, vegetable presentations, and healthy sauces and dips. Sometimes I plate the food; other times, I serve buffet-style.

I can also make healthy brownies or muffins as an added treat, but frankly we eat our desserts at restaurants or other people's homes, so we don't keep high-fat temptations in our fridge. I don't think any guests have left our home dissatisfied with the food choices, taste, or variety. In fact, most people remark on the fresh

PLANNING FOR HOLIDAYS

There are a lot of holidays to celebrate every year: from Halloween through New Year's Day, it's almost one continuous food fest of parties, dinner parties, office gatherings, and family get-togethers. You can really lose track of the amount of overeating that goes on as one celebration blends into the next.

Try some of these tips to help you keep control and perspective:

- Look at buffets strategically. Use a small plate and scan the selection first, picking and choosing the bites you want to try. Your second small plate should be just salad.
- Portion out two mouthfuls of each starchy or high-fat food, and surround them with veggies and healthy dip.
- Choose wine or champagne over hard liquor and have a small glass of water between drinks. Also try wine spritzers (one part wine to one part seltzer).
- If you go overboard one night, cut back for the next few days, even if there are more celebrations. Bring salad or fruit salad for your own benefit.
- Decide whether your calorie splurge should be spent on food, dessert, or a bit of both.
- Steer clear or don't be heavy-handed with creamy or cheesy salads and dishes.
- Don't stand by the buffet and don't linger at the celebration dinner table to nibble.
- Chat more—eat less.
- Increase your exercise, and do it daily during the holiday season.
- Weigh yourself daily during the holiday; if clothes start getting even a little bit tight, cut back.

taste of the foods and the fact that I can create sweet potato fries that rival the "real deal." My friends expect to eat healthy food when they come to my home and they expect to leave pleasantly but not overwhelmingly full. If I'm celebrating a birthday, anniversary, or other special event, I'll often buy a fat-free or low-fat ice cream cake.

The next time you entertain, use this checklist to plan your event:

Basic Entertaining Menu Checklist

1. Optional veggie broth to start meal
2. For hors d'oeuvres, a crudités platter with salsa/bean dip/hummus
3. A themed salad:

   - Spinach, mandarin oranges, cucumbers, jicama
   - Arugula, cherry tomatoes, cucumbers, peppers, shredded carrots
   - Bibb lettuce, radicchio, eggplant tomatoes, yellow and green squash, cauliflower, sun-dried tomatoes
   - Romaine, hearts of palm, corn, cherry tomatoes, celery, cucumbers
   - Mixed lettuces, broccoli, sliced Roma tomatoes, shredded carrots and cabbage, topped with roasted peppers

4. Protein (one or two choices and beans or veggie burgers on hand for vegetarians)
5. If kids are invited, baked chicken tenders, turkey hot dogs, or pasta
6. Steamed vegetable(s)
7. A grain (rice, pasta, corn/peas/potatoes, whole grain)
8. Optional grain-based salad like wheat berries with fruit berries
9. Flavored waters, seltzers
10. Enough fruits to create a fruit salad or fruit parfaits or dip in chocolate sauce

A Final Word about Planning Snacks

Snacks can be tricky to plan. Remember that their purpose is to help stabilize blood sugar levels, provide energy between meals, and keep you from going too many hours without eating. Some people need to address specific cravings or taste preferences, while others will find that they just need a between meals pick-me-up.

You do want to be calorie-conscious with snacks because this is one of the areas where mindless eating can get you in big trouble calorie-wise. You also want to decide if you are truly hungry or just need an energy boost to get you to your next meal comfortably.

Take advantage of seasonal fruit and vegetable options. The summer is a great time to enjoy cherries, watermelon, fresh corn, asparagus, mangoes, plums, peaches, and apricots. Use them as a base for your snacks. Be wary of frozen food snacks: they can be especially high in fat and sodium. Also remember that after-dinner snacks either mean you didn't eat enough during the day or you are seeking a solution to boredom or unchecked emotions. The kitchen door needs to close after your last meal. Creating a "mini-fast" till the next morning means you will wake up with a true hunger for breakfast.

For emotional eaters or people with binge or compulsive eating disorders, snacks can be especially challenging. In some cases, people find it easier simply to eliminate all but the most healthy snack options from their homes, to only stock snacks in small quantities, or to limit daily snack times. It's important that every family find the balance that works best for them.

CHAPTER 6 QUICK-SUMMARY

1. Planning is the most important HFL tool for eating mindfully and maintaining a healthy weight. It may seem time-consuming at first, but the rewards are amazing (and soon it will be second nature).
2. Healthy families are organized, with easy-to-navigate, well-stocked pantries and refrigerators.
3. Use your Yes, No, Maybe So Food Lists and HFL Meal Plan formats to create healthy shopping lists for the week.
4. Never shop without a plan—and stay in the Safe Zones of your supermarket!
5. Have a plan for eating out, entertaining, holidays—and every other possibility you can think of. Remember, it's not about following a rigid plan exactly—it's about having a plan that will guide you generally to make healthier choices.
6. Yes, even plan your snacks—there are lots of good choices that are both tasty and relatively healthy in moderate amounts.

Tips for Kids

1. You need to model the behaviors you want to see in your kids.
2. By age three (sometimes younger), a child can easily indicate the menus they prefer and the new items they are willing to try.
3. If kids seem reluctant or unwilling to participate in choices and menu planning, let them know the menus are firm—but there are "standbys" (add protein to a salad, a wrap with premade tuna or egg salad, etc.—nothing that requires major prep).

4. Let them write the actual list with you, go through a cook-book with you, or taste test foods—involve them in any age-appropriate tasks.
5. Take them shopping with you and let them taste, touch, feel so they become part of the experience.
6. Use color games with them, especially when choosing fruits and veggies so you bring home a "bouquet of colors."
7. This is a great time to teach them hands-on label reading—make it a math game.
8. Play the "Yes, No, Maybe So" game with them while shop-ping—if it adds to your shopping time, remember this is quality time spent with your kids.
9. Be patient and remember changing habits with kids used to high-sugar, high-fat foods is a slow and steady process.

Tips for Teens

1. Find out their favorite foods (which you probably know) and start discussing healthier versions or alternatives (air fries, turkey burgers, whole wheat buns, lower calorie bever-ages, etc.).
2. Let them start to help you cook so they'll be more willing to shop and choose ingredients.
3. If they don't understand how to decipher the elements of a food label, now is a great time to teach them.
4. Let them plan a menu or meal of the day.
5. Take them to a farmers' market and alternative shopping locations to encourage their interest.
6. Discuss the impact of these changes on their health, their energy levels, their school performance, and their athletic performance. Give them three easy-to-understand reasons why this is important (for example, you'll have more energy to run faster, you'll see school performance improve, your complexion may improve).
7. Don't make it a battle or a series of arguments—sometimes just introducing the new HFL habits and sticking with them consistently will lure them over.

8. Keep offering to include them, hear their voice and suggestions, even if their contributions are small.
9. Keep reminding them to add to the list as they think of new items they want.
10. Assign them one shopping day a month so they feel "in charge."

7

Healthy Habit #2:
Prepare Together

Easy Family Meals, Smart Snacks, and Tasty
Tips for Healthy Eating Every Day, Everywhere

The second Healthy Habit of the HFL program is *preparing* healthy food together as a family. Don't freak out—I know this idea sounds about as realistic as flying to the moon for many modern families. But I have seen all kinds of families make big changes in their kitchens without spending too much extra time and energy. (Remember, if you've planned well using tips from Chapter 6, you've got all the ingredients on hand, and you've decided most of what you'll be eating in a given week, so the action in the kitchen should be very focused and efficient.)

Families that work on *any* project together often work out confounding personality clashes along the way. What better way is there to work out some family issues than near the chopping block where you can channel your emotions as you hash out issues? And there's something special about preparing food with your family, whether you're boldly experimenting with an exotic gourmet meal or just making sandwiches and salad. You're creating memories that your kids can take into their own kitchens someday, you're teaching healthy skills, and perhaps most of all, showing them the joy and value of preparing and sharing food with love and mindfulness (lessons that no one will learn in a fast-food drive-through.)

HFL Food Preparation Rules

There are four "rules" for HFL food preparation:

1. Preparing food is **included in everyone's schedule.** If you don't set aside time for it, you'll all be tempted to reach for whatever is fast and convenient, and no one will ever develop new habits.
2. Preparing food means **choices should be mindful**. That means you're not just making whatever you feel like it, whenever you feel like it, without thinking about it. Sure, you can have treats once in a while, but they're part of your overall plan to be responsible for your health. It's not "anything goes" with eating.
3. Preparing food means **everybody gets involved**. Teach all family members to participate; not everyone has to be a talented or enthusiastic cook, but everyone should be comfortable with making some favorite selections.

SILICONE SAVVY

Silicone has entered the kitchen scene in a big way. Here are my favorites: baking mats, colanders, cupcake pans, egg poacher, mitts, ice tray, pastry brushes, spatulas, splatter screen, warmer/steamer, whisk. Go more traditional when it comes to cutting boards (they scratch easily), measuring cups, cake and loaf pans, garlic peelers, lemon squeezers.

4. Preparing food should mean **keeping it simple** and **making it fun**. If you don't, you'll find yourself alone in the kitchen.

Amy's Weekly Prep Plan

I promised that your HFL food preparation time wouldn't overwhelm your schedule, and here's why: your food prep commitment will probably ultimately take you about one morning a week, plus one quick midweek fill-in shopping trip, and thirty minutes before larger meals (most breakfasts and lunches typically can be ready in fifteen minutes or less.) In reality, you're probably already spending a similar amount of time eating out, ordering out, going to the drive-

---

FOUR QUICK LUNCH IDEAS PLUS SNACKS

- **Wraps/Pita Sandwiches/English Muffin Sandwiches**: Layer on tuna, turkey, soy meat, shredded chicken, or beans plus veggies, mustard (make creamy by mixing with non-fat mayo), relish.
- **Pasta Salad**: Toss any whole grain or high-protein pasta plus broccoli and cauliflower florets, cherry tomatoes, bell peppers, red onions, in olive oil and vinegar dressing.
- **Rice and Beans**: Mix together brown rice with rinsed canned black beans, grilled veggies, and fresh cilantro.
- **Asian Noodles**: Combine buckwheat noodles (tossed) with a bit of sesame oil, soy sauce, scallions, and cooked veggies, including snow peas.
- **Afternoon Post-lunch Snacks**: Try natural nuts (small handful), string cheese, and an apple; air-popped popcorn and soybeans; baby carrots and a small handful of sunflower seeds; cubed fresh fruit and fat-free yogurt.

through, and making do with other unplanned, less-than-healthy, or last-minute meals. The HFL program shows you how to use that time in a more organized and productive way at home to help your family develop healthy new habits that will eventually seem like second nature.

Here's a typical Sunday, based on my own experience, with the family pitching in. Keep in mind that I've been doing this a long time so it may take you some time to get your own ideal prep schedule together.

9:00–10:00 A.M.: Shop supermarket with list and my teen.

10:15–10:45 A.M.: Unpack and separate out food groups, stock fridge and pantry with my younger one.

10:45–11:45 A.M.: Separate, season, and pre-cook or freeze three entrées with everyone pitching in.

11:45–12:45 P.M.: Clean, chop, prep, and put veggies and fruit into sandwich bags, serving bowls, and sealed containers. Also

---

MIX UP YOUR SWEETENERS AND FLAVORINGS

Here are some great ideas for boosting taste and not calories:

- Honey (use sparingly)
- Stevia (a sweetener)
- Hot sauce
- Jelly, fruit-based, no sugar added
- Mustards, all kinds
- Salsas
- Soy sauce, low-sodium
- Syrup, low-sugar
- Vinegar, balsamic and flavored
- Worcestershire sauce

HEALTHY DRINK TRICKS

When preparing alcoholic beverages, try these calorie-cutting tips:

- Add club soda to red or white wine to create a wine spritzer and reduce calories.
- Choose light beer over regular full-calorie beer.
- Pack lots of fruit into a glass of sangria.
- Dilute champagne with a bit of low-sugar orange juice.
- Have your margarita on the rocks for fewer total ounces (and calories).
- Squeeze out vodka with sugar-free cranberry juice as a base.

pre-bag snacks, labeling all containers and sorting dry snacks in pantry into portioned sizes. This one is mostly my job, but the kids do pitch in.

12:45–1:15 P.M.: Make fruit salad and veggie salad to start the week. I have this down to a science.

1:15–2:15 P.M. (optional or later at night): Further prep, such as putting together the week's lunch bags with snacks and storing them in the pantry to add the main part of the meal later, making muffins or other "special dishes," and setting the table for dinner that night or for breakfast the next day. Kids help set the table for the next morning and help pick their lunch bag contents.

Sunday night: This is usually a "buffet" night so all the ingredients are ready to go from items you've prepped earlier in the day. It might be a make-your-own pizza night (with whole grain tortillas as your base) or salad bar and bean night. Set the table for breakfast the next day and tackle "orders" for the next day's lunches.

Wednesday or Thursday: This is usually shopping filler day for buying or refilling any needs like fresh fruits and veggies, dairy products, and any additional weekend meal items, plus the ingredients for a special dinner to be prepared fresh that night.

What Is Your Style?

It may help you plan your meal preparation to choose one of the following "Prep Profiles" that describes the kind of cook you are:

- **Quick and Easy.** You choose weekly menus and recipes that require few ingredients and follow a consistent meal plan; little variation can still mean great meals. You'll see a selection of my own favorites at the end of this chapter.

FIVE RECIPE TIME-SAVERS

For quicker, easier cleanup:

- Measure ingredients onto waxed paper; you'll use fewer measuring spoons.
- Use aluminum foil to line cooking dishes and pans; you can just toss out (or recycle) the lining when you're done.
- Rinse measuring cups and utensils with very cold water before using sticky ingredients for faster washing.
- Always beat eggs in the mixing bowl first and then add other ingredients, so you use fewer bowls.
- Rub cutting board surfaces with lemons on a regular basis so odors like garlic don't linger and become impossible to remove by washing.

- **Adventure in the Kitchen.** You have decided really to embrace this experience and truly explore a new and exciting relationship with food and your kitchen. You know it may be "hit and miss" until you get the hang of cooking with less fats and being more creative with rubs, marinades, and seasonings, but you see it as an exciting journey.
- **One Day at a Time** with planned menus. You've decided to cook mostly easy and healthy recipes but have one or two days a week when you explore cooking a bit more in depth and challenge your creative juices and cooking skills.

Remember that you can switch between profiles whenever you want: you may want to be adventurous during vacation or summer break and go "quick and easy" during the school year (or vice versa).

How quickly and smoothly preparation goes really depends on how well you've shopped, stocked, and planned recipes and menus for the week, as well as which prep profile you're using. Here are some examples:

Quick and Easy

- Preparing white meat chicken breast three different ways— initially bake and then finish by grilling, marinating in tomato sauce, and stir-frying with veggies.
- Planning a salad bar one night with tuna or beans as the protein, and pre-made turkey burgers and pre-made turkey meatballs for other nights.
- All of these can be accompanied by a large vegetable salad, large fruit salad, steamed veggies, and a healthy grain (all pretty easy).

Adventure in the Kitchen

These menus can get prepped on shopping day, and require more assembly and cooking time on the individual evenings they're served:

- Bean soup or vegetarian (bean) chili
- Healthy lasagna

TO PLAN YOUR GRAINS, KNOW YOUR GRAINS

If you can grab a pot and boil water, you can cook grains. And if HFL is anything, it's a program that encourages you to step out of your "food box" and explore new, tasty, healthy options.

Kids will especially love the funny-named grains and experimentation offers an opportunity for all of you to decide which grains click for your family and which don't quite measure up. Here's how to prepare these fun choices, so you don't have to pass them up because you don't know what to do with them when you get home:

Amaranth: It's fluffy, slightly sticky and has a "mild popcorn taste." For every cup of grain, use 3 cups of water. Boil 20 minutes until tender. (Yield: 2-1/4 cups with a 1/2 cup serving providing 129 calories, 2g of fiber, 5g of protein, 1.5g of fat.)

Barley: Creamy-tasting and with a chewy texture, it's great topped with diced, cooked veggies. For every cup of grain, use 3 cups of water. Boil 60 minutes if it's pearlized, 90 minutes if it's hulled. (Yield: 3 cups; each 1/2 cup serving has 100 calories, 3g of fiber, 2g of protein, 0.5g of fat.)

Buckwheat (also called kasha): It's light textured, with a coffee-like taste, and makes a great side dish, especially with gravy. For every cup of dry buckwheat, add 2 cups of water. Boil 15–20 minutes. (Yield: 3 cups; each 1/2 cup serving has 105 calories, 3g of fiber, 4g of protein, 0.7g of fat.)

Millet: It tends to have a fluffy texture with a slightly buttery flavor. It's a great topping on salads or combined with bananas, steamed soymilk, and raisins as a whole grain hot cereal. For every cup of grain, boil 3 cups of water. Boil partially covered for 30 minutes. (Yield: 3 cups; each 1/2 cup serving provides 103 calories, 1g fiber, 3g protein, 1g fat.)

TO PLAN YOUR GRAINS . . . , *continued*

Oats (rolled): These have a creamy texture and are slightly sweet. You can serve rolled oats as a cereal topped with berries and nuts or use them in whole grain muffin or nutrition bar recipes. For every cup, use 2 cups of cold water and simmer for 5 minutes. (Yield: 2 cups; each 1/2 cup serving has 111 calories, 3g fiber, 4g protein, 2g fat.)

Wheat Berries: This is a chewy grain with a roasted nut flavor. Add it to soups or make a rice-like dish out of it (add fruit or berries). For every cup of grain, use 3 cups of water. Boil partially covered for 45 minutes. (Yield: 2-1/2 cups; each 1/2 cup serving provides 160 calories, 6g fiber, 5g protein, 1g fat.)

- Cornmeal-crusted fish and roasted corn (served fresh that night)
- Ground turkey and tofu meatloaf with sun-dried tomatoes
- Asian chicken wraps
- Homemade pizza topped with chicken strips and grilled vegetables

One Day at a Time

Just mix menus, using both easier and adventurous recipes. (But again, much of the prep work can be done on the weekend—even for more complicated recipes.) Just create a schedule such as:

- Easy meals: Monday–Thursday
- Adventurous selections: Friday and Saturday
- Buffet night: Sunday

Knowing what you want to serve and not having to take time to shop and prep each day will be an incredibly helpful and time-saving asset. Leftovers are also perfect for some brown bag or home lunches the next day, saving even more time. I'm assuming that you'll follow some of my suggestions later on for finding recipes that appeal to your family, but in case you need some inspiration, I've included a selection at the end of this chapter. These are basic recipes that I've come to love over the years—they're easy, require few ingredients, and most of them are kid-friendly and fast to prepare and cook.

Family Affair in the Kitchen

In earlier chapters, I've talked about you how you can involve the kids in the HFL program in an age-appropriate way. Studies show if they are involved, they will be more likely to eat what you prepare. After all, they'll feel like it's their creation, too. Make sure to offer

TIPS FOR THE "PICNIC" SIDES (YEAR-ROUND)

Just because we love potato salad, coleslaw, and macaroni salad, it doesn't mean we have to be unhealthy by eating the high-fat versions. Here are some great prep tips that preserve flavor but get rid of some calories and fat:

- Use mustard, fat-free mayo, and pickle relish to dress potato salad with less fat. Boil potatoes and refrigerate them overnight, and use vinegar in the salad recipe to neutralize the starch's blood-sugar-raising effect.
- Make coleslaw with flavored vinegar as dressing and use a variety of shredded cabbages as well as carrots.
- In pasta salad, use whole grain or high-protein macaroni and lots of veggies, chopped fine, with non-fat mayo in the dressing.

FOUR DELI MEATS IDEAS

- Buy very low-fat and very low-sodium if you are going to use them as Maybe So Foods.
- Consider soy meats as well because they come in a variety of flavors now.
- Substitute garden burgers and soy and turkey bacon.
- Keep pre-measured (two- and four-ounce) packages handy for sandwiches, wraps, whole grain pita pockets (just add veggies, hummus or relish/sauerkraut) and to shred on salads or add to cooked whole grains or soups.

words of encouragement and praise because positive reinforcement is at the core of the HFL lifestyle program. Let everyone find new seasonings, marinades, and cooking methods, and even create their own new personal favorites.

It's also important to remember that each individual family member has a different stake in this lifestyle makeover. So in the preparing phase, you want to remember what each member's goals are. If your teen is trying to lose weight, get him or her involved in creative salad and vegetable prep activities—don't have them prepare favorite foods they're trying to avoid!

If your husband simply wants to lower his cholesterol, let him weigh in on some of the plant stanol–based margarine spreads (which one's taste does he prefer?), and do some research on which specific food ingredients help lower cholesterol.

Preparing by age group is part of what makes this program unique. No family member gets a pass on participation. However, effort, time involvement, and satisfaction levels need not be equal. There will be family members who are slim and perceive themselves as healthy and think this is all unnecessary, or who are in denial about their weight; there will be teens who want you out of their

WHICH OIL WORKS BEST?

Ethnic Foods: For most Italian and Mediterranean dishes, use olive oil. For Thai or Asian, use sesame or peanut oil. For French cooking, substitute canola or soybean oil for butter. Using small amounts is the key.

Salad Dressings: In vinaigrettes, use a minimal amount of neutral oil, like canola or olive oil, to spotlight a vinegar or use a bit more oil to showcase the oil flavor. Extra virgin olive oil makes a distinctive Italian dressing while a little sesame oil is great in an Asian ginger dressing. If you use walnuts or almonds in a salad, use a bit of similar nut-flavored oil to boost that flavoring.

Sautéing: Try canola, corn, safflower, or soybean oils to add mild flavor—they're great for cooking vegetables. Keep heat at medium and use just enough oil to prevent food from sticking (flavored cooking sprays can also do the job without all the calories).

Baking: It can be done without butter or margarine: substitute three tablespoons of oil for every four tablespoon of butter or margarine (for example, three-quarters cup of oil for one cup of butter). Canola oil is a good choice because it cuts the amount of fat even further (one-quarter cup of oil can replace one-half cup of margarine.) Sometimes, if it won't interfere with flavor, I'll also add apple butter to help use less oil or to replace butter or margarine completely (works in brownies and muffins). If you feel you must use shortening (such as in a pie crust), make sure it has zero trans fats.

More Must-Knows About Oil:
- Monounsaturated oils work best for heart health. They decrease your total cholesterol, as well as decreasing the bad cholesterol (LDL) and raising the good (HDL).

WHICH OIL WORKS BEST?, *continued*

- Polyunsaturated fats lower total cholesterol but not LDL. Saturated fats raise total cholesterol and LDL.
- Trans fats raise LDL and lower HDL.
- When describing oils, the word *light* means *light in flavor,* not in calories.
- Most oils are a mixture of fat types but often have more of one specific fat type:
- Monounsaturated fats—almond, canola, olive, safflower, sesame, soybean, peanut.
- Polyunsaturated fats—walnut, corn, sesame, soybean.
- Saturated fats—all of the above have a small amount of saturated fat.

---

lives and do not want you messing with their fast food; there will be hovering friends and family members who think you are crazy to try this. (They may actually be afraid you'll be successful. What's their excuse then?)

Fine. Just be the captain, take charge and have all menu decisions made only by those who want to participate in the decisions. In most cases I've seen, believe it or not, everyone ultimately climbs on board the HFL bandwagon, because it's fun, creative, and challenging but user friendly, and because frankly, they'll want their own food preferences incorporated.

Three-Step Prep for Shopping Day

The first big secret of Healthy Food Prep is to do as much of it as you can right after you shop. The food's already out as you're unpacking, you know what you've got and what you need to do. You can divide your prep into three primary steps:

ADDING IN CALCIUM VALUE

All family members benefit from calcium, no matter how old they are. And we now know calcium is absorbed far better from food sources than from supplements. So try to include some of these calcium-rich "Maybe So" foods in your daily meals:

- Calcium-fortified juice in smoothies
- Fat-free milk, yogurt, cottage cheese in breakfast and lunch foods
- Canned salmon with bones as a lunch or dinner entrée
- Broccoli in salads, stir-fries, steamed veggies, soups, and stews
- Cooked spinach in lasagna, as a veggie side dish, and in pasta dishes
- Oatmeal as a regular breakfast food
- Fortified soymilk as a coffee creamer, in cereal, and smoothies
- Fat-free cheese/evaporated skim milk in mac'n'cheese made with whole grain pasta

Some other superstar calcium snacks: reduced-fat cheese and baked whole grain crackers, chocolate syrup in skim milk, fat-free yogurt and berries or a splash of maple syrup, calcium-enriched, low-sodium V8® juice and baked crackers or a small string cheese, Skinny Cow® ice cream sandwich.

1. *Prep Your Yes Foods (Fruits and Veggies):* This is the Big One—make sure salads, veggies, and fruits are both appealing and easy to access for all. This will mainly involve cleaning, chopping, cutting, and bagging.
2. *Prep Your Maybe So (Portion-Controlled) Proteins:* This means getting your meats, fish, bean, and veggie protein (tofu, soy, etc.) ready for easy meal-making. Creating marinades and

rub-ons ahead of time helps make this step easy. If you buy proteins in four- and six-ounce portions, they're already individually sized.

3. *Prep Your Maybe So and No (Portion-Controlled) Sides, Grains, and Treats:* The time required for this depends on your food choices—just make sure you do whatever you can in advance, so your meal comes together as smoothly as possible.

Here are some more tips for Three-Step Prep:

1. Yes Foods: Chopping and Cutting

- Chop different herbs and store in airtight containers or Ziploc® bags.
- Chop onions, scallions, peppers, and garlic, and store these as well.
- Cut up a variety of veggies and store in airtight containers for dipping as snacks.
- Cut up a large salad and fruit salad to start the week.
- Chop up any recipe veggies and herbs, then label and store.
- Grate zucchinis, squash, and carrots for salad garnish and to add to dishes.
- Buy ingredients pre-cut if you can afford it and need extra time-savers.
- Create salsas, marinades, and healthy dressings because their shelf life in the fridge is about a week.
- Wash all fruit ahead of time for easy grabbing.
- Freeze berries (including cherries). To freeze berries, wash and let dry completely, then place on single layer sheets to freeze. Once frozen, gather, bag and store in freezer.

2. Protein Prep: Marinating, Entrées, and Quick Meals

- Prepare and portion out meats, fish, and tofu ahead of time.
- Make burgers, pound meat, and section off portion sizes per family member.

- Pre-cook and flash freeze when possible.
- Start the week off by making a chicken salad, bean salad, and tuna salad for easy sandwiches or as toppings for vegetable salads.
- Pre-make lasagna and turkey meatloaf, then refrigerate and cook it on evening you plan to serve it.
- Use a Crock-Pot®. Throw pre-cut and prepared ingredients into it in the morning of so it's ready when you come home.

3. Grain (and Bean) Prep Tips

- A towel under the lid of cooked fluffy grains will absorb excess moisture that gathers while you wait to serve it; otherwise, the grains or rice will get too moist).

QUICK AND EASY (NO COOKING NEEDED) DIPS

Quick and Easy Families, take note: you don't have to make your own to get great dips. You can buy some ready-made dips for veggie snacks and appetizers. These superstars are low in calories (up to forty calories per serving), sodium (less than 200 milligrams per serving), and fat (no saturated fat) but high in flavor. Just don't forget to take note of serving sizes:

- Grande® grilled and roasted salsa (two tablespoons)
- Ortega® black bean and corn salsa (two tablespoons)
- Marina® cocktail sauce (two tablespoons)
- Wegmans® tzatziki dip (two tablespoons)
- Fresh Food Concepts five-layer party dip with guacamole (two tablespoons)
- Fritos® bean dip (two tablespoons)

- Think double boiler when preparing hot cooked grain cereals—water on the bottom, cereal on the top. You won't have to spend a lot of time stirring. Twenty minutes and cereal is ready.
- Take cooked pasta and add it directly into the pan you've cooked the sauce in, allowing a bit of the pasta water to drip in as well. The starch in the pasta water will help the sauce stick.
- When buying dried beans, make sure they are intact and not cracked or chipped (a sign they are old and will take longer to cook.)
- Think red and green lentils, little navy beans, and split peas for soup; sauté onion, add veggie stock, carrots, celery, bay leaf, and parsley plus the lentils or beans and season with umeboshi vinegar (pickled plum-based/sweet and sour flavor).

Try These Rub-Ons

Part of protein preparation is coming up with creative ideas to make your entrées tasty. These rub-on recipes for six to eight pieces of skinless chicken breasts, boneless pork chops, or small turkey cutlets will do just that.

Paprika-Garlic Spice Rub

1 tablespoon dark brown sugar
1 tablespoon paprika
1-1/2 teaspoons ground black pepper
1-1/2 teaspoons garlic powder
1 teaspoon salt

Fennel-Garlic Spice Rub

1 tablespoons dark brown sugar
2 teaspoons coarsely chopped fennel seeds
1-1/2 teaspoons paprika
1-1/2 teaspoons garlic powder
1 teaspoon salt

Cumin, Coriander, and Turmeric Spice Rub

2 teaspoons dark brown sugar
1-1/2 teaspoons garlic powder
1-1/2 teaspoons ground coriander
1-1/2 teaspoons ground cumin
1/2 teaspoon ground ginger
1/2 teaspoon turmeric
1 teaspoon salt

Ginger, Cinnamon, and Cloves Spice Rub

2 teaspoons dark brown sugar
2 teaspoons paprika
1-1/2 teaspoons garlic powder
1-1/2 teaspoons ginger
1 teaspoon salt
1/2 teaspoon cinnamon
1/2 teaspoon ground cloves

Prep Your Refrigerator

We discussed refrigerator strategies in Chapter 6, but here are a few more ideas to reinforce the idea that the more organized you are, the healthier you will eat overall.

Create "ethnic folders" in the pantry so you have the ingredients grouped together for easy meal-making when the time comes:

- **Asian:** ginger, five spice, oyster sauce, dry mustard, rice wine vinegar, sesame oil, chili paste, dried shiitake mushrooms.

- **Italian:** balsamic vinegar, basil, oregano, rosemary, bay leaf, Italian mixed spice, sun-dried tomatoes, pine nuts, capers.
- **French:** thyme, five spice, savory, bay leaf, chives, tarragon, whole cloves, Dijon mustard, champagne vinegar, shallots, walnut oil.
- **Middle Eastern:** tahini, kalamata olives, mint, oregano, cloves, raisins, dried figs, cinnamon.
- **Southwestern:** chili powder, oregano, tamarind, cumin, garlic, salsas.
- **Scandinavian:** dill, cloves, horseradish, sweet mustard, cloves, white peppercorns, cardamom.

In rubs and other recipes, herbs and condiments can mean the difference between "blah" meals that send family members back to fast food, and great-tasting meals that make them come back for more:

- Crumble dried herbs to release flavor.
- Add dry herbs at the beginning of the cooking process, while fresh herbs should be added toward the end because they are more volatile.
- Make sure to clean sandy herbs like parsley well.
- Not all fresh herbs dry well. Ask questions at your supermarket.
- Use smoked paprika, black pepper, curry powder, Herbes de Provence, and/or coriander to add a "kick" to recipes.
- Think *dried and preserved veggies*, which are flavorful and can be kept on hand without perishing quickly, to add in small amounts (due to sodium) to sandwiches, wraps, salads, sauces:

  – pickle relish
  – artichoke hearts
  – dried mushrooms
  – sauerkraut
  – marinated mushrooms
  – pickles
  – roasted red peppers
  – sun-dried tomatoes
  – dried fruit

HEALTHY SUBSTITUTION MAGIC

The following food substitutions can help you shift your food and preparation choices into the healthy zone by cutting calories and fat while still offering great taste. The purpose of this list is to familiarize you with healthier options. Particularly when it comes to cooking, substituting apple butter or cooking sprays for oil, apple butter for jam, evaporated skim milk for cream, egg whites and Egg Beaters® for whole eggs, skim milk for whole milk, and non-fat half-and-half for regular half-and-half will have a dramatic impact on overall calories and fat intake but still offer palate satisfaction.

Think about using the following ingredients in addition to fresh and dried herbs to add even more flavor:

Fat Saver Guide

Use this chart for tasty low-fat substitutes for everyday foods and ingredients. Many small changes can make a big difference. Making lower-fat substitutions just twice a week for a year could result in weight loss and health gains!

Breakfast Items

Instead of:	Substitute:
Two regular pork sausages	Two non-fat sausages
One Danish pastry	One bagel with non-fat cream cheese
Two slices toast with one tablespoon butter	Two slices toast with one tablespoon jam
Two eggs	Three egg whites or egg substitute
One bagel with regular cream cheese	One bagel with non-fat cream cheese
One muffin	One bagel with non-fat cream cheese
Cereal with one-half cup whole milk	Cereal with one-half cup skim milk

HEALTHY SUBSTITUTION MAGIC, *continued*

Sandwiches and Burgers

Instead of:	Substitute:
Three ounces roast beef	Three ounces sliced turkey breast
Three-ounce beef hamburger patty	Three-ounce ground turkey breast burger
Three-ounce beef hamburger patty	Three-ounce veggie burger
Three-ounce croissant	Two slices whole wheat bread
Three ounces tuna salad with regular mayo	Three ounces tuna salad with non-fat mayo
Three ounces chicken salad	Skinless chicken breast
Three ounces ham	Three ounces fat-free ham

Side dishes

Instead of:	Substitute:
Salad with two ounces regular dressing	Salad with two ounces non-fat dressing
Four ounces french fries	Four ounces fruit salad
Four ounces french fries	Four ounces oven fries or baked potato
Potato salad with regular mayo	Potato salad with non-fat mayo
Four ounces buttered vegetables	Four ounces steamed vegetables

Butter, Oil, and Margarine

Instead of:	Substitute:
Two tablespoons oil for sautéing	Two tablespoons broth or wine for sautéing
One tablespoon butter, oil, or margarine	Two sprays vegetable oil

Dinner Entrées

Instead of:	Substitute:
One fried chicken breast (breaded)	One skinless roasted chicken breast
Three ounces roast beef or steak	Three ounces roast turkey breast

HEALTHY SUBSTITUTION MAGIC, *continued*

Dinner Entrées, *continued*

Instead of:	Substitute:
Two slices veggie pizza with cheese	Two slices veggie pizza without cheese
Three ounces regular ground beef	Three ounces ground turkey breast
Three ounces regular ground beef	Three-ounce Boca® burger
Four ounces breaded fried fish	Four ounces baked fish (not breaded)
Eight ounces spaghetti with meat sauce	Eight ounces spaghetti with marinara sauce
Three ounces regular ground beef	Three ounces extra-lean ground beef
Eight ounces chili con carne	Eight ounces vegetarian low-fat bean chili

Dairy Products

Instead of:	Substitute:
One-half cup whole ricotta cheese	One-half cup non-fat ricotta cheese
One ounce heavy cream	One ounce evaporated skim milk
One ounce regular cream cheese	One ounce non-fat cream cheese
One ounce regular grated cheese	One ounce non-fat grated cheese
One cup whole milk	One cup skim milk
One cup whole yogurt	One cup non-fat yogurt
One ounce sour cream	One ounce non-fat sour cream
One-half cup whole cottage cheese	One-half cup non-fat cottage cheese

Snacks

Instead of:	Substitute:
One ounce roasted peanuts	One ounce whole grain pretzels
Six cups oil-popped popcorn	Six cups air-popped popcorn
One ounce regular potato chips	One ounce baked potato chips
One ounce regular potato chips	One ounce rice cakes

HEALTHY SUBSTITUTION MAGIC, *continued*

Snacks, *continued*

Instead of:	Substitute:
One ounce regular tortilla chips	One ounce baked tortilla chips
One ounce regular crackers	One ounce non-fat crackers
One tablespoon nacho cheese dip	Two tablespoons non-fat bean dip

Dessert

Instead of:	Substitute:
One-half cup ice cream	One-half cup non-fat frozen yogurt
One ice cream bar	One frozen fruit or non-fat yogurt bar
One regular chocolate brownie	One fat-free chocolate brownie
One serving regular pudding	One serving fat-free pudding

Source: Manufacturer's Data. USDA Handbook B. Nutritionist IV Database

MORE SO-LONG-FAT SUBSTITUTIONS

Try these substitutions to take more fat out of your foods:

Ingredient	Substitute
Creamy soups and sauces	Non-fat strained yogurt, evaporated skim milk, soymilk, puréed roasted vegetables, cooking rice in soup then puréeing it
Oil in baked goods	Applesauce, puréed bananas, puréed cooked prunes
Oil for sautéing	Vegetable stock, wine, vinegar

Source: www.vegetariantimes.com

Amy's "Quick Attack" Meal Prep (Because We Moms Need a Battle Plan)

This is a quick approach to preparing your three daily meals ahead of time, using foods I know my family loves. "Throwing together" a few ready-made ingredients can still yield a quick and nutritious meal.

Breakfasts: Boil one dozen eggs; buy three containers of yogurt per family member, two boxes of high-fiber cereal, one box high-protein cereal, one box of frozen whole grain waffles, peanut butter, fruit, and skim milk.

Lunches: Whole grain tortillas, English muffins, pre-made tuna and egg salad, shredded white meat chicken, low-sodium deli turkey, cut-up veggies, shredded part-skim cheese, fruit.

Dinners: Grilled chicken breasts, pre-made turkey burgers, homemade lasagna, veggie chili (Crock-Pot®), salad and fruit salad, sweet potatoes, pre-made taboulah, cold high-protein pasta and veggie salad.

Snacks: 100-calorie puddings, 100-calorie South Beach Bars®, homemade trail mix, cut-up veggies (pre-made) and hummus, cut-up apple slices (sprinkled with lemon juice) and peanut butter.

Final Health, Sanity and Timesaver Tips

- Make sure each family member is weighing in on entrée options. As I mentioned before, have back-up tuna salad or beans always on hand for anyone who thinks dinner is a strikeout and not a home run. No drama, no preparing a new and different menu: just an easy alternative.
- When you make a dish, always ask yourself, what can I do with leftovers? Chicken can be shredded for wraps, turned into chicken salad, added to a veggie omelet, or cut up to be added to a mixed salad or rice dish the next day.
- Use leftover frozen dinner trays to create refrigerated and ready-to grab meal kits (serving of main dish, cooked veggies, grain) or refrigerated ready-to-grab assembly kit (tor-

tilla, sauce, shredded low-fat cheese, and veggies for pizza creation). Your kids will love it and can weigh in on suggestions. And portion size is built in to these trays (which may be a shocking revelation). If you're still hungry, you can always add salad or fruit.

- Try to "multi-purpose" food. Grilled chicken breasts that are cooked ahead of time can be added to salad, stir-fries, or soup. They can also be ready for a quick wrap. Marinating tofu ahead of time in several different sauce preparations (tofu acts like a sponge with marinades) means you can cube it and use it in a salad, stir-fry, or soup as well.

- Consider portion size within your food menu plans to help your family members target their goals (some may need weight loss, others weight maintenance, so portion sizes should be consistent, but some family members may get *more* portions of some of the Maybe So foods in a day. Protein, fats, and carbohydrates are the foods that fall into the "be wary of portion size and number of servings" category.

- Another important part of prep is food substitutions. You can find an array of "light," "high-fiber," "nutrient-dense," "low-sodium," and "low-fat" substitutions that will still punch up taste and provide creaminess or other necessary textures while saving you calories. (See page 216.)

- Be aware that many boxed rice products that call for butter or oil taste fine with the specified fat cut in half or omitted completely.

- Consider always including three or four "super-fast" recipes in your weekly meal plans for the days you come home tired and hungry, and want the food ready fast.

- Invest in certain appliances if you can afford it: a food processor, blenders (and new ones have food processor attachments), specialty blades and choppers, specific knives, a Crock-Pot (with removable liner), a scale, a timer, a variety of measuring cups and spoons, a steamer, a wok and a good set of cookware with non-stick surfaces are totally worth the investment.

These time-savers are worth their weight in gold and will also help you get even more creative with healthy, tasty creations.

CHAPTER 7 QUICK-SUMMARY

- Yes, believe it or not, even YOUR family can learn to take the time to prepare healthy food!
- If you've planned and shopped the HFL way, food preparation will not require too much extra time.
- Preparing food needs to be included in everyone's schedule for the week.
- Prepare by plan, not by "anything goes."
- Nobody gets a "pass"—everyone helps out with something.
- Keep it simple and make it fun.
- Your meals can be quick and easy, more adventurous and ambitious, or a combination of both—it's up to you.
- Remember—organization is the key to the HFL plan and to life.

Tips for Teens

- Be prepared to let teens work a recipe from beginning to end independently, especially if your relationship is a bit tense. They'll actually learn a life lesson from managing a recipe from start to finish and probably ask for help (maybe grudgingly—but they will ask) if a technique or ingredient is unfamiliar—with luck, you'll get to the point where working together becomes an "acquired taste."

- Use every opportunity to talk about why changes needed to be made, why eating fresh foods when possible is healthier, how to read and decode labels, even explaining important buzz words like antioxidants, trans fats, fiber, healthy oils, whole grains, and plant stanols, as well as continuing the dialogue about Yes, No, and Maybe So foods.

- Explain healthier versions of foods, better drink choices, and why you are starting to limit fast food and stay on top of snacking. This is even your chance to point out what you didn't know before that is now making you rethink how you want to eat and how your family should be eating in order to embrace a healthier lifestyle.

- Encourage them to remind you when ingredients are running out and what ingredients they may want to see in recipes. Keep a handwritten or running computer "fill-in" list.

- Use this as an opportunity to explain science principles wrapped in cooking demos (what happens when you don't attend to rice), how to avoid burning food, what ingredients thicken, what ingredients don't work well together. This is also a great opportunity to taste new foods.

Tips for Kids

Preparing meals by age group includes setting up safety standards so that younger children know they can never prepare or cook without supervision. It also needs to address what is reasonably within the child's abilities from an age group perspective. Three-year-olds can tear up lettuce, but they can't chop safely yet. A six-year-old can mix ingredients together but should not be cooking over an open flame. There are too many dangerous appliances and situations that can happen in the kitchen, so revisit the safety discussion constantly.

One approach I love is to allow kids to go on Web sites (with supervision when needed) and to choose recipes from the recipe section here or from kid-friendly sites. The popularity of the Food Network means there are thousands of HFL-friendly recipes online.

I think it's also very important to lighten up when it comes to messiness in the kitchen. The kids are learning math and techniques and how to work as a team—all invaluable lessons while learning to prepare healthier food options—so I think of the kitchen as a classroom. But that doesn't mean you can make a mess and leave without cleaning it up; involve the kids in cleanup, too. That's an important life lesson and they'll catch on after a while: it's fun to *make* a mess but not to *clean* it!

- *Ages 3–6:* Gather ingredients, stir ingredients, scrub and wash fruit, tear lettuces, arrange veggies and fruits, measure ingredients and spill them into the bowl (with help), mash bananas or potatoes, cut with cookie cutters, garnish foods, help close storage containers, be taste testers, help make pizzas, help pack lunches, help prepare breakfast, etc. Practice math with them on making measuring decisions, such as: "If the recipe needs to be doubled, then . . . ")
- *Ages 6–8:* Fill and level measuring cups and spoons, gather all ingredients for recipe, grease pans with cooking spray, set the table, beat ingredients with a wire whisk, set up and serve simple breakfasts, peel and slice eggs (with an egg slicer), peel oranges, make healthy trail mix, help create pizzas, make a salad, use a rolling pin, help pack lunches.
- *Ages 8–10:* Use a can opener, use a microwave oven, prepare simple recipes themselves, set up a buffet, help pack lunches, prep bagged pre-measured snacks, spread peanut butter or other spreads, make kabobs of all kinds, use an electric mixer with supervision.

- *Ages 10–12:* Use an oven, use a knife with supervision, grate cheese and veggies, use a blender, set up a steamer, make wraps, help pack lunches, handle preparing a soup recipe, fill a Crock-Pot® (make sure to go over handling meat and keeping surfaces clean), set up and blend a smoothie.

Utensils kids can use: egg slicer, brushes (for marinades), apple slicer, blunt scissors, rolling pin, ice cream scoop, plastic scrub pads, handheld grater, cookie cutters, pizza wheel, bouncy whisk, silicone baking trays, stools with rubber base tips (to grip the floor so it doesn't slide), plastic measuring cups, measuring spoons, bowls with counter grip bottoms.

8

Healthy Habit #3: Portion Together

On the TV show *What Not to Wear,* fashion experts make it very clear what you shouldn't do when it comes to clothing: don't walk around in sweats, loud paisley colors, jumpsuits, overalls, teen trendy wear, etc. The list goes on forever. But one of the biggest gaffes is wearing "camouflage wear"—loose, baggy clothing meant to hide a larger body or too tight clothing intended to "hold the mass in." Don't wear something too big or too small. Ever.

Well, when it comes to the obesity epidemic and food problems, you can point your finger at the media, schools that don't offer enough physical activity, Hollywood and the modeling industry with their unrealistic images, advertisers beckoning with their tempting food messages—this list goes on as well. But the bottom line is, generally speaking, if you eat too much, you are going to gain weight. Just as with clothing, there is a right "size" of food for your body to be healthy. If the food you eat is too "big" for you, your body will eventually expand to match it.

Lately, many families have fallen into a serious portion distortion trap. We've become accustomed to giant, outsized portions, and we end up wearing them in the form of fat, like an extra, unneeded layer of clothing. We're so used to "big" food that smaller amounts— amounts that would fit our healthy bodies perfectly—seem odd and downright unsatisfying.

HFL Habit #3 is about changing the way we think about portions to achieve a better fit. We'll give you lots of tips in this chapter to help your family change habits, but perhaps the most important tool is awareness of the problem.

Let's look at the typical American consumer. We eat out—a lot. In fact, many of us spend half the dollars we spend on food eating away from home.[1] We are surrounded by eating opportunities and the food is convenient, cheap, tasty, and served in large portions. The average person eats 159 fast-food meals every year, and many of those are "super-sized" (the meals and, consequently, the people).

Even if we were to try to create one portion standard at home (because we're in control, so to speak) and one portion standard outside the home, we would still face a major challenge. That's because our kids would be begging for the gargantuan/fat-laden choices typically available. Over time—and research bears this out—we begin to blur the two environments and we ultimately end up eating larger portions in both environments. Studies have shown that the more food you are served at a given meal, the more you want to eat.[2]

We tend to eat the same portions every day, but we also tend to eat what's put down in front of us. So, if you serve larger amounts of cereal in the same bowl to people who routinely take an exact portion size, they won't take the time to measure the amount visually and consider its consequences. In general, we tend not to evaluate many of the serving sizes placed before us— we just assume it's the same portion as usual and eat more. Our basic ability to judge fullness and satiation is easily blurred by portion distortion.

Portion sizes have increased inside and outside the home.[3] The place where we see this the most is in the fast-food industry (high-fat/high-calorie/high-sodium/highly refined food), which is marketed as giving you the most for your dollar. Unfortunately, the two types of food most consumed are high-calorie sugary drinks and fatty foods (burgers, fried foods). So we get the double unhealthy whammy of bigger portions and poor quality foods. In this case— two strikes and you're out.

We also know now that if you consume numerous portions of foods high in processed sugars on a regular daily or even weekly basis, you will be at higher risk of developing type 2 diabetes.[4] So imagine consuming numerous large portions of the food and the impact it has on heightening the risk factors.

PORTIONS MADE SIMPLE WITH THE ROYALTY DIET

I stand by a motto that helps to clarify the importance of the amount of food or portion sizes you are eating *and* when it makes sense to time the size or amount of food in these portions, so you are sustained through out the day:

Eat Breakfast Like a King/Queen: Have an ample portion of a protein, a serving of a (carb) grain, a serving of a (carb) fruit, and a small serving of fat.

Eat Lunch Like a Prince/Princess: Have one serving each of protein, fat, and (carb) fruit, and two servings of (carb) veggies.

Eat Dinner Like a Pauper: Eat a small serving of protein, double serving of (carb) veggies, one serving of (carb) grain or fruit.

Hungry between meals? Fill in with fruit and/or fat-free dairy snacks.

Big Servings, Big Problems

It's gotten a bit crazy. We've become so used to seeing gargantuan steaks, fries, muffins, pizza, ice cream splits, and soda cups that we feel disappointment and perceive hunger when we are served reasonable-size portions. We commonly get three servings of pasta and meatballs equal to three to four servings of meat during an Italian meal served in an American restaurant. A typical "serving" of sticky white rice in an Asian restaurant is actually three to four servings of rice. Snacks have followed the same pattern; they are often meals unto themselves.

And when we take in liquid calories, our bodies very often do not register satiation or "feeling full" in the same way. We may actually eat more food overall in a day when one of our meals is a smoothie. And unfortunately, our bodies often don't register satiety at all when we consume soda and juice calories, regardless of the portion size. They just get added to the day's heavy calorie tab.

We know that most fast-food eaters underestimate the number of calories they eat.[5] They don't do it intentionally; there's just a perpetual bias in how they perceive how much they are eating. It's typical human nature to minimize the bad ("I didn't eat that much today," "That piece of pie was really small," "I only had a small burger and fries") and overexaggerate the good ("See how small my plate is"—never mind that the food was stacked nine inches high). As we've become accustomed to the super-sizing concept, it seems we are no longer able to estimate what we should eat in order to feel satisfied but not sickeningly full.

Well, what if you start by setting up guidelines to take less? "See less, eat less" is a true phenomenon that research has proven to exist.[6,7] Avoid seeing more food than you need or want to eat and you will eat less. See more, and you will likely eat more. And remember that portion control is harder with trigger foods, so deciding how you will keep these foods out of your life or how you will create a portion-specific way to handle them is an absolute in the HFL guidelines. You can't wing it when it comes to tempting foods— ever.

A good reference when it comes to the importance of portion and weight control is the National Weight Registry, which tracks individuals who have successfully lost an average of seventy-three pounds and kept off at least thirty pounds for more than six years. The registry notes that, regardless of the plan used to lose the weight, all of the registry members:

- Limit calories to around 1,800 per day by using portion control and counting calories per serving.
- Exercise daily—they never miss workouts.
- Watch less than ten hours of TV weekly.[8]
- Some of them use the "Five Pound Max Rule," meaning if they regain five pounds, they immediately reinstitute the dietary plan they lost weight on until the five pounds are gone again.

The moral of the story is that in order to achieve weight loss and health gains, you *need* portion control. And in order to *sustain* those accomplishments, you *still* need portion control.

That is why I've repeatedly referred to awareness of eating in earlier chapters and why I emphasize that, even when it comes to the healthier Yes and Maybe So Foods, portion awareness is paramount. If you only remember one formula—remember that: **Mindless eating + portion distortion = weight gain**. You cannot have a food free-for-all, even with healthy foods! A calorie is a calorie, and too many calories will be a problem, regardless of the quality of the food from which they come.

Changing Your Family's Portion Perception

How much food you take in should relate directly to your level of activity. (See Appendix 8A, "My Pyramid Food Intake Pattern Calorie Levels, U.S. Department of Agriculture.") A sedentary person should probably eat around 400–500 calories *less* than an active person, as a general rule. A sedentary person who eats 2,200 calories per day could be slowly gaining weight daily or weekly, and it could be quite insidious—just kind of creeping up. A total of 1,800 calories might be better, or if that leaves someone hungry, 1,800 calories plus extra calories in the form of Yes fruits and veggies. These foods are high in water content and fiber, so they fill the stomach with minimal calories per portion. Thanks to their fiber content, there's also a better chance some of the excess calories from these foods will be digested and eliminated.[9]

It takes time to change any habit, and portion perception is probably one of the toughest. It can seem challenging, but remem-

SWITCH IT OUT

It may help to make some food switches; when you swap an unhealthy food for a healthier one, you can sometimes eat a larger portion without increasing calories OR get greater health benefits for the same calorie amount:

- Switch out milk chocolate for dark chocolate.
- Switch out white wine for red wine.
- Switch out soda for unsweetened iced teas.
- Switch out whole milk and cream for evaporated or condensed fat-free milk and skim and 1 percent milk.
- Switch out high-calorie flavored drinks for low-calorie flavored waters.
- Switch out meat (some of the time) for lentils/beans.
- Switch out meat for fish.
- Switch out regular dairy products for fat-free dairy products.
- Think one teaspoon olive tapenade instead of mayo.
- Use unsweetened applesauce instead of butter.
- Think three tablespoons cocoa + one tablespoon fat-free condensed milk instead of baking chocolate.
- Add fruit and shredded veggies to bump up the volume and flavor of entrées.

OUTSMART DESSERT PORTIONS WITHOUT SACRIFICING PLEASURE

- Flip your dessert. Top fruit with a treat instead of topping a treat with fruit.
- Always share really decadent desserts.
- Try fondue. Dip fruits into dark chocolate sauce instead of crackers or bread into a cheese sauce.
- Make lighter versions of banana splits (with fat-free ice cream), cheesecake (with ricotta and fat-free cream cheese), pie with low-fat pudding fillings and whole grain crust, fresh non-fat yogurt-based desserts (add fruit, nuts, shaved dark chocolate).
- Embrace sorbets.
- Create thin crepes filled with fruit.
- Use melon halves as shells for the dessert presentation.

ber that as your family makes the changes we've already discussed (better food choices, more activity, etc.), your new habits will help tremendously to calm down cravings, shift food preferences, and get you into a healthier zone of eating. Foods high in fiber and water content will also fill you up. You or your family may easily drop weight just by eating less sodium-laden, sugar-laden, fatty foods.

But in most cases, portion control is also necessary. You will need to gain control of overeating, even if you're overeating healthy foods. Mindless eating, or eating for the wrong reasons (emotional eating), will sabotage your results. Noshing while at home all day, while watching TV or while in your car, mindlessly eating at work, taste testing during cooking, as well as nibbling as you clean leftovers off the dinner plates—these are all practices that can let unwanted calories slip in, because there are no boundaries in place.

Maybe you remember that famous line: "It's 10 P.M. Do you know where your children are?" Every parent was affected by that public service announcement slogan because it forced us to stop and think about the safety of our children, especially if they were new drivers.

Well, here's another slogan you need to keep in mind: "It's dinner time. Do you know how much you are actually eating?" A full plate arrives at the table and we think, "It looks delicious and I'm really hungry and this must be how much food I need to feel full, right?" and we eat it all. Our eyes may have said, "Wow, that's a lot of food," but we don't heed that message because there's a disconnect. Too many of us don't use our eyes-to-brain measuring stick, which quite often screams at us: "Large food plate coming down—go easy," especially when it comes to enticing foods.

For years, I have been retraining my clients' eyes so they actually see the portions within typical servings both inside and outside their homes. In the confines of your own kitchen, it's easier to serve appropriately plated portions. I ask all families to adopt one habit: never serve foods family-style except for tossed salads and fruit salads. Plating food means portion control is already in place if you follow the protein/grain carbohydrate/vegetable format and if you end with a piece of fruit—not a second round of entrées.

Ten Tips to Encourage Family Portion Control

Use Small Plates

One of the most effective tools for retraining your family is to serve portions on somewhat smaller plates. A four- to six-ounce portion of protein, plus a baseball-size serving of grain, and lots of cooked veggies will look extremely satisfying on an eight- or ten-inch plate. On a large twelve- or fifteen-inch plate, it may seem paltry.

Communicate Your Downsizing Plan

Be sure to prepare your family. Let them know that super-size portions are not reasonable or healthy, and that you don't want to fall into that trap, so you plan to rebel. All family members may not get on board right away, but that's OK. They will probably respect your commit-

GET PORTIONS UNDER CONTROL

- When eating out, start the meal with an undressed salad (spoon dressing on yourself or dip the vegetables sparingly into the dressing).
- Put aside half the entrée immediately and ask for a double portion of steamed veggies.
- Consider ordering a large salad and an appetizer (they're usually smaller) as your main course.
- Stick with water, diet soda, tomato juice, or skim milk.
- Order entrées baked or broiled with sauces on the side.
- Make sure steamed means *without butter* so you avoid extra fat calories and you get a true calorie-sized portion of vegetables.
- Order berries with a bit of chocolate dipping sauce as a dessert treat. This provides a portion-controlled Yes Food with only a little bit of caloric decadence from the sauce.
- Try to avoid buffets. Otherwise, create a salad base on the plate, then position small amounts or tastes of entrée selections.
- Use salad plates instead of the large dinner plates.
- Ditch the "clean plate mentality" and substitute the "healthfully full" mentality.
- Talk in between courses; it slows down eating.
- Avoid reading or watching TV while eating; you lose satiation awareness.

ment, even if they don't show it. And you probably have more influence than you know. If nothing else, just employing this concept in the home will have an impact on the quantity of food you eat, even if old habits die hard outside the home. Habits outside the home can affect the habits you're trying to develop inside the home, but the habits inside the home can impact eating going on outside the home, too. Changing portion perception will take time and there may be perceived or real hunger as you acclimate. Be patient, and don't give up!

Slow Down

Anything that forces you to take more time with your meal will help contribute to portion control. Remember, we're deciding to put a certain measure of food on our plate that's reasonable for enjoyment and satiation, but if we shovel it in—instead of slowing down and savoring it—you will more than likely want more. The eating will happen way too fast and you may not have given your stomach a chance to start to feel full and send the appropriate signal to the brain. Encourage family discussion with involvement by every family member. Everyone needs to understand this physiological mechanism. Make your meals positive, fun experiences for everyone. Emphasize that what matters most are the people, the companionship, the sharing, and the togetherness. Make sure there's no TV watching, put your fork down occasionally, and get up between courses just to slow the whole eating process down a bit. You won't just be encouraging better portion control—you'll be establishing solid eating patterns (priorities) that may continue to pay benefits into future generations.

Teach and Model Measuring by Hand

Show your family how to use hand measurements, and start using them yourself: a fist to represent bread carbohydrates (rice/pasta/potato/peas/corn), a thumbnail for fat, an open palm for a thin slice of chicken breast or fish, two hands (palms down, thumbs underneath) with fingers outstretched and touching to visualize how much space your meal should generally cover on your plate.

Don't Forget to Portion Drinks

If it's water or unsweetened tea, drink as much as you want. Otherwise, pour any liquid with calories into tall, skinny glasses to make the amount look as large as possible; it is a practice that has been tested and found to help retrain the eyes-to-brain measuring stick I mentioned earlier. You'll actually see a larger portion in this case, thanks to the shape of the glass, so you will be more likely to feel satisfied.

Make It Hard to Get To

When designers reconfigure kitchens, they look for ways to mini-mize steps for cooks, so less time is wasted tracing and retracing steps. You need to do the opposite when you "design" where to put treats and No Foods that you want to limit. Extra steps will give everyone extra time to reconsider their food choices.

Treats Need Special Portion Treatment

For many people, treats can be too tempting to resist (this can be true not only for kids, but for adults too). The best solution is either not to stock them at all, slowly shift some of the treats in your pantry and fridge to healthier treats, or pre-portion snacks and treats, either by dividing them into portions yourself or buying them that way. Remember you need to decide how many outright

CONTAINER AND PORTION TRICKS

Sometimes your kitchen tools can encourage or discourage great portion habits. The trick is to turn to the sizes of contain-ers (or bowls and cups) that can offer you individual measures of food, hold multiples of portions, or give you visual cues. Try these container tricks:

- Bowls that are sized for measured amounts, such as half-cup or one-cup bowls (great for yogurt). Available at http://www.yumyumdish.com.
- A sugar dispenser that portions out a half-teaspoon of sugar at a time. Available at http://www.wrapables.com.
- Plates that show (with lines sectoring the plate area) appropriate amounts of protein, vegetables, fruit and whole grain carbs. Available at http://www.theportionplate.com.
- A cereal dispenser that releases six-ounce portions at a time. Available at http://www.containerstore.com

decadent treats your kids will have in a week and then you can shift to some foods that feel like treats but are whole grain or calcium-rich. If you are going to buy pre-portioned snacks, use common sense when bargaining with your children. A six-ounce Yoplait Light® 100-calorie snack is a great selection, while typical potato chips have very little nutritional value, and a 100-calorie portion of them is really quite small. If they still want the chips, you need to be clear that the small bag is a "treat portion size" and if they want more food at snack time, more must now be a Yes Food. A banana is a really satisfying fruit snack; you can make it more desirable by offering a bit of dipping chocolate as the "treat part." Other kid-friendly snack choices include string cheese or a small serving of nuts (beware nut allergies). They do satisfy quickly. Here are some other portion-controlled options for *healthier* treats that are low in fat and sodium:

- Jell-O® fat-free pudding or tapioca, 100 calories
- Jell-O® fat-free puddings, various flavors, 60 calories
- Skinny Cow® low-fat ice cream sandwiches
- A small square of dark chocolate
- Oreo® thin crisps 100-calorie pack
- Nabisco® Honey Maid® thin crisps 100-calorie pack
- Fudgsicle® frozen treats (low-sugar)
- South Beach® 100-calorie snack bars
- South Beach® Diet Whole Wheat Crackers 100-calorie packs
- South Beach® Diet oatmeal chocolate chip cookies 100-calorie packs
- 100-calorie rice cake packs + 1 teaspoon of peanut butter

Give Label Lessons

Reading labels is another great habit you can pass on to your family. They need to be able to tell how many portions are in a food container, the numbers of calories and the kind and amount of fat in each serving, and the sodium and sugar content per serving. They also need to be able to assess just how highly processed the product is. That's how kids will learn to tell a "true No Food treat" from a treat that may have some better-quality ingredients (such as

PORTION RED ALERT

Some foods need tighter portion control than others:

1. Oils
2. Salad dressings
3. Dips
4. Nuts
5. Desserts/treats/processed carbohydrate foods

those listed previously) from a Yes Food. We've included a basic food label breakdown here (see page 246). For more extensive label information, see "Labelman" at www.cfsan.fda.gov/labelman, which offers a series of online exercises to help you understand portions, calories, saturated fat, sodium, fiber, and calcium content on food labels.

Learn as Many Visual Cues as You Can

One of the best ways to control portions is to learn as many visual cues that correlate to actual portion sizes as you can. When you're eating out, you can't measure precisely, so visual cues and comparisons give you an approximate association of portion size to some easily recognizable items. Here is a list of common cues:

Grains:
- Three-quarters cup cereal = a small fist
- One pancake = CD
- One-half cup cooked grain (pasta/rice/potato) = half of a baseball
- One slice of bread = cassette tape
- One piece cornbread = bar of soap
- One grain serving = three-inch make-up compact

Dairy/cheese:
- One ounce of hard cheese = two stacked dice
- One-half cup ice cream = half of a baseball
- Six-ounce yogurt = cell phone
- Two-ounce serving of cheese = 5-piece pack of gum

Fats:
- One serving = one die (from a pair of dice)
- One serving nuts = ping-pong ball
- One serving of baked chips = ring of keys laid out

TWO APPROACHES TO PLATING FOOD

Here are two convenient methods for determining your meal portions:

The New American Plate (based on the Swedish plate method used in Finland, France, and Canada):
    Take an eight- to nine-inch plate.
    Fill two-thirds of the plate with fruit, veggies, whole grains, and beans.
    Fill one-third of the plate with seafood or poultry or lean red meat (occasionally).

The Idaho Plate Method (based on the Swedish plate system):
    one-half plate: non-starchy veggies
    one-quarter plate: grains or starchy veggies
    one-quarter plate: protein

Note that in both cases, the height of the food should not exceed one-half inch (width of your little finger)—food shouldn't be stacked.

Source: American Institute for Cancer Research

Veggies/Fruits:
- One cup salad greens = baseball
- One small baked potato or ear of corn = computer mouse
- One-half cup fresh fruit = half of a baseball
- One-quarter cup raisins = hard-boiled egg
- One fruit serving = small change purse
- Medium potato (starchy veggie) = gift card

Proteins (Meat, Fish, Beans, Tofu, Chicken):
- Three ounces = deck of cards or checkbook
- Burger = PDA
- Serving of nuts = box of Altoids®

Watch and Weigh

One of the best things you can do to get portion-savvy fast is to weigh foods on a small kitchen scale so you become accustomed to true food amounts. You will probably not need to weigh foods for very long in order to familiarize yourself with normal (not giant) portions. But it will do a lot to help you develop an eye for amounts and calorie counts, so that you and your family never have to suffer the consequences of portion-mad eating again. As I've also repeatedly emphasized, try to buy foods that are pre-measured (for example, raw fish and chicken in four- to six-ounce portions, dairy products in sixty- to eighty-calorie packs, deli meats in two- and four-ounce packages). This will also help accustom you to proper portion sizes because it provides repetitive exposures to exact measured amounts. The portion sizes you see on a regular basis are what you will get used to if you really do it consistently.

Amy's Sample Day Menu with Portions

Just to give you an idea of how portion amounts work in a daily food plan, I created this sample daily menu that I have used for myself:

HFL QUICK-TIPS TO HELP YOU END THE MEAL

Portions are very important when it comes to considering daily food amounts, but just as you're required to put a period at the end of a sentence, you still need to put a final end to the day's eating. It's especially important when you are trying to cut down on mindless munching. Here are some helpful techniques:

- Brush your teeth after dinner.
- Chew sugar-free gum after dinner.
- Sip a hot, low-calorie beverage like tea after dinner.
- Agree to avoid the kitchen until the next morning and physically close the door. (Oprah tries to do this).

Sample Daily Menu

Three grain servings, two dairy servings, two large protein servings (ten ounces total works for my particular frame and fitness level), three fruit servings, six veggie servings, two fat servings.

Breakfast
One-half cup of GOLEAN Crunch™ high-protein cereal
One-quarter cup Bran Buds®
One cup of fat-free vanilla yogurt
One-half cup berries
Two teaspoons crushed nuts
(One serving dairy, one serving cereal, one serving fruit, one serving fat)

Morning Snack
Plum
(Second fruit for the day)

Lunch
Two cups mixed greens
One quarter of a large cucumber
One-half cup shredded carrots
One quarter of a jicama
Two eggplant tomatoes
One-half cup shredded cabbage
One-half cup mushrooms
Four ounces soy deli slices, shredded
Two teaspoons of olive oil/vinegar dressing
Four baked crackers (second grain serving)
Iced tea
(Three servings of veggies, one four-ounce serving of protein, second bread-like carb serving for the day, second serving of fat)

Afternoon Snack
One peach
Small fat-free latte with sugar-free vanilla syrup
(Third fruit of the day, second dairy serving)

Dinner
Six ounces low-sodium V-8® vegetable juice cocktail
Six ounces of grilled fish
Two cups of steamed veggies with a bit of tomato sauce
One-half cup couscous (third grain)
Iced tea
(Second serving of protein, three total servings of veggies [that's my six servings], third serving of grains)

What Works for Me

The sample daily plan shows you what I would typically eat on a day during which I exercise quite intensively for about one hour. I have two days a week when I do a longer cardio and weight-training session; on those two days, I have a fourth grain serving and an additional fruit serving to help with replenish my energy reserves.

TEEN/ADULT DAILY BEVERAGE PORTION GUIDELINES

- Water: Unlimited.
- Unsweetened black coffee: Up to four servings.
- Unsweetened tea: Up to eight servings.
- Skim milk/unsweetened soymilk: Up to two 100-calorie servings (count as dairy).
- Diet soft drinks: Up to four servings/day.
- Whole milk, 2 percent fat milk, sports drinks: Limited, if at all.
- Soft drinks, juice: Very limited.

This outline follows the new Daily Health Beverage Guideline you'll find at http://www.beverageguidancepanel.org/. Until recently, there was only a food pyramid.

I consider the eating plan outlined above my "maintenance" eating program. It's about 1,500–1,600 calories (I no longer measure precisely because I really have the visual cues ingrained in my brain. I really do know when I'm spooning too much out on the plate or sizing my protein portions too large). When I want to drop a little weight, I lower my protein a bit (down to six to eight ounces daily) and drop a grain serving, taking me closer to 1,400 calories, while also increasing my cardiovascular training effort just a bit.

My personal assessment of my metabolism is that it runs a bit slow and I am also moving into perimenopause, which tends to affect women from the perspectives of metabolic rate and muscle mass. That's why I've chosen my somewhat low daily maintenance calorie plan. I know myself well, and even though I am very active, even though I weight train to keep muscle mass on, aging is having an impact—I begin to gain weight easily when I move closer to 1,700–1,800 calories/day. Part of the HFL philosophy is "know thy-

HFL QUICK-TIP: DRINK OR DEVOUR?

It's important to differentiate between thirst and hunger. Always try downing one or two cups of water or iced tea to see if you still feel hungry before munching on a food snack. One great liquid snack that kills two birds with one stone is low-fat chocolate milk.

self, regardless of what your blessed neighbor can eat." I can honestly say I'm not hungry on this plan.

I always hesitate to give precise calorie amounts to individuals trying to lose weight because, though there are general ranges that most nutritionists agree upon, based on current weight, gender and the goals you are targeting, sometimes you do need to play a bit with the numbers.

PORTION QUICK-TIP

When considering portion sizes for most proteins, try using a 50–60 calories per ounce guideline (to which most lean proteins will conform). So four ounces of fish, seafood, and white meats (skinless) would weigh in at around 200–240 calories (typically four to six ounces is an average, healthy-size portion of protein if you are following the HFL outline and adding a salad, fruit, and sometimes a whole grain carbohydrate to round out the meal). Use the same *calorie* guideline for other sources of protein, such as dairy products, tofu and soy products, eggs and egg whites, peanut butter, and lean meats (given that we're establishing the fact that 200–250 calories for the protein part of a lunch or dinner meal is a pretty good serving size for the average individual).

LABEL READING 101

This label and an in-depth discussion of deciphering a food label can be found at http://www.cfsan.fda.gov/~dms/foodlab.html.

Label Basics

Take immediate note of the serving size and the number of servings/package (in this case, two servings).

Note the calories/serving (in this case, 250 calories per serving, 500 calories for the whole thing).

Note the number of grams of fat, whether there is any trans fat and saturated fat (the presence of those two should be sufficient for you to want to make a better food choice)

How much sodium? If it's more than 300 milligrams/serving—it's a lot.

How much sugar? Is high-fructose corn syrup (HFCS) present in the ingredients list?

Doing the Math

One gram of fat has 9 calories—so you multiply the number of grams of fat by nine. You can then tell the percentage of fat. In this case, $12 \times 9 = 108$ calories, which means that almost 50 percent of this serving (250 calories) is fat—way too high.

We also know that 27 (9×3) of those fat calories are from trans fat, and 27 (9×3) of the fat calories are from saturated fat.

Protein is 4 calories per gram, so in this case $4 \times 5 = 20$ calories—not a lot of protein to this food.

Carbs also gets multiplied by four calories, so $4 \times 31 = 124$, so this product has about nine teaspoons of sugar (one teaspoon has 16 calories).

Sodium is well over 300mg (470mg to be exact).

LABEL READING 101, *continued*

Overall assessment: This food has trans fat and saturated fat present, is high in fat, has a lot of sugar and sodium—so it does not qualify as an HFL Yes or Maybe So Food.

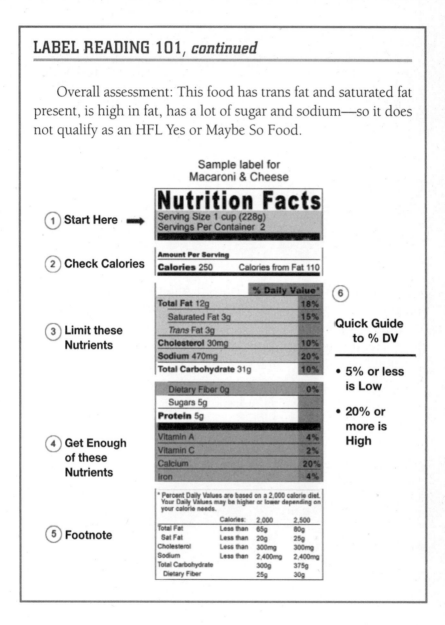

Sample label for
Macaroni & Cheese

I find that making better food choices and just paying attention to portions (without severe restrictions) is often enough to produce some weight loss and better "numbers" (cholesterol, blood sugar, blood pressure) over time. If you do choose to eat more under those circumstances, it's intentional; you're taking an additional portion of one of the food groups because you're experiencing true hunger and you're addressing it with a healthily portioned choice. So you're now eating extra food with *mindful awareness*. Just add portion control to your current eating plan and your whole eating profile will shift, usually to a downward calorie trend. You will also find that you are more aware of what you are eating.

KNOW YOUR SWEET STATS AND SALTY FACTS

The average American consumes a minimum of twenty teaspoons of sugar/day; the World Health Organization recommends a target of about ten teaspoons of sugar daily.

A teaspoon of sugar has sixteen calories; a twelve-ounce can of soda has ten to eleven teaspoons of sugar.

Americans should shoot for 2,000mgs of salt or less/daily; deli meats, canned foods, frozen meals, and snacks are notorious for high levels of sodium (sometimes more than 900mgs of sodium per item).

CHAPTER 8 QUICK-SUMMARY

- Portion distortion is running rampant and families today are wearing "big" food on ever-expanding bodies. Your family needs to buck the trend and find portion sizes that are just right for you.
- Managing portions is not just a good idea, it's essential for good health and successful weight management. Even healthy foods can't be eaten free-for-all style.
- "See less, eat less" is a proven strategy—so you need to help your family retrain their portion perceptions by getting smart about how you present and stock food.
- Portion retraining will take time and requires patience, but these are lasting habits we're building.
- Meals should be about quality and quantity, so focus on getting family meals on the table that are shared together and portion controlled—meaning you plate the food and only the salad and fruit come to the table family-style. Use the time together to enjoy a true family meal.

Tips for Teens

There is no easy way to take teens already conditioned to super-sizing and teach them to reduce portion sizes. In earlier chapters, I've talked about how teens may be motivated by athletic performance, dating pressure, or clothing styles to shift their eating patterns to healthier ones. Peer pressure and self-esteem issues are other incentives. It can also really help if your pediatrician weighs in on the health and weight issues.

The discussion of portion size is of paramount import when it comes to modifying teen eating patterns. They need to understand the best food combos, appropriate portions of snack vs. full meal selections, and the need to hydrate adequately with the least caloric liquids. If they are on the constant fast-food/candy/soda track, this is going to require patience, a lot of dialogue, and possibly the involvement of a health professional if they are seriously overweight. If they have really outrageous patterns of eating oversized portions of fast foods and processed foods, and they *are thin*, you still need to talk about food choices and portion size from a health perspective. Too many "thin people" hit a huge metabolic swing in adulthood; those with no concept of portion control or understanding of true hunger/satiation are surely on the road to serious weight gain later in life. And of course, as I pointed out, large portion of high-sodium or high-fat food can create health problems in thin people.

Teens do need to be able to decipher a label so that they can make independent food selections in portion-sized amounts. They also need to be willing to check out nutritional info when it's available at fast-food restaurants so they really understand how much they are eating from a caloric perspective and gain control of their food choices and portion sizes in general. Remember, these teens will soon be young adults, out on their own, and eventually parents one day. It may be reasonable for them to "test out" different daily calorie amounts so they can learn about energy vs. weight loss needs through self-discovery. If they're involved in sports, a coach can offer support or advice as well. An athlete needs balanced meals/adequate calories. A growing teen also needs adequate calories to support a still growing body.

Tips for Kids

Understanding toddler or kid portions is important so you don't literally train kids to want more and eat more. Remember that force-feeding a child the portion size you think is appropriate is a behavior that undermines a child's feeling of satiation or hunger and their natural, built-in control. Let them graze or eat solid portion sizes that they themselves determine. If it's a healthy HFL Yes Food or Maybe So Food, then you have little to worry about. If you've already "trained" your child to love too many treats or too much food then, yes, you will have to work diligently to get them to play more to offset calories and work with them so they choose more Yes Foods when snacking. Over time, I do encourage you to downsize portions that you know are too adult-size or too big. I don't encourage you to force-feed a child who stops eating when he or she feels full and who is growing well. These measured amounts are (also) important so you have some gauge of reasonable portion sizes integrated into meals for smaller individuals with smaller tummies.

Here are some examples of appropriate meals/snacks:

- One-half whole grain mini-bagel with one tablespoon nut butter and four ounces milk
- One-half slice of pizza with four ounces of calcium-fortified orange juice
- Four ounces of low-fat fruit yogurt and a small slice of whole grain toast
- Fruit and yogurt smoothie made with four ounces of low-fat yogurt, one-half banana, one-quarter cup frozen berries
- One hard-boiled egg with four baked whole grain crackers
- Two tablespoons hummus or nut butter with four baked crackers
- One whole grain waffle, folded and cut up, with one tablespoon nut butter, and four ounces low-fat milk
- One-half cup cereal plus one-half cup low-fat milk
- One-half cup thinly cut veggies plus one-quarter cup bean dip
- One-quarter cup low-fat cottage or ricotta cheese with cinnamon and four baked crackers

9

Healthy Habit #4: Play Together

How To Get the Whole Family Moving with an HFL Family Activity Makeover

Okay, your family is planning, organizing, shopping healthier, and eating healthier, and at the sight of the title of this chapter, you're likely thinking, "Are you kidding me? We're all supposed to exercise, too?"

In my office, I also hear the reverse. People want to know why they can't just exercise more—do they really have to worry about nutrition, too? Unfortunately for those of us who would prefer single-focus solutions, maintaining a healthy weight is not a single-factor challenge. But very little in life is. Think of the child who asks, "Why can't I just learn math because I'm good at it, and I hate English and science and all these other subjects?" As a parent, you explain that all the subjects are necessary to get a solid foundation for success in life, although eventually we can specialize in areas that appeal to us.

HFL STRATEGIES FOR ADDING ACTIVITY

One of the biggest challenges families face is trying to engage in activities that are appealing to everyone and finding the time to fit them in. How can you easily increase it? Look at every activity you do and see where you can build in more exercise: walk the dog longer, walk the golf course, walk your child in a stroller to the local food mart, park your car further away from locations, have your kids walk or bike to school if it's safe. (By the way, on average. if you've only got a couple of floors to go, it takes less time to use the stairs than the elevator.)

Imagine a day where you and family members rack up 10,000 steps by accumulating exercise minutes throughout the day: going grocery shopping, walking through the mall, vacuuming and cleaning (going up and down home stairs), walking the dog twice for ten minutes each time, going up and down basement steps to keep the laundry going—it all adds up. And if you're a golfer, it's time to start walking the fairway instead of riding around on the golf cart. Walking can rack up an average of 13,145 steps vs. only 6,200 steps when using a golf cart. I might also add that dog walkers who walk what is considered the minimum amount of time still walked about a total of two and one-half hours/week, which meets the thirty-minute commitment minimum the American Heart Association recommends.

Here are some ideas for sneaking more activity in:

- Take every opportunity to walk (to and from work, park your car a distance away from work and walk, take lunchtime and after-dinner walks).
- If you use public transportation, get off one stop early and walk.

HFL STRATEGIES FOR ADDING ACTIVITY, *continued*

- Walk your dog, a friend's dog, or volunteer to walk dogs.
- Wash your car by hand.
- Take care of your garden, weed and prune and plant.
- Run or walk fast when doing errands.
- Pace the sidelines or walk at your kid's games.
- Do home repairs and maintenance yourself.
- Do less e-mailing and more walking to people's offices at work.
- At the mall, walk stairs. Never use an escalator.
- Window shop non-stop for two hours.
- Plant flowers.
- Rake the lawn.
- Vacuum the house.
- Play tag.
- Barbecue.
- Bathe the kids.
- Walk with a portable phone while talking.
- Shovel snow.
- Wash windows.
- Jump on a home trampoline.

Weight management works that way, too. Initially, we need a solid foundation in all the basics (assessing our health needs, planning and preparing food, portion control, and physical activity), but eventually we may focus a little more on areas that we enjoy. Some family members may spend more time at food planning or preparation; others may excel at sports or physical activity. Ultimately, every family member will need to find the balance that works best for him or her. But to get to that point, everybody needs to understand that physical activity is essential to reach health and weight goals.

PREGNANT? IT'S OK TO BE ACTIVE

I have two children. During both pregnancies, I exercised consistently. I went from running to jogging to brisk walking as I progressed through my nine months. I continued to weight train with little modification (except I abandoned some machine-based exercises due to my very large belly in the eighth and ninth months). I also modified my abdominal crunch work and added in some back exercises to help with carrying the added weight. I monitored my heart rate and kept it at or less than 130 beats per minute. I had done enormous research on the benefits of exercising and the downside to adopting the sedentary (do what you want, if anything at all) advice of many obstetricians.

I knew that exercising would help with maintaining my core muscle strength, help with my growing appetite and weight gain, allow me to prepare for the marathon known as labor, keep my energy levels up, and help prevent gestational diabetes. Lifestyle and health experts, including cardiologists and diabetes specialists, mostly agree that being sedentary during pregnancy is a poor lifestyle choice.

I DO NOT advocate a marathon or doing intensive, strenuous exercise while pregnant. However, if your doctor says it's okay (and he or she should), I would seek the help of a fitness professional educated on safe exercise regimens for pregnant women. It's worth going the extra mile! Too many obstetrician/gynecologists are simply not up to date on the current fitness and activity recommendations for pregnant women and may even have exercise aversion. Pregnancy is a wonderful time to be active and healthy. Let a positive pregnancy test motivate you to give up bad habits (smoking, for example) and adopt or continue good habits, such as a reasonable and safe exercise program.

WINTER OUTDOOR WORKOUT TIPS

- Dress in layers to maintain body temperature.
- Wear inner layer fabrics that wick moisture away from the body.
- Wear socks that wick away moisture.
- Cover your head, ears, and hands.
- If you have any disease (diabetes, for example) that can put you at risk for frostbite due to compromised circulation, talk to your doctor.

For one thing, once you start to lose weight, you'll be supporting a smaller body mass and your metabolism will wise up, as it's now forced to burn fuel more efficiently in order to supply energy. You may need something else to nudge weight loss along because dieters often hit a weight plateau.

Plus, regardless of your weight goals, exercise offers health benefits that nutrition alone cannot. It gets frustrating for me to see my clients desperately looking for a silver bullet for their health and weight loss efforts but resisting the idea of exercise. Although they often don't want to believe me, the simple truth is that *exercise is the silver bullet.*

Several exercise studies released in October 2007 at the annual meeting of the Obesity Society confirms that if you were to commit to a solid sixty minutes of exercise daily—it could be brisk walking, a couple games of tennis, swimming, or even a combination of two or three activities that add up to an hour—you would have the key to losing weight and keeping it off. Researchers speculate that it could be the effects of the actual workout, or spending time being active that is typically spent eating, or the reduction in stress that reduces emotional eating, or the fact that exercise suppresses appetite or at least offsets some of the eating in which you sometimes indulge.[1]

Exercise is, by far, the easiest, cheapest, most accessible, and effective tool we know of for preserving health and maintaining

EXCUSES, EXCUSES

Just as families come in all shapes and sizes, so do they vary greatly in their activity levels and attitudes. Here are some of the most common situations I hear about in my office. Which one describes your family?

- We all hate exercising. We're slugs most of the time!
- We're an academic family. Who has time?
- Superman, Superwoman, or Superkid lives among us. The rest of us just sit back and watch!
- We're weekend warriors: we actually do active stuff on the weekends, but without any activity goals or plans.
- Mom and Dad remember playing sports long ago— really long ago. Our kids do like sports, though.
- Our kids try to get us to play with them, but most of the time, we're just too tired.
- Our kids play sports regularly after school and on the weekends, but for us, just getting them to and from their activities is exhausting.

Sound familiar? Don't worry. No matter where your family is today, you can learn to become more active to support your HFL health and weight goals.

weight goals.[2] If you aren't teaching your children to be active, you are neglecting one of the most important lessons you could possibly ever pass on to them.

Why Move Your Family to Move?

If you are asking this question, it's time to wake up to the fact that *physical activity is the most effective, least expensive medicine you can give your body to help achieve better health and lose weight.*

According to the Centers for Disease Control, this is the current situation in the United States:[3]

- Approximately 13.5 million Americans have heart disease.
- Roughly 1.5 million people suffer a heart attack annually.
- About 20 million people have type 2 (once called "adult onset") diabetes.
- Ninety-five thousand are diagnosed annually with colon cancer (new cases).
- A quarter-million suffer a hip fracture each year.
- Fifty million people suffer from the "silent killer"—hypertension.
- More than 60 million people are overweight or obese.
- Major depressive disorder affects approximately 14.8 million American adults or about 6.7 percent of the U.S. population eighteen years or older in a given year.
- More than 25 percent of the population have metabolic syndrome.

Many experts expect the situation to get worse before it gets better. Now, consider the benefits of exercise as proven conclusively by research:[4,5,6]

- Reduces the risk of premature death
- Reduces the risk of developing or dying from heart disease
- Reduces high blood pressure and the risk of developing high blood pressure
- Reduces the risk of developing high cholesterol and the risk of developing that condition
- Raises HDL, the good cholesterol
- Reduces the risks of breast and colon cancer
- Reduces the risk of developing pre-diabetes
- Helps reduce body weight and maintain it
- May improve metabolic rate
- Builds and maintains bones and muscles
- Reduces depression/anxiety
- Improves psychological well-being
- Enhances work, recreation, and sports performances

- Helps you to sleep better
- Exercise can delay age-related brain fogginess that often develops by age sixty-five

Still wondering why your family should exercise? Very few families haven't been affected by one of the health challenges in this list, and very few couldn't benefit from more activity. As I said, exercise is *the* silver bullet when it comes to thinner, healthier, and more productive families.

HFL SEVEN-STEP INTERVAL JOGGING WORKOUT FOR HOME OR TREADMILL

Sample:

- Warm up for five minutes, slowly increasing your speed.
- Jog lightly for two minutes. Recover for two minutes walking slow and steady.
- Walk-lunge for one minute and then break into a run for one minute. Recover for two minutes walking slowly but steadily.
- Jump rope for two minutes (just keep starting if you catch the rope). Recover for two minutes walking slow and steady.
- Jog for two minutes. Recover for two minutes walking slow but steady.
- Walk-lunge for one minute and then break into a run for one minute. Recover for two minutes walking slow and steady.
- Jump rope for two minutes. Final recovery for three minutes walking.
  Total time: thirty minutes

BEWARE EMPTY PROMISES

Marketers know how badly you or family members want to get healthy and lose weight, and they are experts at appealing to your wishful thinking. Always be on the lookout for these false promises in exercise equipment ads:

- Long-lasting, easy, no-sweat results. **Reality:** you can't get the benefits unless you put in the time and effort.
- You'll lose pounds and inches in days. **Reality:** water weight comes off easily, but *nothing* works in days.
- You will eliminate fat in particular body locations. **Reality:** sorry, there's no such thing as spot reducing.
- Before and after testimonials and photos show miraculous results. **Reality:** you'd be amazed at how deceptive these usually are—they're often not the same people, or the photos have been enhanced (*very* common).
- Just the machine alone will produce amazing results. **Reality:** very often the fine print will reveal that a diet is also suggested.
- Money-back guarantee. **Reality:** be alert to the fact that the company may keep the shipping charge, which is often inflated.

What makes exercise work so well? According to scientists, a variety of factors contribute to the enormous impact exercise has on our health:[5]

- It increases blood flow, which stimulates the release of certain chemicals that relax the walls of arteries and reduces blood pressure.
- It burns calories to shift weight downward or maintain weight.

- It lessens inflammation, which lowers the negative impact of stress, namely free radical formation.
- It may stimulate the release of an enzyme that improves cholesterol balance by driving more of the good HDL and less of the bad LDL.

Before I forget, add anti-aging to that list of "silver bullet" benefits. Starting at around age fifty, there is a natural decline in muscle mass of about 10 percent, as well as a significant decline in aerobic capacity. Recent studies show that aerobic exercise, weight training, and functional exercise (or workouts that include moves similar to those we use in daily life) can offer substantial benefits to quality of life as we age.[4,7]

How Much Is Enough?

Despite the overwhelming evidence of exercise's benefits, everyone has an excuse, or a list of excuses, for why they don't have the time or need to exercise. Nearly half of all Americans don't get the minimum exercise amount necessary to confer some health benefits (thirty minutes or more most days of the week). Twenty-five percent of Americans are classified as sedentary, meaning there is little if any activity in their daily lives.[8]

Experts recommend a baseline of thirty minutes of aerobic exercise most days for adults to get basic health benefits, and sixty

SHOULD KIDS LIFT WEIGHTS?

Contrary to popular belief, weight training will not stunt growth. In fact, one study revealed that nine-year-olds who did strength training with five-pound weights and resistance bands three days a week developed more bone mass than kids who were active but didn't lift weights.[9] Remember, it helps if you do it together and model the behaviors you want your kids to emulate.

to ninety minutes most days if you are targeting serious weight loss.[10,11,12]

Aerobic exercise involves the big muscles of your body and means that you raise your heart rate so that your body burns calories or uses energy to accomplish the effort. The number of calories burned is just as critical as the intensity of the exercise, but both contribute to achieving heart health and additionally weight loss (time factors heavily as well). You can break up the thirty minutes, but each small effort has to have the same calorie-burning intensity as the full thirty-minute session.

THE POWER OF EXERCISING WHEN YOU'RE OLDER

There's a big difference in how you work out in your twenties or at least in the effort you can physically exert, and a workout in your thirties, forties, and beyond. But I have seen many people in their fifties who are far fitter than their counterparts in their twenties and thirties.

That's the magic of fitness and working out. Over time, even extremely sedentary individuals can literally turn back the clock. I myself can lift weights at a level that compares with exercisers in their late twenties or early thirties. I've also been able to maintain significant muscle mass and maintain a bone density of greater than 2 (on a bone density scan), which is extremely important for a woman entering perimenopause because of typical muscle and bone loss related to aging and the loss of estrogen.

If you are an older parent or grandparent, you can get even more exercise tips by ordering the free 100-page booklet: *Exercise: A Guide From the National Institute on Aging and NASA.* Call 1-800-222-2225 or log on to: www.nhlbi.nih.gov/health/public/heart/obesity/phy_active.htm.

HFL HOME WORKOUT WITH FREE WEIGHTS

Looking for a basic weight routine you can do at home with free weights? For a typical weight workout, you train different muscle groups with sets (usually two to three) of twelve to fifteen reps (unless you're doing super slow reps, which involves heavier weights, very slow movement, and very few reps). Beginners will typically use two-, three-, and five-pound free weights, more advanced individuals will use five-, eight-, and ten-pound weights. You can always use a heavier set of weights for the first set and go lighter on the second set.

You should allow twenty-four to forty-eight hours of rest or recovery for a given muscle group. If you are weight training properly and using adequate weights, to exhaustion (meaning you really struggle to lift on the last two or three efforts), you will cause little micro-tears in the muscle. Usually, if the last three to five reps are difficult and you are struggling but able to finish them, you will succeed in causing these micro-tears. The rest or recovery period allows those tears to heal and form new muscle tissue, which means you increase your muscle mass, the ultimate goal of a successful weight-training program.

Here's a sample overall home workout you can do with free weights:

Upper Body: Two Sets of Fifteen Reps

- Bicep curls
- Shoulder press
- Front raises
- Side raises
- Triceps pushups
- Chest presses
- Chest curls
- Back pulls (for rhomboids or back muscles)

HFL HOME WORKOUT WITH WEIGHTS, *continued*

Lower Body:

- Lunges in different directions (forward and backward)
- Squats (static and active, where you step out and into squat position)
- Plié squats (with feet turned out; options include heels flat and then raised off the floor)
- Step-ups (onto a step) with weights (one-step height for beginner, two-step height for more advanced)
- If you have a multi-station gym, you can also do these lifts:
  - Leg raises or extensions
  - Leg curls
  - Heel raises
  - Inner/outer thighs

Abdominals:

- End workout with crunches (flat on the floor or on a large inflated ball)
- Stretch all body parts that you've worked out, gently

I usually perform two sets of fifteen to twenty reps, although sometimes I'll also do one long set of each exercise to exhaustion. After many years of weight training, I know my body and what level of exercise training works for maintenance or will yield weight loss or muscle gain. Sometimes, for variation, I only work my biceps, shoulders, and triceps one day; back muscles and chest muscles another day; and legs a third day. I then repeat the cycle so I cover six days, and on the seventh I rest (or just play a fun activity like tennis). On four of the days, I add thirty to sixty minutes of cardio as well.

These are the health benefits you can expect according to researchers:[13]

For thirty minutes of aerobic exercise every other day:
30 percent reduction in heart disease
20 percent lower risk of stroke

For thirty minutes of aerobic exercise every day:
40 percent reduction in heart disease
27 percent lower risk of stroke
63 percent lower risk of colon cancer

America on the Move (www.americaonthemove.org), a national initiative dedicated to helping individuals and communities across the nation make positive changes to improve health and quality of life, says that most Americans barely meet a 5,000 or 6,000 daily step goal. The most recent report from the Surgeon General confirms that too many American children, teens, and adults are overweight and sedentary.[14] Research has shown that if previously sedentary diabetics walked 4,400 steps daily (about 2.2 miles), they reduced their A1C level, cholesterol, triglyceride levels, and blood pressure, even if they didn't lose weight. The study showed the greatest health achievements when the subjects targeted just over 10,000 steps or 5.2 miles (which on average was an investment of eighty-three minutes/day). Most impressively, these patients needed less insulin and they saved on their yearly health bills. So the most basic lesson this study revealed was that even an extra 2,000 or 2,500 steps daily (the 4,400 steps mentioned in the study plus an additional 2,000 so that they meet the minimal 5,000-6,000 minimal requirement) will impact health positively.[15,16]

More Is More

As you can see from the benefits associated with exercising daily vs. every other day, and 4,400 vs. 10,000 steps, bigger efforts yield bigger results. More exercise for your family simply means more health benefits, and more savings in health costs, both now and years from now.

FIGHT BOREDOM: THINK OUTSIDE OF THE (EXERCISE) BOX

Boredom is a natural human response, but not an excuse to stop exercising! There are lots of things you can do to change it up (and you'll probably find that some family members need more variety than others).

- Cross train by doing different exercises each time: walk one day, do a DVD another day, take a class another day, or switch off on different cardio machines.
- Keep changing the workout itself: if you only like to walk, walk hills and valleys one day, do speed walking another day, climb stairs and jog a third day.
- Try something new: dance, circus trapeze classes, boot camp, kickboxing, personal training sessions. The idea is to keep variety and different types of challenges ongoing so you stay really engaged and enjoying exercise.
- Get a workout buddy. If your family is not on the same page in embracing exercise, then having a supportive friend who will keep you on track, as you do the same for them, is a powerful tool. This person can also help to spot you during your weight routines so you can lift heavier weights more safely because someone is nearby to assist in the lifting or lowering phase.
- Add another discipline to your exercise routine. If you only run, add some yoga; if you only do weight training, add jumping rope; incorporate something that's a polar opposite to what you normally do.

MORE WAYS TO TRAIN

Consider these great training options as you plan your physical activity:

Continuous training allows for a greater calorie burn by keeping your heart rate at a certain level throughout the workout. A long, steady-paced walk or run is an example of this.

Interval training, which can help you to improve your conditioning and performance levels. You alternate fast-paced with slow-paced activity, so you could do a brisk walk for five minutes and then follow it with a jog or run for five minutes. Or you could walk on a treadmill for five minutes and then add an incline or hill effect for five minutes. One study found that after two weeks of interval training, six out of eight college men and women doubled their endurance or the amount of time they could ride a stationary bike at moderate pace before exhaustion.[17]

Circuit training combines stations of weight training for specified amounts of time followed by timed cardio efforts. Sometimes people choose just to circuit weight train (no cardio intervals), but because they are moving with little rest time between stations, their heart rate remains elevated and they get an aerobic benefit as well.

I like circuits and intervals because you can create goals and it helps to avoid boredom. It's also quite helpful in allowing you to progress to more challenging forms of training.

That's why I'm not a big supporter of targeting the minimum amount when it comes to exercise—it does a disservice to the true benefits of physical activity and how they are actually achieved.

It's fine to get started with a "lower dose" of exercise (and it is indisputable that some activity—practically any activity—is better than none). But a year from now, if you aren't pushing yourself to achieve higher goals, you're missing much of the value of exercise, and you're still in denial about how much you really can do to make positive health changes for yourself and your family. Since I became an avid exerciser, I always try to push myself to climb one more flight of stairs, take a parking spot that's one spot further away from my target location, extend that after-dinner walk even ten minutes more, or simply replace familiar exercise with a new challenge. I want to get all the benefits I can from exercise in my life.

Your Family's HFL Activity Program

What does your family need to do to change activity habits and become a Healthy Family for Life? My basic HFL guideline is to:

Plan thirty to forty-five minutes a day of activity on most days for all family members over the age of four.

Younger kids should be allowed to crawl, not left in playpens or swings for too long, or be allowed to run and play actively, not plunked down in front of a TV. They should enjoy active living as much as possible by playing with other family members frequently.

Some families prefer to count daily steps, in which case we recommend 10,000 steps daily. The easiest way to target 10,000 steps is to wear a pedometer and walk whenever possible—in other words, simply to be aware that every situation offers an opportunity to add extra steps or movement.

I know that thirty to forty-five minutes of activity a day for everyone in the family sounds simple enough, but putting the recommendation into practice can be pretty challenging! That's usually why I tell most of my adult clients to put it in their calendar every day so they see it, and try and get it done in the morning, then add to it during the day if possible. They can do it with the kids or set up "playtime situations" that involve lots of movement.

HFL Family Activity Guidelines

Here are some detailed HFL Activity Guidelines for you to follow to achieve your "family activity makeover":

Discuss your family plans for becoming more active by having a family meeting where you create a list of activities; then keep revisiting the issue, so you delete the things that don't work and add new ideas. Make a monthly activity commitment together by creating a calendar with family and individual activity times penciled in. (See Appendices, Appendix 9A, page 462.)

Create individual plans to achieve thirty minutes or more of activity most days of the week. This will differ for every family member: some of the activities can easily include sports or school activities, Mom or Dad may take an exercise class or have personal training sessions, etc. (See Appendices, Appendix 9B, page 463.)

Make sure that activity times and locations are practical, clear, and planned into everyone's schedules. This means you should decide:

- If you want to create a home gym, get a health club membership, or bring in a professional (personal trainer, yoga or Pilates teacher, etc.) or a combination of these options.
- If any family members need to make schedule rearrangements so that you (or they) can sneak in exercise opportunities. Maybe you can arrange a carpool pickup to buy you thirty minutes of exercise time before the kids come home.
- If any family members can help others with issues such as transportation, experience in a particular activity, etc. A teen driver can get himself to an activity or pick up younger siblings so you can squeeze in a workout.
- If the best ways to get fit include exercising with DVDs at your convenience at home, or if a trampoline in your backyard would be a good buy, or even if the cul-de-sac you live on has lots of families who can join together to play. Whatever route to fitness you take, there are ways to strategize and include affordable home workouts that get all family members involved. Touch football, anyone?

HFL GYM WORKOUT FORMULA: TWELVE MACHINES FOR AN OVERALL WORKOUT

As a certified personal trainer, I have many years of experience training clients with a wide variety of goals on a variety of exercise equipment. If I had to choose a list of machines to give you an overall workout, it would include the following twelve machines. You can talk to a trainer yourself, as well as check out books and other resources for the correct way to perform these common exercises:

Leg extension
Prone leg curl
Leg press (squat position, plié squat position, one leg each)
Seated or standing calf raise
Inner and outer thigh machines
Lat pull-down
Bicep curl
Triceps extension or press
Chest press
Seated row
Shoulder press
Crunches

Note: Many of these machines can be replicated by using free weights, so do not be deterred if you can't afford a gym membership or home gym setup. The purpose of the list was simply to offer a basic "suggestion list" of machines that would challenge your upper and lower body muscles.

FORMULAS FOR MONITORING TARGET HEART RATE

"Target heart rate" is a very important health assessment parameter that every age group needs to consider. You want to raise your heart rate to around 50–85 percent of maximal heart rate. A doctor's cardiac evaluation can help you determine safe parameters. Exercises that can help you to target these goals are: brisk walking, hiking, stair-climbing, aerobic exercise classes, jogging, running, bicycling, rowing, swimming, soccer, basketball, and singles tennis.

This American Heart Association table below uses the formula 220 minus your age and then percentages of that number to show you target heart rates for different age groups.

Age	Target HR Zone 50–85%	Average Maximum Heart Rate 100%
20 years	100–170 beats per minute	200 beats per minute
25 years	98–166 beats per minute	195 beats per minute
30 years	95–162 beats per minute	190 beats per minute
35 years	93–157 beats per minute	185 beats per minute
40 years	90–153 beats per minute	180 beats per minute
45 years	88–149 beats per minute	175 beats per minute
50 years	85–145 beats per minute	170 beats per minute
55 years	83–140 beats per minute	165 beats per minute
60 years	80–136 beats per minute	160 beats per minute
65 years	78–132 beats per minute	155 beats per minute
70 years	75–128 beats per minute	150 beats per minute

Your maximum heart rate (HR max) is about 220 minus your age. The figures above are averages, so use them as general guidelines. Of course, if you were sedentary it is probably best to target the 50–60 percent range of maximal heart rate initially. But over the course of weeks and months, as you get fitter, you may find yourself more comfortably at the higher end of your range, and that's a fabulous achievement!

FORMULAS FOR MONITORING HEART RATE, *continued*

Another More Specific Formula for Target Heart Rate

220 minus your age = HRmax

Now, subtract your resting heart rate (that's a sixty-second pulse rate count) from HRmax to get your HRR or Heart Rate Reserve

(Heart Rate Reserve is the difference between your Maximum Heart Rate and your Resting Heart Rate.)

Multiply your HRR by the percentage you want to train at (0.50, 0.60, 0.70, 0.80)

Now add back your resting heart rate

Amy's Notes: So, for example, I'm 48. 220 minus 48 = 172 (HRmax). 172 minus 60 (my resting heart rate) is 112 (HRR). 80% of 112 is 90. 90 plus 60 (my resting heart rate) is 150, and frankly that is my usual target heart rate for aerobic exercise.

Perceived Exertion

Another way to gauge your heart rate (this is general, not specific) is the talking or singing test that we mentioned. As a rule, if you can talk comfortably and walk, then you need to up the effort a bit so that talking while you exercise is a bit challenging. If you can walk and sing—you're definitely *not* in the zone.

Heart Monitors or Self-Monitoring

You can also wear a Polar® heart rate monitor (or the Mio™ heart rate watches) or simply take ten-second counts (and multiply by six for a sixty-second count) to check out these ranges during your workout.

Note: A few high blood pressure medications lower the maximal heart rate of patients and thus the target zone rate in those cases should also be in the lower range. If you're taking medication in general, call your physician to find out if you need to use a lower target heart rate.

PERFECT PRE-WORKOUT SNACK

A small bite about thirty minutes before a workout will boost energy without weighing you down. Just be sure to keep it small so your exercise efforts aren't competing with your digestive efforts. The best combination is a protein and a healthy carb. Consider:

- A small yogurt, plus a few baked crackers (or berries)
- Apple slices and peanut butter
- Turkey slices and some hummus
- Veggies and bean dip
- A handful of nuts and half of a banana
- Non-fat latte and a few baked crackers

Also remember to hydrate with water before, during, and after workouts.

As a family, discuss how you will help motivate each other (see more about this in Chapter 10), when you will have weekly check-ins to discuss how your activities are going, and how you will reward yourselves (see "Using Goals To Spur the Exercise Experience" on page 294).

You can achieve your thirty minutes (or more) of daily committed exercise in a variety of ways. You can specify a fifteen-minute morning workout before leaving for work, a twenty-minute lunchtime walk, and an after-dinner yoga session in one given day; after-dinner bike rides or walks that last thirty minutes are also great if you live in a safe neighborhood. Accumulating time through three separate but smaller workouts is a way to fit adequate exercise time into your life, allowing for snippets of exercise that accumulate throughout the day. A recent study suggests that fifteen-minute "bursts of activity" can dramatically reduce your child's risk of diabetes.[18] Just remember that you do have to get your heart rate up, even when it's a short exercise experience. And I am personally a firm believer that you do need to keep changing your workouts to stay engaged and reap the benefits; you also need to look for more creative ways to sneak exercise into your life. For myself, I find it easier to set up a planned weekly schedule so I exercise for a set amount of time on weekdays, and on the weekend I can let loose and have fun doing a variety of activities.

Throughout the rest of this chapter, I have provided a wide variety of tools to help you and your family change your activity habits, including sample walking and jogging workouts (pages 260, 285), sample weight-training workouts (page 264), and a list of family

GREAT DVD WORKOUTS

You can find more than 700 workout DVDs with excellent descriptions and fitness level ratings at www.collagevideo.com. Some do require free weights, elastic tubing, a step, a large inflated ball, or other inexpensive exercise equipment. Some of the best include:

- Crunch series
- Kathy Smith series
- Leslie Sansone series
- The Firm series
- Tae Bo Series
- Christi Taylor Fantastic Four Workouts
- Tracie Long Training Endurance for Movement
- Winsor Pilates series
- Shiva Rea Yoga Trance Dance
- Ten-Minute Solution Rapid Results (Pilates)
- IntenSati with Patricia Moreno
- Sergeant Weichert's *START Fitness—Operation Living Fit* DVD series

GYM CHOICE CHECKLIST

When you decide to join a gym or health club, it's important to make sure it's a good fit, meaning that the money you spend will not be wasted. For example, I actually love going to the gym, even though I have a full gym studio at home. It helps me to see gym buddies, take classes I enjoy, and just change my exercise surroundings. For me personally, the main attraction is several instructors and the wide variety of classes. My gym is a little run-down and some of the machines are older, but I don't mind because it's not too busy and the price is right for me after assessing how much it would cost to take classes just three times a week at a private studio. This way I get classes, a large gym with machines, and the opportunity to work out with other exercisers. However, different factors matter to different people. A pool or track may be important to you, or childcare facilities, certain types of classes, or a particular location close to home or work.

Here are some of the questions you need to ask before committing to a gym:

- Are we really ready to make the membership worth the investment?
- Should we buy a family membership?
- Do they keep the gym clean?
- Is the equipment new? Well-maintained?
- During the hours we plan to go, is there a wait for every machine?
- Do we fit in with the other members? Will we feel comfortable?
- Is the gym open during the hours we need?
- Are there clean and adequate bathroom facilities?
- Does this gym offer childcare?
- Does the gym slant to a specific gender?

GYM CHOICE CHECKLIST, *continued*

- Are there gender-separate workout areas?
- Do they have a variety of classes?
- If I want to hire a personal trainer, is it affordable? Do I like the approach that many of the trainers have?
- Do they offer any membership specials?
- Is it a national chain (if I travel a lot)?

The best option is a one-week trial membership (or even a month, if you can get it). Then you can observe the positives and negatives over time and not just on a given day or two. If you're thinking of a family membership, consider that local YMCAs have actually become rather hip hangouts. Also, certain gyms specifically cater to families, while others (like Curves®) specifically cater to women.

I like gyms because they will often help you find like-minded people who don't need to become your best friends, just exercise friends. It may also be the answer to reluctant family members, because you can look for a gym that offers basketball, racquetball, or other "sports options" rather than just traditional weight machines and treadmills. You can also choose smaller studios or trendier clubs like Equinox® Fitness or Crunch, which offer a constantly evolving roster of innovative classes. For some families, it works well to have several gyms—Mom may like Curves® and the kids may like the Y, or Dad may like a place closer to work. By watching carefully for promotions, discounts, and bargains, you can find smart ways to make a gym membership(s) fit into your family budget.

For most families, the amount of money they spend on a gym membership is much less than they typically used to spend on junk food (pizza and fast food), too many non-exercise activities (like movies or trips to the mall), weight-loss solutions that don't work (diet products), and health care consequences (the eventual medications and interventions you will need if

---

GYM CHOICE CHECKLIST, *continued*

you don't take charge of your health).

In short, health club memberships can be money extremely well spent for your family. But (and this is important because many gym memberships go unused each year) if your family does better with options such as community sports teams, area tracks and hiking trails, a home gym and/or at-home personal training, go for it. The important thing is that you get active in the way that works best for your family.

---

activities (page 289). Remember, every family member's physical activity journey will be different. Everybody will progress at a different pace and find different ways to fit exercise into their lives. It may be a challenge to juggle the different ages, ability levels, schedules, and interests of various family members. Just remember that the important thing is to become active people, not just for a week or a month or a year, but for a lifetime. And again, parents need to model the desired behaviors for older kids who are already somewhat sedentary. Who wants to listen to someone who doesn't practice what he or she preaches? They want to see you doing it and then over time they'll be more likely to "do as you do," especially if they see your results (less yelling, more energy, more willingness to play with them).

How To Change Your Family's Attitude

We call Healthy Habit #4 "Playing" because activity can be just that. Too often as adults we have lost the art of play: one of the great joys of having children is relearning what play and fun are all about from the masters. One of the unique aspects of becoming healthy together as a family is that you have more opportunity to have fun than people who are working on health goals on their own.

Dancing in the den with little kids to their favorite pop songs is a blast. Taking a hip-hop dance class with a pre-teen, a surfing lesson with a teen, or a family hiking trip at a national park are just a few of the endless ways that families can get healthy creatively by being active together. As a family, it's up to you to figure out what would be fun and to make "fun" a higher priority if it's something you've been putting at the bottom of your "to do" list lately.

Now let's talk about attitude, because it's one of the biggest factors I see in clients who want to become more active. If you really are determined to "suffer through" your daily exercise and hate it every step of the way, fine. That's an attitude choice that some people make. You may, for example, find a family member who simply refuses to be positive about exercise. Again, that's a personal attitude choice. However, as an adult and a role model for your family, make sure you consider how your attitude impacts the people you love. If

WHAT SUCCESSFUL COMMITTED EXERCISERS DO TO STAY COMMITTED

- They make daily exercise (sometimes with planned days off) a priority.
- They actually put it on their daily calendar like any other important event.
- They habitually do it at the same time every day.
- They do it even when they don't feel motivated.
- They miss it if they have to skip a day when they would usually exercise.
- They find the exercise formula that clicks with their personality and work schedule.
- They look for ways to squeeze in more activity.
- They don't look for a quick fix.
- They understand the value and impact on their health, vitality, and weight.

HOME EQUIPMENT

The great thing about exercise is that it can fit all budgets. Walking is free—it just requires a really sturdy pair of walking shoes. The most elite treadmill can cost as much as $9,000, but there's an awful lot of price options in between. So here's a list of equipment that can help you create anything from a simple to the ultimate gym setup. But you do have to use it to get the benefits! You also want to do price comparisons, check out warranty options, and determine the best buy for your price range.

Simple setup:

Step (which can also act as a bench), some sets of free weights, elastic tubing, mat, large inflated ball, DVD player.

Want to add in?

Add one piece of cardio equipment, such as a treadmill, recumbent bike, elliptical trainer, or stair climber.

Too expensive?

A jump rope or trampoline can provide a great cardio workout as well and you can add more variety: weighted medicine balls, a weighted vest, Pilates ring.

Additional elements you might consider:
- Pedometer
- Strap-on hand weights
- Boxing bag
- Barbell set or weighted bars
- Pilates reformer
- Multi-gym workout weight station
- Incline/decline bench
- Ballet barre
- Mirrored wall

HOME EQUIPMENT, *continued*

Other items you may not know about in various price ranges include: TRX® suspension trainer (www.fitnessanywhere.com, BOSU® balance trainer (www.bosu.com), Hula-Hoop® (www.hoopnotica.com), Gliding Discs (www.glidingdiscs.com), the Bean® (www.bean.com) or the BodyWedge™ (www.bodywedge21.com). Also consider investing in a Polar® heart rate monitor if you don't want to be bothered with taking your pulse for targeted heart rate workouts. Remember, these items may help you to stay engaged, but don't just waste your money. Do some research and see if these fitness products will improve or jazz up your workouts effectively; equipment can help to battle boredom.

activity is a tedious chore for you, it is unlikely to appeal to your kids or your grandkids or perhaps even to your spouse. Remember, *exercise is life-saving medicine*—and how you approach it may literally have a life-and-death influence on the people around you. And though exercise has to have some rules (targeting heart rates, sustaining it for a specific amount daily, engaging in aerobic and strength training), I find most adults who "hate it" are simply setting goals that are too difficult to achieve or they're trying to accomplish too much too fast (or expecting too much from too little effort).

Am I telling you that you have to LOVE getting on that treadmill or trail everyday or doing those free weight reps? No! Just try to fit in as many fun activities in as you can and avoid negativity by maintaining an attitude of awareness regarding all the good things you are doing for yourself and your family when you are active. I still think the biggest gift is taking on an exercise that seems hard initially and then finding that you have progressed well beyond that difficult starting point over several weeks; the memory actually puts a smile on your face.

EXCUSES: ARE THEY REALLY WHAT'S HOLDING YOU BACK?

I've heard the best and worse excuses. These are the most common ones that have been told to me over the years:

"I don't have time." Yes, you do. Exercise can be done in small spurts during the day, during TV commercial time, or by doing extra prep work the night before so you can use the extra time the next day to get moving.

"I never see results." Maybe you're not assessing the situation properly or you have unrealistic expectations. Are you stronger, do you have more stamina, has your face thinned out a little, are you sleeping better, can you walk longer without feeling tired? Your waistline is not always the best indicator of results, although if you are combining exercise and good nutrition, you'll see results there too. Just give it time!

"I don't have a convenient place to exercise." There's no perfect way to exercise: it's what fits with your schedule: a morning workout with a DVD, a gym membership for after work, a lunchtime walk, a weekend activity. They all work.

"I have an injury or illness." Have a pulled muscle in your leg? You can still work out your upper body until it heals. Sore elbow? You can still walk and train your lower body. Need rehab? A physical therapist can help the injury heal and put you on a great post-injury program.

"I'm a gym dunce: when I walk in, I don't know what to do." Most gyms will offer one free personal training assessment and training session. You can ask the person to walk you through the equipment and make some recommendations. Take notes and bring them with you when you work out.

EXCUSES, *continued*

"I'm too fat." Once you start exercising, you may be surprised to find that there are people of all shapes and sizes in health clubs, walking at malls, in water fitness classes, on tracks and trails. Look for locations that make you feel comfortable.

"I'm too old." You're never too old (research proves it) to get incredible benefits from exercise. As you age, you actually may see more dramatic results—and you may find that you exercise "smarter" than younger counterparts. Think of it as exercise to function.

"My back hurts." The right exercise can actually help—just make sure to get appropriate medical guidance.

"It's not fun." Well, actually it can be. What may not be so fun is your attitude. Besides, lots of things in life aren't fun (brushing your teeth, maintaining the safety of your car, cleaning your house, etc.) but you do them because the results of not doing them are worse.

"I hate doing it alone." Great idea—get a buddy!

"I can't keep up." Just because you couldn't keep it up in the past doesn't mean you won't be able to now. You might surprise yourself! Make it personal—make the initial goals small and achieve those personal goals.

"My kids get in the way." If you have kids, there's no more important reason to exercise regularly. They will learn from you. Strollercise®, a national exercise program that allows women with babies in strollers to walk together and then briefly stop for short weight-training routines, is just one approach to exercising with kids.

EXCUSES, *continued*

"I'm already thin." Thin is not healthy; thin is just thin. You may be surprised at how much better you feel when you become active.

"I don't know how to begin." Ask someone—there are plenty of people in the medical and fitness fields who will be happy to help. Or ask an active friend or family member to buddy up.

"I'm already sick, so what's the point?" No matter what your health condition, exercise can often improve your quality of life, including how you feel, diminish your risk factors or illness itself, and improve your ability to function optimally in your daily life.

Sure, sometimes it will be boring, you'll feel too tired to get going, your schedule will seem too full. But just as we have to take medicine, clean the house, go to the dentist, do homework, take tests, do less-than-pleasant tasks at work—we need to exercise to achieve a basic level of health. And most people will tell you if they meet their exercise goal of the day, it just feels so good when it's over and you've stayed committed to your health.

Tips for Family Activity Success

Here are some suggestions to help you change your activity habits:

- Family members with similar tastes can buddy up, work out together, and inspire each other; or you can team up together and all agree to try something new—boating, bicycling, swimming are just some of the activities that can include all family members.
- Everyone can set personal goals and cheer each other on.

HFL SIX-STEP INTERVAL WALKING WORKOUT FOR HOME OR TREADMILL

Using intervals is a great way to increase calories burned. You alternate fast and slow aerobic paces in an effort to increase the total number of calories burned without fatiguing yourself excessively. This also helps to strengthen your heart and improve your overall fitness. You'll find over time that it also help to increase walking pace or work up to jogging from a walking program.

Sample:

- Five-minute warm-up (light, easy walking).
- Walk up a hill for two minutes at a pace that leaves you a bit breathless. Walk down as a recovery for two minutes.
- Do a light jog for four minutes. Recover for two minutes by walking.
- Walk a very fast walk for two minutes. Recover with a slower pace for two minutes.
- Walk up the hill for three minutes and then one minute down the hill.
- Recover for two minutes with a slow steady walk.
- Light jog for three minutes. Recover for three minutes with a paced walk.
- Total elapsed time: thirty minutes.

Over time, you can extend some of the intervals, or increase the effort during the more challenging parts of the intervals. As a beginner, you can shorten the more challenging intervals and add more of these shorter intervals in, making it an eight- or ten-step interval program. As you get fitter, use fewer intervals and make each one longer or keep slower intervals short and increase the timeframe of the more challenging phases (walk for two minutes, run for ten minutes and that's your new interval for four repeat cycles).

- Change the scenery by using *active picnics* to engage the family—plan a family sport and pack an HFL lunch for the entire family.
- Create family competitions with fun in mind—who can do four days in a row of thirty minutes of exercise—you get a gold star—four gold stars get a prize. Make the goals about meeting daily activity levels for everybody and not just about weight loss or game scores.
- Take family vacations that incorporate land and sea sports, hiking and biking, and a more (active) varied approach to the getaway.
- Track progress by having a family powwow and notice if individuals are feeling stronger, more energetic, getting better grades, sleeping better, exhibiting better moods. Comparing notes can be a "can you top this" game.
- Pump up the volume by sharing music choices on iPod® media players and create companionship and camaraderie by exercising to DVDs together. Help by spotting for each other during weight training to improve performance and progress to heavier weights, while giving support.
- Make sure exercise clothing and footwear are always clean and available. Surprise each other with new workout wear—those are feel-good gifts that enhance workouts.
- Follow the most important rule: Be verbally positive and share positive observations. People need to hear praise and encouragement, even if they are seeing and feeling physical changes.

A Word About Strength Training

The virtues of weight training for all ages cannot be overemphasized. It will give you a variety of benefits:

- Allow you to do more work with less effort
- Maintain or increase your metabolic rate
- Give you a fitter, healthier appearance
- Increase energy levels (because calories can be efficiently burned for fuel)

SIGNS OF DEHYDRATION

Knowing these signs is very important, especially if you're exercising for long periods in the heat and/or with children:

- Noticeable thirst
- Muscle cramps
- Weakness
- Decreased performance
- Difficulty paying attention
- Headache
- Nausea
- Fatigue
- Lightheadedness or dizziness
- Amber or dark yellow urine or little urine output

- Increase balance and preventing injury through shock absorption
- Build bone and muscle mass

I'm a true believer in weight training. I believe it has provided me with a way to maximize my physical assets, increase my caloric intake (which means a lot in my case because my resting metabolism is a bit on the low side), and make me look and exude a healthy vitality.

My recommendation is to find a program that suits your goals. You can buy a book with strength training formulas, go online and join a community that offers daily workouts, or follow televised workouts. Why not take classes at a local gym? Classes range from traditional strength training to boot camp; being in a group can be a great motivator. Choose podcasts or hire a personal trainer, even for a short time to get some sample programs. Many gyms across the nation offer classes geared to families. Spouses can train with each other or set up circuits that the whole family can do. Some free

MOST COMMON EXERCISE MISTAKES

No warm-up before starting aerobic or weight training. You have to warm up your muscles for either of these disciplines. Tight, cold muscles can mean injury. A warm-up is usually five to ten minutes and involves gentle calisthenics or brisk walking, anything that gets your upper and lower body literally "warmed up."

No cool-down time. Cool-down time is necessary, especially after cardiovascular exercise. You want to allow your heart rate to recover, and also avoid blood pooling in the lower extremities (which can cause you to feel faint) due to stopping abruptly.

No stretching. You need stretching after a workout to allow muscles to relax, increase blood flow to the areas you worked out, help increase range of motion, and help prevent injury. Do not stretch cold muscles. The best time to stretch is after a ten-minute warmup or after the cooldown.

Training the same muscles day after day. You want twenty-four to forty-eight hours of rest after you've trained a specific muscle or muscle group, or you'll minimize your training gains and increase your chance of injury.

Overtraining. If you exercise too much (more than several hours a day every day, for example, though overtraining amounts can vary), you'll actually diminish the benefits of exercise, lower your immunity, and increase injury risk. Stress fractures and pulled or strained muscles are often the result of overtraining. Most people know when they are too gung ho or adding in additional exercise too fast, training multiple times in a day, or going for time spans that are too long. Even if you're training for an event like a marathon, there are clear training guides to help you get to the long runs before the event; about four to six months is needed for preparation. Excessive daily soreness, repetitive sprains and injuries, and an impact on eating patterns (becoming less hungry) are all signs of overtraining.

weights, a step, a jump-rope, a large inflated ball, even a Hula-Hoop® can all be used to set up fun stations the whole family can use—and the beauty is you can make each station fit the person's ability level. Just put different size weights at stations or have higher and lower steps or a range of elastic bands for different ability levels.

Combining Weight and Aerobic Training

As you become more proficient and familiar with consistent exercise, you will want to find ways to combine aerobic or cardio training with weight training and other integrative exercise modalities such as yoga, tai chi, Pilates, etc.

FAMILY FITNESS MAKEOVER GUIDE BY AGE

Here's a list of age-related ideas to build in workouts during the day that are fun for everyone:

Ages three to eighteen months: Take them for a dip in the pool and get them moving their legs and arms.

Ages eighteen months to five years: Dancing, tag, and red light/green light can be free form and fun.

Ages five to eight years: Backyard treasure hunts can involve clues with jumping jacks, hopscotch, roller skating, beginning soccer moves, and other fun movement games. Also, try basketball with a lower hoop.

Ages thirteen-plus: Water fights, Frisbee®, and Capture the Flag are fun for everyone.

All ages: Walking is great, no matter what your age!

WHEN TO CONSULT WITH A DOCTOR

- If you've had a heart attack or stroke, you do want medically supervised exercise (and possibly exercise rehab first).
- If you feel breathless after mild exertion.
- If you feel any chest pressure or pain while or right after you exercise.
- If you've experienced chest pain when not exercising.
- If you haven't ever exercised or exercised in a while, get checked out first and get guidance.
- If you are on medications for diabetes, heart disease, or other conditions.
- If you have bone, joint, or muscle issues that could be made worse with exercise (usually a physical therapist can guide you so that you can successfully exercise).
- If you or family members are seriously overweight.

Unless you are extremely fit and a long-term exerciser, there are general recommendations for fitness that adjust for typical age-related wear and tear. Here are some guidelines for age-related training programs, based on age groupings for general safety:

In your twenties: Do thirty minutes of cardio (70–80 percent maximal heart rate), thirty minutes of weight training for three days a week; forty-five to sixty minutes of cardio for three days/week. Consider adding some yoga, too.

In your thirties: Circuit train for forty-five minutes for three days/week, interval cardio train for forty-five to sixty minutes two days/week, do one day of cardio for sixty minutes, and take one day of rest. Include static and active stretching. If you are postpartum, add Pilates as you slowly work back after giving birth.

In your forties: One hour of full body weight training three days a week or two thirty-minute cycles of upper body and two of lower body (four total days of thirty minutes), plus five days of forty-five minutes of cardio (cross training so you incorporate challenge and use different muscles so you are less likely to incur injury). This is a good decade to use a trainer for getting some guidance, learning new programs, and avoiding injury.

In your fifties: Weight train incorporating balance exercises four to five days a week for thirty minutes. Add Pilates for fifteen minutes two days a week. Do only two or three muscle groups at a time in the upper body and one or two in lower body. More forgiving cardio (recumbent bike, brisk walking, jog/alternate walking, elliptical, rowing, Hi-Lo impact classes) forty-five to sixty minutes three days a week, and then thirty to forty-five minutes another three days a week.

In your sixties: Daily walking program of thirty to sixty minutes, tai chi two days a week, weight training for thirty minutes three to four days a week with balance and flexibility exercises included.

WAIST CIRCUMFERENCE GUIDELINES FOR ADULTS

Women with a waist measurement of more than thirty-five inches or men with a waist measurement of more than forty inches may have a higher disease risk than people with smaller waist measurements because of where their fat lies.

To measure your waist circumference, place a tape measure around your bare abdomen just above your hipbone. Be sure that the tape is snug and is parallel to the floor but does not compress your skin. Relax, exhale, and measure your waist. [20]

For your sixties and beyond, I would get an evaluation and recommendations from a trainer or health professional, again for health safety reasons. You do want to get moving—but you want to "move smart."

Calorie-Burning Reality Check

If you choose to work out on exercise equipment, it's important to avoid what I call *calorie-burning delusion*. Clients will sometimes swear to me they are working out on a treadmill or stationary bike and its readout is showing at least 600–800 calories burned, or they take a really tough class and the instructor assures them that on average they are burning about 1,000 calories per class.

I am here to tell you—as I've already told them—that these numbers are probably not accurate. In fact, they're probably not even close. Often, machines are calibrated to male individuals of a specific weight and ability level so the readouts are just not realistic for most people. Calorie estimates from exercise classes are very speculative and too generalized to be accurate.

If you are a beginner and just starting out, then there is a chance that for a short period of time, you may actually achieve close to some of these numbers. And if you are an advanced exerciser doing a very advanced workout, you may burn a high number of calories. For most people, though, the only way to evaluate your actual calorie-burning efforts is to have an exercise test performed at a Fitness Testing Lab, where they will hook you up to a face mask that will measure your oxygen consumption and then translate that into METs or metabolic equivalents.

A great place to get well-researched information is the My Pyramid Food Intake Pattern Calorie Level chart (Appendix 8A), which categorizes men and women separately and then does an age breakdown with "Sedentary," "Moderately Active, and "Active" categories. Using this chart, you can target your calorie intake to complement your activity level.

Of course, if you are following the HFL plan, then sedentary just doesn't cut it anymore for you and your family. You'll see that if you go from sedentary to active, you can usually eat about 300–400

TIPS TO CALCULATE YOUR HYDRATION NEEDS

Weigh yourself before exercising. If you weigh less afterward due to excessive sweating, drink more next time. Your target post-exercise weight should come within 98 percent of your starting weight (If you weigh 130, then target 127.5–130). If you weigh more post-exercise, then drink less next time.

Water is the best source of hydration (or zero-calorie flavored waters, iced tea) unless you exercise intensely for more than an hour. Then you can also hydrate with small amounts of electrolyte replacement beverages such as Gatorade®. Rarely do you need these kinds of drinks if you are adequately nourished and hydrated and exercising for sixty minutes or less.

more calories and still maintain your weight, if you're eating HFL foods. If you're trying to lose weight, you may want to steer your daily *calorie intake* to the "sedentary range" or even a bit lower, as long as you are not suffering physical symptoms that indicate you are not eating enough to sustain daily activities plus exercise comfortably. The most common complaints of someone who doesn't eat enough are: fatigue, dizziness, inability to complete a workout, change in bowel habits, feeling cold all the time, and inadequate perspiration. As a rule, never go below 1,200 calories a day, which is not enough for anyone doing a serious workout training program, even when trying to lose weight (unless you are being supervised by a physician who has made this recommendation for morbid obesity). Remember my 300/400/500 meal calorie plans plus one or two snacks, which would put you around 1,500 calories. These menu choices were set up to be balanced and provide adequate calories for an individual engaged in a regular exercise program.

CALCULATE YOUR BMI

A BMI chart is provided in Appendix 2C, but you can also calculate it yourself. BMI measures your weight in relation to your height and is closely associated with measures of body fat. You can calculate your BMI using this formula:

$$\text{BMI} = \frac{\text{weight (pounds) x 703}}{\text{height squared (inches}^2)}$$

For example, for someone who is five feet, seven inches tall and weighs 220 pounds, the calculation would look like this:

$$\text{BMI} = \frac{\text{weight (pounds) x 703}}{\text{height squared (inches}^2)} = \frac{154660}{4489} = 34.45$$

A BMI of 18.5 to 24.9 is considered healthy. Someone with a BMI of 25 to 29.9 is considered overweight, and someone with a BMI of 30 or more is considered obese.

Using Goals to Spur the Exercise Experience

Absolutely use goals and rewards to encourage yourself and other family members—just make sure food is not the usual goal or reward! If everyone meets a weekly goal, then maybe you can reward yourselves on the weekend reward with a family outing to a theme park or a special hike and picnic or a weekend movie outing. On occasion, you may add in some exercise because you know you want to splurge at a party or restaurant that evening, or you're on vacation and really want to enjoy dinners, so you'll up your walking or activity during the daytime. In this case, you know the reward coming is a food reward or extra calories at a special event so you pre-pay the price with extra calories for the "reward" you're giving yourself later. It's a good habit to "pay before" with exercise as a proactive move rather than punish extra calories with exercise after the fact.

Choose age-appropriate rewards for short-term and long-terms goals to inspire your family to stick with the exercise recommendations. It can be anything from a new outfit or a spa treatment to a new book, toy, or game or a family special event like a weekend getaway or beach day. You can also use fitness events to spur on your exercise progress: target a 5K run, a marathon, a triathlon, or just being able to make it around the local high school track several times.

For your kids, it might be being able to jog a certain distance or do a certain number of chin-ups or pushups. Write the goals down and chart progress for all to see and cheer for and then decide when and if a reward is appropriate.

The whole point of the HFL program is to make healthy habits a regular part of your life so that they feel natural and habitual— so that you actually miss them if you get off track. Exercise, like nutrition, has to be integrated into your family life so it feels like it's a daily priority.

Make it a habit that you feel is necessary; when you are forced to compromise or skip it, you should really miss it.

10

The Right Way (and Wrong Way) to Support Each Other

It's funny how you remember certain things from your childhood. For example, I had a skinny, chain-smoking aunt who would ask me every time I saw her: "So, when are you going to drop those extra pounds, honey?"

She'd say it so casually that it became her opening comment at every greeting, but those casual words cut through me like a knife. Sometime after my weight loss, I had a family wedding to attend. I credit my mother because, even on our very tight budget, she convinced Dad to splurge and let me buy a dress worthy of my new figure. I couldn't wait to wear the dress and have my aunt see the new me.

When she finally recognized me, I'll never forget what she said: "Honey, what happened to you? You look like one of those starving African refugees."

My mouth just dropped open. I learned a very important lesson in that moment—make lifestyle changes *for yourself*. Don't ever make them for others or for their feedback (it will often disappoint). It's not about them, it's about you—your health, your happiness.

The truth is that I didn't get a great deal of healthy support when I was a kid struggling with my weight, but today my job is supporting people as they work toward changing their lifestyles. As I've worked with many different kinds of families, I've seen how important family support is—and I've also seen every possible form of family sabotage.

Most families who have food fights—and I don't mean the kind where you're tossing food across the room—live in very stressful, unpleasant environments. When a child or adult is struggling with weight, and everyone is pointing fingers (even out of love)—instructing him or her what to eat, what not to eat, and even humiliating them—it's a gruesome experience for everyone.

When every mouthful is being scrutinized and every treat indicted, the home becomes a battlefield. As the well-intentioned family members are ganging up (because that's how it feels to the person trying to change), the target of their attention is wondering: "Why do you get to eat one way and I have to live this miserable existence?" Often, the negative attention creates frustration and defiance that aggravate the very behaviors the person wants to change.

Nothing feels worse than thinking, "I'm all alone, they're all against me, no one gets what I'm going through." One of the most challenging aspects of family weight management is that family members aren't all the same: some are more genetically blessed and so can eat in much the same way as the more weight-challenged individual without the consequences of their poor health habits showing up as extra weight.

The worst thing that can happen is for families to make weight-challenged individuals feel even more isolated than they already do by adopting different standards for different family members. Nor is it kind to keep the pantry one way for the skinny people and expect the person struggling with weight issues to just deal with it.

Rule #1 of HFL Family Support: We are all in this together. Everyone in the family can benefit, everyone can change, everyone needs to support each other for the individual and the greater good—even though everyone will have distinct goals to set and meet.

There are some things a supportive HFL family does not do:

- Isolate an individual's needs
- Denigrate individual members
- Tempt each other
- Battle over food
- Refuse to take the time to incorporate changes slowly
- Reject attempts to find solutions creatively
- Continue on an unhealthy lifestyle path rather than embrace possibilities

A supportive HFL family addresses problems very differently:

- Recognizes individual goals and works together
- Recognizes the weight loss struggle with empathy and supportive words
- Responds in a reasonable way to each other's needs
- Works on new and easy menu plans creatively
- Works on planning, preparing, playing, and portioning out together
- Knows how to celebrate without food always being at the center of the celebration
- Enjoys treats with respect and timing
- Makes the effort to be active both individually and together
- Eats together as often as possible

Threatening the Status Quo

A recent study[1] showed a link between your weight and that of your closest friends. According to the study, people who associate with heavy people tend to "gain weight as well." It might be that we think,

"If they're okay with their weight, then it's okay for me to let loose, gain weight, and be large, too," or "If they are successful and like me and are large, then I'll be like them, too—in every way." Although the connection is unclear, one thing is certain: peer pressure is powerful in most groups; when one or more people break away from the typical behaviors of the group, it can be threatening. Your friends may feel you are judging their behaviors because you are choosing to change.

The same holds true with family, where you don't just share habits and experiences, you share genes. Breaking with family norms for eating and exercise often leads to negative reactions and sabotage rather than support.

So how can you break through bad habits and suggest or encourage change in your family? The trick is to stay positive and avoid negative judgments or overtones. Now, let's agree that a "reality check" is not equal to criticism. A doctor pointing out that you are seriously overweight is not a criticism, it's a fact. When your wife points out that your pants are four sizes larger than when you got married, it may feel really confrontational, but it is also the truth. On the other hand, slapping someone's hand as they reach for an extra serving of pie is humiliating, as is any comment that judges or labels someone unkindly.

Here are some fair ways to point out the need for a lifestyle change without being negative or critical:

- I am worried about your health.
- I notice you are struggling to keep up physically.
- You seem to be suffering from the extra weight. Can I help?
- I am concerned that you are at risk for _____ (fill in the blank).

Positive vs. Negative Comments

Let's take a look at more examples of how your choice of language can change the impact of a statement. Here are comments made in a very unkind way:

- Your being overweight makes me sick.
- You really can't take just one, can you?

- You must be dying from the effort of carrying around all that weight.
- You know you're going to suffer a heart attack or a stroke and die.

Now here are some contrasting positive statements:

- I would love to help you if you want to try to improve your health.
- You know we both have slowed down a bit. Maybe we should take a class together or hire a personal trainer and partner up. It'll be fun!
- I love you so much and it scares me to see that extra weight creeping on. Can we do something about it together?
- I am worried about both your health and mine, so can we try to change some habits together?

Notice how the positive comments offer love, encouragement, or a willingness to be part of the solution. These supportive factors are enormously important when it comes to lifestyle change.

Spousal Sabotage

Men and women are different in so many ways, and this can play heavily into the success or failure of a lifestyle change. Women are often raised to be nurturers, so if their spouses want to get back in shape, their attitude will typically be supportive. They'll change the shopping list, buy light beer, work on serving healthier dinners, try to provide better snack choices, and generally go along with the program, even if they do not want to embrace those changes personally.

Men can be quite a bit different in how they respond to a mate's efforts. They are less likely to see these efforts to change as something that should concern them, too. Some will certainly offer support but without participating in the process. Many will not want to deal with losing their favorite foods or snacks, or even no longer having a buddy to eat and enjoy the same foods with them. In general, losing weight or eating healthfully may not be a priority for them.

These are generalizations, of course. Women are just as capable of being uninvolved, and men are just as capable of offering meaningful support. And both men and women can take their reluctance about their partner's efforts a step further—into downright sabotage. They may get nervous when they see that their beloved has accomplished a goal, is feeling more attractive and confident, and may be getting more attention.

So though Eve tempted Adam with an apple, your spouse may be more inclined to tempt you with a caramel-dipped apple, Godiva® chocolates, or decadent ice cream.

What he or she is really saying is:

- This change in you makes me feel uncomfortable and threatened.
- I like me just the way I am—I want you to stay that way, too.
- I don't like the attention you're getting; I no longer feel worthy.
- I feel like I'm not moving forward in my goals the way you are, and that really upsets me.
- By taking control of your weight and health, you make me feel like a lazy loser.
- I feel like you are leaving me behind.

Here are some strategies for handling the challenge of spousal sabotage:

- Let your partner know that this is important to you and explain why calmly and clearly.
- Make it about "health" as opposed to looks; you may meet with more acceptance and less antagonism. Get your doctor's help to clarify the health benefits.
- Express that you are lucky to have your partner love you "just the way you are," but that you don't want food to rule your life or the life of your household. You need to put better habits and healthier practices in place.
- Let your spouse know that you feel differently about the excess weight than he or she might—for you, it represents a roadblock to your happiness and self-esteem.

- Let your partner know you would love him or her to join you in your efforts, but if not, you would prefer demonstrations of love that are something other than gifts of food—maybe new kitchen tools and appliances, fitness equipment, or fitness wear?
- Let your spouse know that if you have kids or are anticipating having kids, you really want them in the best health, and that means better food options inside and outside the home.
- Reward your spouse with new tasty meals that incorporate HFL principles.
- Demonstrate that you appreciate your spouse's support both verbally and physically.

Remember that you bear responsibility as well. If your husband or wife persists in bringing home treats, it is still your choice whether to eat or not, to nibble or not. Don't throw in the towel and eat, only to feel miserable later. Give your partner the pleasure of eating the treats while you whip out some substitute treats like frozen yogurt, frozen fruit, or fat-free pudding. You can share the snack time without sharing the actual snack!

More Tricks for Dealing with Sabotage

Realize there will be times when temptations from inside or outside the family are unavoidable. Every member of the family needs to be prepared with these simple coping skills:

- Be mindful and responsible. This is an ongoing "state of being," so be prepared with your own food plans and choices instead of getting caught off guard. For example, when going to dinner at someone else's home, you can make a pre-emptive strike by bringing a dish you know you can eat and letting the hostess know your challenges so she can have a veggie platter or fruit for your benefit (everyone else benefits, too).
- Never let yourself get too hungry or you'll be vulnerable to impulsive choices, which tend to be high in fat/sodium/ sugar.

- Remember that the goal is not perfection; it's a better lifestyle that incorporates better choices. Succumbing to an occasional treat is not the end of the world.

Here are some of my favorite verbal responses to people who challenge you or tempt you:

- I already had my treat for the week, but go ahead, enjoy it!
- I'm just not hungry right now, but I'll let you know if I want some later.
- I'm working really hard on breaking some difficult relationships with food so I just want to say No tonight and feel good about that.
- Could I just have fruit instead?

When someone becomes truly pushy, you may need to take them aside and speak to them directly, making eye contact and conveying how important it is to you to embrace these behavior modifications.

Just remember that, if you love your friends, you will give them time to work out their discomfort with the changes you're making. My experience is that most of them will adjust. If not, it may be time to re-examine the relationship.

Buddy Up for Support

The buddy system is one of the most effective tools available when it comes to successful weight loss or lifestyle shifts. I'm not sure why people always think they have to go it alone. Isolation does not breed success. Family members can really provide the love, empathy, and encouragement required to support successful change. Spouses can be buddies, siblings can be buddies, or parents and kids can buddy up. Every member of your family can act as buddy for every other member. It just depends on who is willing to participate.

Remember, there are no real rules to having a buddy except the ones you decide on for yourself. Maybe you want your buddy to stop you when you are overeating or to tell you a bad day is just that—one bad day. Maybe you want him or her to be your exercise partner.

One strategy that works well for buddies is the "check-in." Here's how you can use it to prevent the derailment of your efforts:

- Set up regular check-ins by phone. Agree in advance on what is fair game to talk about and share. Decide if you want your buddy's input or not so you are clear on the roles you will play. The Internet can be used the same way.
- Set up activity check-ins after workouts, perhaps by having a coffee or snack break for chat time.
- Try e-mail check-ins. That way, if your or your buddy's schedule is hectic, you can check in any time of day or night. Or use instant messaging if you want an immediate response.

With or Without a Biological Family

Maybe you're a single person or a widowed grandparent or a single mom or dad or someone whose family is not nearby. Perhaps you are in a traditional family, but other family members aren't ready to embrace the program yet. In any case, you can find support, regardless of your family situation.

- Find a friend who's willing to be your buddy. He or she doesn't have to work the program personally—just be understanding.
- Journaling can serve as a check-in of sorts if you use it to write your food and exercise, but also your feelings, struggles, and moments of challenge. Depending on your comfort level, you can share this journal with a friend.
- Also consider support groups that are available at religious institutions, hospitals, local Y's, and community centers. Remember, the people in these groups don't need to be on the HFL plan—they just need to share similar circumstances.
- A number of Web sites, like ivillage.com and sparkpeople .com, have community centers you can join and message boards where you can find support.

How to Handle the Skeptics

It's critical to avoid the negative emotions that critics or naysayers can evoke. Quite often, your response will be an attempt to defy them by being stricter than is reasonable with your eating or exercise. This is a setup for disaster because you won't be able to keep it up or you will get frustrated and overeat in response to your own emotions. Remember, this isn't about what others think or want you to do or their opinion of what is best for you. This is about your decision to change habits that lead to weight gain, health risk factors, and health issues for yourself and your family. I cannot tell you how often I've watched people adopt the HFL plan successfully in spite of "caring" friends and family who offer them "relief" or a "quick treat that won't hurt" or a "rest from discipline."

The reality is that you can't change people; you can only change yourself. The individual trying to derail you is probably grappling with his or her own emotional and lifestyle issues. Very often, while saboteurs are making an unkind comment or observation or trying to entice you, they are actually feeling a bit crummy about themselves. Your achievements make them feel inferior or out of control.

Remember, it's your responsibility to set firm but gentle boundaries so that people both within and outside your family understand that you need them to support you or simply leave you alone. You can use the following comments as samples of what you might say to someone who is not aware of how important the lifestyle change is:

- This effort is really something personal I decided to do and I can really use your support and your blessings.
- I have always loved your cooking and there will be times when I choose to enjoy the full menu, but right now I need to watch my choices.
- My health and my self-esteem have been suffering for some time and I hope you'll understand and support me. If I choose only some of your great menu selections, it's because I need to watch my weight and my health.
- I am trying to change some family habits inside and outside the home because I am realizing the kids and I might be developing some health issues. I hope you won't take offense

if we're a bit selective about what you're offering. We are so glad to be here.

I do think it's important to always include "health" in the discussion because most people will be reticent to challenge you on the health issue; when it comes to weight, they may be a bit more likely to ask you to indulge and "then go back to your diet." Do not be surprised if close friends take it personally; again, they may define their own value in the food they cook. Another option is to call the person ahead of time and discuss your HFL program and see if they would be willing to have a salad or a fruit salad or make an entrée that is HFL-friendly. Just be gently persuasive and complimentary as you stick to your HFL habits.

Celebrating Success

Celebrating achievements is a vital part of lifestyle change. You need to reward your own efforts and those of family members who take small or big steps forward in shifting their habits to healthier ones. Fitting into smaller sizes, seeing a face in the mirror that doesn't look quite as full and chubby as before, noticing clearer skin, finding physical exercise easier, fitting into an airline seat, and seeing a child's height grow into his or her "girth" are all reasons to celebrate.

Physical and emotional gains are exciting, but sometimes external rewards are important, too. Based on age, choose little gifts to reward the goals achieved. Here are a few examples:

- A book
- An inexpensive toy
- A visit to the zoo for a child
- iPod® music or movie downloads
- A DVD
- A new lipstick
- A movie gift card for teens
- A new exercise outfit
- A scarf
- A massage
- A manicure
- Golf balls or other sports equipment

TROUBLESHOOTING

If support is ongoing, then troubleshooting is just an extension of that principle. Here are some typical situations that will require a plan or response. It helps if you can anticipate a situation so you are armed to deal with it.

Only one family member needs to lose weight and still feels "isolated," even if the whole family has agreed to follow the HFL plan. It's pretty understandable that if children or teens are the ones grappling with weight loss, they are still going to feel like the deck is more stacked against them. Or they feel like everyone is scrutinizing their every move to see if they are "cheating" or eating more than they should. That's not the intent of this book.

It is quite obvious that portion control and calorie counting have to happen if someone is to lose weight; so does exercise. But the idea is that if you are truly working the program as a family, then even healthier food choices, participation in the four P's, and other habit changes are being celebrated and rewarded. You'll notice less "poor me syndrome" because everyone is participating, evolving, and adopting the changes. There is less likely to be an isolation issue.

One family member or participant may give up and go off the program. This is a really common situation. More than likely, some family members will be judgmental, others will feel tempted to do the same, and others will want to be supportive but feel resentful. That's why family dinners and powwows are so important: they defuse the possibility of an escalating situation. Have patience, make sure to have an ongoing dialogue, and try not to be judgmental.

One family member says, "I've tried it for a while and it feels too rigid." They're probably specifically referring to the controlled

TROUBLESHOOTING, *continued*

treats and maybe the exercise parameters. My attitude on this one is: when you're at home, you do as we do. When you're away from home, I can't control your decisions.

A family member persists in sabotage. If it's a spouse, you need to communicate how important these changes are for both you and the children. It's not unreasonable to enlist the help of a physician or other health professional to emphasize how important and necessary these changes are. If it's a teen or young adult, then it's again within your parental scope to set the rules inside the home and hope that over time they'll come around and join the family effort.

Plateaus are quite challenging. A weight plateau merely means the scale stopped registering change for a while, but the tape measure, the mirror, and the fit of your clothing can still show signs that things are happening. And let's not forget that for the first several days, weeks, even months, a lot of habit changes are going on, so at any given time, there may be a plateau in one area while progress is going on in other sectors.

Bigger family gifts can be voted on or raffled off (i.e., you can exchange responsibilities for a bigger vote) or planned far in advance of large milestones the whole family achieves.

Quieting Your Inner Saboteur

What do you do when the saboteur is you? I can hear that nasty little voice now:

- There are those leftovers in the fridge—go ahead, nosh a little.
- There's ice cream in the freezer, have just a scoop . . . or two . . . or three . . .

- Let's stand here in front of the fridge (or pantry) and just *see* what's here . . .
- I'll just eat these little tastes as I clean off the plates.
- It doesn't count if I eat it behind closed doors at home.
- I'll just nibble a little as I watch my evening shows.
- I have to taste as I cook so it tastes good for my family.
- I need something to make me feel better NOW!
- I'm thirsty—NO—I'm hungry.
- This diet is making me so hungry and frustrated, I just have to give in and . . .
- I exercised really hard today, so I can have anything I want.
- I can't think straight and eating will help.
- They're just little tastes, so it doesn't matter.
- I am so _____ (angry, depressed, lonely, anxious, etc.). I deserve a little something to make me feel better.

The answer to this saboteur is . . . a reality check. You've got to ditch the inner voice by coming clean—calmly and with control and reason. Yes, some desires need to be met occasionally. That's just the way it is. But just as you can't purchase every piece of clothing you might want, you can't indulge your food urges every time they strike. The "I want it now" mentality has to be replaced with a calculation of "Do you really need it? Do you really want it? Does it have to be now or can it wait? Is it worth the impact it will have on my weight or my health?"

The habit of appeasing your emotions with food has to be replaced with stroking your emotions with evaluation, redirection, or even therapy when appropriate. A buddy or support group inside or outside the family can be incredibly helpful as you struggle with these issues.

Here are a few simple ways to respond to your inner saboteur:

- *Distract yourself* with some other behavior: call a friend, go outside and do a chore, run a bubble bath and soak, get in the car and do an errand.
- *Wait it out*, which can be tough, but it does allow you to have an inner dialogue and figure out what's really bothering you;

then it allows you to choose to cope with an alternative other than food.

- *Analyze your feelings* and what moments lead you to reward yourself, stroke yourself, or simply overindulge with food.
- *Say consequences out loud* so you acknowledge them: "This will undo my exercise effort. This will affect my health parameter (blood pressure, cholesterol level, blood sugar level). I've already had treats this week, so it's not like I've been deprived."
- *Avoid telling yourself "just one won't hurt"* because the truth is that it's almost never just one; this is a daily game people play; by the end of the week, just one becomes several, a dozen, many. I'm a big believer in moderation, but ongoing daily "justifications" in the name of moderation will not work.
- *Don't eat something just it because it's a freebie.* A lot of business professionals do this on the lunch circuit scene with clients. You don't need to have a steak or dessert or rich dressings at lunch because "the client is paying." Trust me—he won't be around to pay your escalating health bills down the road.

Supporting Success and Making It Fun

At the core of every diet failure is boredom, monotony, too many rules, and too few choices—in short, the fun factor is missing. So, how do you convince yourself and your family that a lifestyle change filled with rules can still be fun?

Well, first of all, a lot of variety and variability is built into the HFL program. Second, having more time on your hands because the plan is so organized means more time to pursue fun. Finally, when each family member begins to see goals accomplished—more energy, better sleep patterns, better grades, weight loss, a more enjoyable home life, more together time, and much less stress around food, family fun is more likely to happen naturally.

Here are some ideas for making things fun or offering support that will increase your family's HFL success:

HOW TO SUPPORT YOUR SPOUSE BY MAKING HFL FUN

- Use new recipes to entice.
- Make a food shopping date—I kid you not—it brings folks together.
- Ask what they want, then find lighter, healthier versions of the recipe and "fake them out" by serving it and then revealing the surprise "lighter aspect."
- Barter with them—if you participate in this, I'll help you with that or make a candlelit dinner or massage those aching feet.
- Create great picnic baskets and a special outing just for the two of you.
- Pose an adventure hiking/eating weekend at a spa to get the process going.
- Offer to take over garbage detail or dishwashing.

- Do a buffet night at least once a week so everyone can create a personalized dish. Vary the entrée salad ingredients and the protein topping options.
- Create nights of "personalized opportunities"—personal pizza, personal wraps, add-to-a-soup (beans, meat, fish), dairy night (healthy omelets, quiches, frittatas, chili bowls topped with a bit of melted low-fat cheese).
- Use fun family rewards to motivate: a weekend movie, a beach day, a picnic, a day trip somewhere special.
- Have the family figure out new ways to "measure portions" by creating their own visual cues.
- Pick a new weekly ingredient and have everyone create a dish around it.
- Check out new cooking classes as a family.

- Subscribe to a cooking magazine that features light recipes or go online to find new recipes.
- Explore ethnic recipes and substitute ingredients to make them healthier.
- If weight loss is a goal, get any family member who hits a milestone a gift certificate to a favorite store.
- Remember the things that were fun in childhood—games, buddying up in sports, cooking with mom, riding a bike with a buddy. Why not recapture them now with your family?
- Be spontaneous and flexible. Sometimes the best-laid plans get ruined and the disappointment can be really overwhelming, so agree to set aside workout time, but be more free-spirited and spontaneous with plans. Kids especially love sudden surprises like a family picnic and hike, a family cooking class, or an outing with members of their extended family to play a sport.
- Surprise your spouse by taking on more of the plan or prep responsibilities one week. That shows love and support more than any other gesture.
- Put a "love note" or "support note" on each plate at the dinner table, in lunch bags and then pay it forward to another family member to do the same. This way, you'll begin to express love and support verbally instead of with food.

Tips for Kids/Teens

- Use shapes (for muffins, mini-sandwiches), use math, use new ingredients.
- Let them know why you're doing this program and how they can help.
- Let them voice unhappiness or rebellion—it's part of the process.
- Use family outings as much as possible.
- Let them choose sports they want to pursue.
- Give them leadership roles whenever possible.
- Let them run the show at the supermarket (at least once in a while).

- Give them a cooking night and let them really experience the role of chef.
- Do taste testing and let them "grade" the experience and the foods.
- Do surprise nights where pitching in to help gets a surprise movie at home or a night out.
- Reward cumulative milestones with something they want. We all reward good behavior and changing habits deserves non-food rewards.

11

Don't Fight the Feelings

Family Strategies for Going to Each Other
(Instead of the Refrigerator) to Handle Stress
and Avoid Emotional Eating Traps

I love my family. I love their quirkiness, their humor, their passion, their optimism—I even love that they love food. I can also tell you that over the years I have noticed that, as with all families, our lives do seem to revolve around food, at least when it comes to special occasions. And because my family is Jewish, food features prominently at holiday time (not to mention birthdays, anniversaries, graduations, weddings, showers, and fundraisers, to name a few).

Food celebrates life and to deny that would be really disingenuous.

But my family knows that if I'm invited, I'll be the one bearing a salad, fruit salad, and healthy main dish. Sure, I could make it a battlefield, a constant clashing of wills, an ongoing sermon, or just a real downer of an experience in order to make a "health point." Instead, I choose to celebrate the joyous occasions with my family—on my terms—without encroaching on their choices.

While I was growing up, my dad seemed to have a natural tendency toward slimness, coupled with the ability to cut back on eating if his weight shifted a bit. Mom, on the other hand, was a whole different story. She had been raised in a very rigid family where food was celebrated but controlled; my grandmother was extremely specific about how much and when to eat and she had managed to battle and successfully control her weight, so she wanted her daughter to do the same. I think my mother figured out young that turning to food for solace would particularly antagonize my grandmother, so she ate on the sly and grew, battling my grandmother's increasing attempts at control with more eating on the sly. I know my mother also probably had clinical depression; as she entered her adult life, she continued to self-medicate with food.

So I learned from a very young age that food was reward and punishment, the answer to emotional highs and lows, the devil among us. It could help me deal instantaneously with any emotion, but afterward I always felt guilty. I wondered: How did I lose control like that? Why am I turning to food to feel better? Why is this pattern now so entrenched in me? How do I dig out?

I looked at my friends at school and sometimes their behavior seemed alien to me: they could be sad over a grade without grabbing a bag of chips or be truly happy without the reward of cookies or a cupcake. I, on the other hand, handled my emotions with food, as I'd learned from my mother.

Here are the top ten emotional reasons people turn to food for comfort, as my clients have shared them with me over the years:

1. Anxiety
2. Fear
3. Anger
4. Frustration
5. Sadness
6. Insecurity
7. Rivalry
8. Boredom
9. Stress
10. Other emotion (you fill in the blank!)

The point is that we can use food as a way to handle ANY emotion, and we often do. Through my own personal experience, and through working with hundreds of families, it's easy to underestimate the importance of feelings in the weight loss equation. For some people, emotional eating is a severe problem that may require the help of therapy or ongoing support groups. The reality, however, is that *most* people have a tendency to turn to food for emotional reasons, including stress, now and again—and feelings can easily create problems for anyone's efforts to change their lifestyle. Emotional eating is a significant cause of weight gain, even in children and teens.

At the end of the day, this is the part of every food or lifestyle plan to which people simply don't pay enough attention. Even the most successful dieters can easily fall off the wagon of healthy behaviors if they haven't worked on the emotional issues that can spur an eating orgy. If you can't cope with daily highs and lows and/or if you are carrying around emotional baggage that is bubbling just below the surface, you are at risk for emotional eating. You won't be truly successful at changing your lifestyle or your weight over the long term unless you face up to any level of emotional eating, and work on new strategies to replace those behaviors.

It's tough to face painful emotional behaviors or past memories that instigate emotional eating or even just habits that have become so entrenched they seem normal and familiar. You will need to tackle these emotional eating issues for yourself and encourage family members to consider their issues as well.

I can offer you the hopeful message that if you tackle this part of your eating dynamics and add it to the HFL program, you will truly be a healthy family for life.

Are You an Emotional Eater?

Here are some questions to help you investigate whether or not you turn to food in emotional situations and how deeply these habits are entrenched. Though some of these behaviors can be caused by other issues or problems, they are often indicators of *in the moment* or *delayed response emotional eating*:

- Do you keep a significantly larger supply of food on hand at home or at work than you or your family need? Why?
- Do you keep large stores of carbohydrate foods in your pantry and fridge?
- Do you find yourself grabbing food whenever you feel mood swings, highs and lows?
- Do you keep food stashed in drawers, your purse, your car?
- Do you eat significant amounts of food after dinner? Why?
- Do you wake up at night to eat? Why?
- Do you reward yourself with food?
- Do you console yourself with food?
- Did you grow up in a household where behavior and emotions were handled with food?
- Do you feel out of control during any eating experiences?
- Do you grab food and eat when no one will know?
- Do you justify larger or additional eating experiences because of your exercise efforts that may indeed burn some calories but not enough to justify eating "extra food"?
- When you become emotional, do your thoughts veer to food quickly?
- Do you eat in secret?

In the questions that end with "Why?" I'm asking you to be honest with yourself, to find out if the motivation to eat is indeed emotional in nature. Were you steaming over something that happened earlier that day or even the day before? Was it a celebration that just kept on giving and giving—food, that is? Is your immediate gut reaction to turn to food as a bandage or coping mechanism or reward?

Finally, there is a very important two-part question that is the unmistakable identifier of emotional eating: (1) If you shared *how you eat* with others, would you feel embarrassed? and (2) Do you want your kids to eat like this?

If your answer to (1) is yes and (2) is no, we both know there is emotional and—to some degree, destructive—eating going on.

Sometimes the light bulb of recognition going off is enough to cause a change in behavior. For others, therapy may be necessary, especially if these behaviors are having an impact on the quality of life and health. Most people fall somewhere in between and need to identify the emotional eating problem, isolate specific habits that need to be changed, and devise new behaviors to replace the old ones. In this effort, patience is a virtue. You may need to develop a variety of emotional strategies and responses to help you replace your old emotional eating habits. Again, the support of a buddy, family and friends, support groups or counseling professionals can help you overcome emotional eating for good.

In order to make progress with emotional eating, you need to ask yourself another question: when you eat with emotion as your

MAKE SURE IT'S EMOTIONAL, NOT MEDICATION

Certain medications can make you more prone to gain weight. It's important not to confuse emotional eating with physiological responses to medications that can make you less active or hungrier or otherwise impact your calorie in/calorie out balance. Talk to your doctor if you believe a medication might be causing hunger or weight gain. Here are the more likely culprits:

- Antihistamines and sleep aids, which can sap your energy, so you move less.
- Antidepressants, which can make you eat more by affecting the neurotransmitters in your brain that modulate appetite and mood.
- Birth control pills, which can make you retain water.
- Migraine medication, which can make you hungrier thanks to its active ingredient.
- Steroids, which are notorious for making you moody and hungry.

impetus, do you really feel the pain? When I say "pain," I mean the insidious weight gain, the slightly shifting blood pressure profile, the increased risk of diabetes? Because you need to use that reality as a source of motivation to break the emotional food bond. Something needs to be *at stake* for you to seize the moment and want change. You need to have clarity about what this habitual emotional eating is doing to you.

The Stress Connection Is Real

One reason that emotional eating is such a universal problem is that stress is naturally associated with eating behaviors. Research indicates that stress can cause increased levels of cortisol; experts believe that higher levels of circulating cortisol may actually enhance fat storage. There may be other effects of increased levels of cortisol:

- Lower metabolic rate and increased levels of gastric acid, which maximizes the calories you get from your food.
- Retention of additional sodium, causing a bloated feeling.
- Release of high-energy fats and blood-clotting agents into your bloodstream.
- Energy being diverted from your immune system.
- Possible increase in cholesterol (research still ongoing).

People under stress may also experience feelings of depression, anxiety, frustration, and fatigue, leading to lower self-esteem and self-confidence, which then leads to eating. There are also indications stress can change the shape of your body. It may partly explain why some people develop an "apple" shape, storing fat centrally in their body. Not to mention that stress can simply increase your appetite.

Researchers have postulated that there may be a bi-directional connection specifically between stress and food.[1] You crave food emotionally, especially carbohydrates and high-fat foods, because these foods actually calm you down. The hormones that stress releases may instigate a physiological desire to treat the "fight or flight" response with calories so your body has an immediately available energy source. Carbohydrates in particular offer that kind of easily utilized energy.

On the flip side, overeating can in and of itself create a feeling of being out of control, and so the cycle continues, with you turning to food because the overeating is actually stressing you out.[2] There is no "fight or flight" response in this case: you are actually immobilized. Because you're not using those immediately available energy stores, your body is tucking them away as additional fat stores. You gain weight—you eat out of misery—the cycle continues.

It's also been theorized that some foods have a calming quality that, in some cases, may be downright addictive. Let's take a food like chocolate, which research indicates may actually cause your body to release small amounts of mood-altering or satisfaction-boosting opi-

ATTITUDE ADJUSTMENT TIPS (EMOTIONAL APPETITE IS ALSO OKAY)

- Remind yourself that emotional eating is not normal unless it is occasional and controlled (we all can have an emotional food moment).
- Explore how the cycle of emotional eating began. Identify mitigating events and childhood situations and behaviors. Get in the habit of talking about your feelings out loud.
- Recognize the difference between mild, moderate, and serious emotional eating.
- Seek out behaviors in others that mirror how you would like to behave during emotional highs and lows.
- Make a list of any health issues you have that derive from stress and stress-eating and post it where you can see it on a regular basis.
- Journal to get a true picture of your eating in relation to your emotional moods.

BEWARE OF BLOWN DIET SYNDROME

Back in the late 1970s, Janet Polivy and C. Peter Herman, PhD, researched and coined the term "blown diet syndrome." They looked at restrained eaters, chronic dieters who carefully monitored their intake because of fluctuating weight issues. Then they compared them to unrestrained eaters, people who ate unthinkingly (no real food issues—regular eaters). When the restrained eaters were given milkshakes in various portion sizes, they then pigged out on ice cream, as if it was an uncontrolled extension of the milkshake, regardless of how large or small the milkshake was. It was as if the milkshake experience unleashed the cravings demon within them. If they had no milkshakes, they were able to remain restrained. The unrestrained eaters drank the milkshakes and behaved proportionately to the portion size. If one milkshake left them some comfortable eating room, they had some ice cream. If, however, they were given two milkshakes, that was it—no ice cream and no feeling of deprivation. So it seems like if they were chronic dieters and went off the "diet track," their next step was to say, "What the heck" and go overboard and indulge. That's the origin of the phrase "blown diet syndrome."

I believe there is something in between called healthy restraint: saying no to a second cookie, having a dessert one night, and saying no the next two nights. Exercising healthy restraint means you stop when you're full—and that's a healthy habit. It does not necessarily mean vigilantly counting every single calorie you eat with utter dedication. Obsessively counting every morsel can be debilitating if you don't eventually shift to a healthier way of tuning into the feeling of satiation. It's important to truly embrace how it feels to be full so you can use it as a healthful gauge and then choose portion sizes that satisfy you.

ates.[3] Sensing this "reward" may very well lead you to gravitate to chocolate repeatedly, seeking to re-experience that instant positive feeling over and over again, especially if you experience a mood alteration. So every time you feel "down" or stressed or anxious—you crave chocolate. Carbohydrates in general may confer a peaceful feeling when you eat them in an agitated state because they calm the "fight or flight" instinct. Put more simply, let's just say that the pleasure of eating seems to help ward off or calm negative emotions.

However, it's important to realize that this soothing effect is temporary. In the long run, the negative emotions caused by the consequences of ongoing emotional eating are likely to trigger as many or more negative emotions as the emotional eating is temporarily warding off—it's a vicious cycle.

Food can also be a distraction. If you're worried about an upcoming event or rethinking an earlier conflict, eating comfort foods may distract you. But the distraction is only temporary. While you're eating, your thoughts focus on the pleasant taste of your comfort food. Unfortunately, when you're done overeating, your attention returns to your worries, and you may now bear the additional burden of guilt about overeating.

Brenda Crawford-Clark, MPH, MS, author of *Body Sense: Balancing Your Weight and Emotions,* urges, "Consider what trauma and loss has occurred, because often that's where food issues begin. Things that most people don't even consider can be the anchor that keeps someone from keeping weight off or getting past a stuck point once they've started to lose." She suggests that the following situations could be the first triggers of a pattern of emotional eating that entrenches itself:[4]

- Miscarriage
- Illnesses or accidents
- A death
- Divorce
- Infertility
- Financial strain
- Feeling like you have to be perfect
- Childhood bullying

- Childhood sexual assault
- Childhood abuse
- Being labeled as different (such as a kid who has ADHD or a learning disability)
- Adoption

She also echoes something I was subjected to in my childhood: a household in which there was an awful lot of yelling and constant criticism. I call it the "den of negativity." I remember one event as clearly today as I did almost thirty-five years ago. My family moved when I was in the sixth grade and I was placed in a new school. I knew that my academic record, of which I was incredibly proud, would probably not get me the middle school valedictorian or salutatorian honor I really coveted. Transfer kids were always at a disadvantage because a record from another school could never be assessed and compared to the new school's standards.

I continued to toil, though, because throwing myself into school was another way to escape my difficult home life. The day of academic award announcements came two years later, in eighth grade. To my utter shock, I was recognized and shared the honor of valedictorian with a friend. I ran to a pay phone around the corner from my school and called home.

When I breathlessly announced my award to my mom, she said, "There must be some mistake. Are you sure? Why would they give it to you?" My response was to assure her tearfully there was no mistake, and then to walk quickly to the local deli, where I stuffed my face with fresh pastries. My best friend, food, was always there to console me. Later on, I felt miserable, overstuffed, unloved, and emotionally spent. I can still remember the pain.

Four Strategies for Emotional Eating

There will always be situations that provoke emotional responses. How you deal with those situations depends primarily on four strategies:

1. Retraining
2. Mindfulness

3. Prepared responses
4. Asking for support

1. Retraining

The first step is to retrain yourself and replace eating in response to emotion with other behaviors. That can involve some serious work. Despite the length of time you've been conditioned to respond to any swing in emotion with food, you must now replace that behavior. Some people can do this with ease once they understand why they have been using this habitual response. For others, it's an ongoing struggle. I assess my clients to decide if they need to work with a therapist, even for a short period of time, to talk it out, heal old emotional wounds, and work on healthier behaviors.

Many people will fall somewhere in between: they are sometimes able to listen to their healthier inner voice saying, "Don't do that" and at other times, the emotional pendulum swings too far too fast and they turn to food. If you can acknowledge this behavior and continue to work on replacing immediate food response with other patterns of habitual behavior like knitting, drawing, journaling,

---

STRESS AND METABOLIC SYNDROME

Ongoing stress and emotional eating can be a serious precursor to metabolic syndrome, a cluster of risk factors that I've mentioned before, and which is being diagnosed in escalating numbers among both children and adults.[5]

People (and children) with metabolic syndrome are at increased risk of coronary heart disease and other diseases related to plaque buildup in artery walls (e.g., stroke and peripheral vascular disease) and type 2 diabetes. The metabolic syndrome has become increasingly common in the United States. It's estimated that more than 50 million Americans have it.[6]

chewing gum, or going outdoors, you will undo a huge source of pain and weight gain. You will also begin to gain a sense of being in charge and choosing to avert these emotional feelings with a choice other than food.

To begin with, the four P's of the HFL plan will help you to select and control your food choices. However, you still need to face your emotional "food demons," so to speak.

Here are some quick tips for retraining:

- Journal to learn if there is a pattern to your emotions. Maybe Monday and Thursday are particularly stressful days because you do mommy duty or have work stress, or perhaps weekends are especially stressful because you're trying to squeeze in so many errands and responsibilities.
- Know your triggers or trigger situations so you can anticipate them and have a non-food solution ready.
- Do get a professional assessment if you think that therapy may help.
- Make it easy for your family and yourself by sticking to the planning and preparation parts of the HFL program. Too many unplanned meals and snacks or keeping unhealthy food on hand just encourages emotional eating.
- Pre-plan the replacement behaviors: everything from having gum on hand to removing yourself from the situation to calling a buddy for support.
- Try out a bunch of new habits and then choose one or two that you turn to consistently, which can become your new "emotional treatment habit."
- Seek comfort elsewhere.
- Don't get down on yourself; it takes time to replace ingrained behaviors.

2. Mindfulness

Being mindful about what and how you eat is a huge step toward changing your food behaviors and responses. Studies at Brigham Young University have shown that intuitive eaters are less likely to overeat because they listen to their internal hunger cues and are less likely to be swayed into eating by external cues, like emotional and environmental stresses.

Mindful eating takes that concept a step further by causing you to assess what you really like and don't like. How often do you find yourself in an emotional moment eating things you don't even like, just to assuage those awful and overwhelming feelings? Being mindful means learning to savor food, eating slowly, and reducing distractions during meals (like TV). And being mindful may help reduce food anxieties, such as when you are so anxious about certain foods causing you to binge that you cut them out of your diet entirely. At some point, that rigid behavior, which only works for a small part of the population over the long term, will be challenged and you will succumb, possibly continuing the binge for several days.

Mindful eating techniques include slowing the pace of eating, being aware of each bite, and talking and drinking water at meals to slow down the whole tempo of the experience. For some people, practices such as mindful exercise (yoga, tai chi, qigong) or meditation can be helpful in creating a more mindful lifestyle in general, as well as in creating more mindful eating habits.

Again, being mindful should make you aware of foods you struggle with, because many of us know that we have little control of eating limits with certain foods like bread, chocolate, ice cream, or french fries. As I mentioned, they may either have a calming association from childhood or they may actually have a chemical impact on your brain chemistry. Ultimately, you need to work on the habitual relationship that food represents in order to gain a healthier emotional relationship with that food.

As a child, I hoarded chocolate and turned to it for comfort; today, it's still a challenge. I now enjoy it under controlled circumstances, as a shared dessert, always outside the home, while keeping track of portion size. I have also found "better choices" that allow me to savor the taste of chocolate without a lot of calories: low-fat chocolate pudding, Skinny Cow® ice cream sandwiches, Fudgesicle® treats, diet chocolate soda, fat-free frozen vanilla yogurt with a little chocolate sauce, diet hot chocolate.

Those foods allow me to manage my craving mindfully so I can truly appreciate a decadent treat less frequently. This kind of mindful eating keeps me from experiencing overwhelming cravings, and it also allows me to control the tendency to turn to high-fat chocolate treats to deal with emotional swings. If I really can't manage certain feelings, at least I'm eating foods that are less caloric!

3. Prepared Responses

One of the lessons that I work with during an HFL transformation is the idea of having a repertoire of responses already prepared or available to be put in place. The art of preparing responses to eating urges is a very personalized experience. Over the years, I have had some clients who, even with therapy, have turned to rather unconventional ways to deal with their emotional eating issues. One woman actually has her husband lock the pantry and puts an alarm on the fridge because she simply can't cope with end-of-day stress without turning to food. Now you may think that's insane, but she will tell you that that this simple technique has allowed her to lose eighty pounds and finally keep it off after more than two decades of cyclical dieting. How can you argue with that?

DON'T BUY INTO THE HEALTHY HALO

That phrase was coined by Brian Wansink, director of Cornell University's Food and Brand Lab. When you eat for emotional reasons, you very often underestimate the amount of food or calorie count of food in your daily diet. Sometimes this is due to a belief that the food choice is "healthy" (for example, Subway's® sandwiches or McDonald's® salads). The term "healthy halo" refers to the idea that we often overeat because we think the food we're eating is healthy. A calorie is a calorie. Overeating will cause weight gain, even when the choice is so-called "healthy" food.

You will need to find the prepared responses that work best for you, but here are some examples of behaviors that can distract you from emotional eating:

- Deep breathing
- Chewing gum
- Exercising
- Physically leaving the situation
- Calling a buddy
- Writing a blog entry or going online to an established message board
- Knitting
- Listening to music
- Playing an instrument
- Cleaning (sounds crazy, but it does work for some people)
- Taking a long shower or bath
- Physically closing the kitchen door (or pantry door) so that you see a physical barrier
- Making your menu plans for the next day so you are actively engaged with a task from the HFL program

4. Asking for Help

For some people, the final step is incredibly hard: asking others for help. It is really hard to state, out loud, that you need someone to intervene if they hear you going down to the pantry at night; it may be really difficult to admit to hoarding food or using food as a crutch to handle overwhelming emotions; it may be extremely intimidating to share with someone the fact that although you appear to be coping, you are actually unhappy and struggling with your eating. And this goes for each family member, even children. If your family is participating in the HFL program, then your family will naturally be discussing food issues, and everyone should feel encouraged to ask for help and support. Just remember that even moms and dads sometimes need to ask for comfort, a listening ear, or someone to take over when they are being challenged by emotions or cravings on a given day.

You May Need an Appetite Adjustment

One of the things you can do to help control emotional eating is to make an "appetite adjustment." Your eating should be driven by appetite or genuine hunger, which normally ebbs and flows naturally during the day. Most of us do need to eat every three to four hours in order to feel energetic and to respond to blood sugar lows or hunger. But emotions can get in the way, fueling an additional eating session or a larger than necessary meal or snack. Here are some ways you can counteract cravings or an emotional food response:

- *Examine the volume of your meal.* Eat those bulky fruits, veggies, and whole grains so you feel fuller.
- *Consider the satiety factor.* Remember to include protein at every meal because it does seem to increase satiation.
- *Don't underestimate palatability.* Just don't equate high doses of sugar and fat with the only way to feel palate pleasure. Fruits and vegetables in season are incredible palate pleasures and have an inherent sweetness. Chicken and fish seasoned with fresh herbs can be delicious. Using small amounts of healthier oils can enhance the flavors of foods.
- *Watch portion sizes and visual cues.* These retraining methods go hand in hand with mindful eating and can help you to understand when you are full.
- *Distractions are a no-no when you're eating.* Studies show you will eat more when distracted by TV, music, nonstop chatter, or the presence of alcohol.
- *Be aware of the impact of variety.* Though I'm all for different tastes and textures at a meal, lots of variety can stimulate false appetite. This is a perfect explanation for still having "room" for dessert, even when you are really full from the meal itself.

How do you prevent situations that provoke emotional eating? Can it really be done on a consistent basis? After all, humans are emotional creatures.

We all deal with emotions differently and perceive stresses differently. Nothing seems to ruffle the feathers of one of my friends. She just seems to glide through life, coping with upsetting situations calmly. In her presence, I feel just a little more grounded, just a bit more able to cope in a rational fashion with even truly challenging situations. She's my "go to" person when I need an opinion. She says she loves my heightened emotions, my zest for life, my passion, my energy. That's why she's attracted to me. I would love to have just a bit more of my friend in me—especially when I feel an overwhelming emotion that threatens to send me right into the embrace of my favorite food. When I'm with her, self-control is a lot easier. When I'm not, I have to follow a somewhat different action plan. I have learned that responding in a more modulated fashion to highly emotional situations is helpful. I also know that simply learning to relax as soon as I feel the upsweep of emotion can be one of the most valuable behaviors to master.

For many people, it is often a question of accepting reality—that although the moment may seem incredibly important at the time, something that food might help you get through, in the end, life will go on without any dramatic impact and eating won't do anything about it, anyway. So I work with clients to imagine situations and we literally role-play ways to avoid them, defuse them, or diminish their impact.

Here are some techniques you can use to avoid the emotional shifts that may induce you to treat yourself inappropriately with food:

- Ask yourself if the impact of the situation is irrevocable. If the answer is no, then troubleshoot a solution calmly.
- Ask yourself if your anger will solve the situation. If not, find a way to convey your feelings to the person and reward yourself for being in control.
- Ask yourself if a do-over is possible and if so, do it over!
- Ask yourself if a little bit of quiet time will give you a clearer perspective.
- Ask yourself if this emotional extreme will benefit the situation. If not, grab a pad and paper and jot down other ways to cope.
- Ask yourself how you'll feel after the emotional onslaught leads to an unnecessary eating experience.

Creating Healthy Behavior Patterns That Last

Anyone can say they are ready to lose weight, ready to get healthy, ready for change. It takes genuine honesty and courage to say "I am willing to face my emotional demons." The HFL 4 Ps can help to create healthy habits and the Yes, No, Maybe So food plan can help you to understand how to eat and get active, but as an experienced lifestyle coach, I can tell you that to achieve long-lasting healthy behavior patterns, you have to conquer the emotional part of the equation too.

MORE STRATEGIES FOR STOPPING EMOTIONAL EATING

- Be willing to get honest with yourself and tackle the emotional component of your eating.
- Seek therapy if these are lifelong, entrenched behaviors.
- Keep a diary and take note of when you are more likely to have an "emotional food fest," what foods you turn to, how often it happens.
- Also note in a diary the replacement behaviors you plan to use and monitor which ones work and which ones don't.
- Stop hiding or hoarding food and be willing to exhibit emotional eating in public. Just eliminating the secrecy may help you cut down on emotional eating habits.
- Remind yourself of the physical complications that come from emotional eating.
- Turn to soft music, meditation, yoga, or deep breathing to calm yourself in the moment.
- Have an emergency buddy to whom you can turn.

Tips for Kids/Teens

When dealing with kids or teens who may be turning to food to handle emotions, you need to be aware of when they are getting agitated, in a good or bad way, and talk to them. Ask them to tell you how they're feeling, and why turning to food seems to be the answer. They're not as sophisticated as you are, and they may initially be resistant to your efforts to intervene. Make the conversation nonconfrontational. Be real and let them know that turning to food instead of dealing with emotions in a more direct and effective way can cause problems. Don't forget to be honest about your own experiences, and share your own struggles with them. Mostly, be patient, be available, be nonjudgmental, and share your own experiences.

12

There Are No Perfect Families: The Art of Making Realistic Goals and Helping Your Family

Stay on Track for Generations to Come

I want the face of Tyra Banks, the body of Heidi Klum, the wealth of Donald Trump, the smarts of Bill Gates . . . and the list goes on and on. Pretty lofty goals, right?

When most of us start a diet or a lifestyle change, we can't help but reach for the stars:

- "I'm going to lose thirty pounds in one month."
- "I'm going to fit into a bikini (or my wedding dress) in two weeks."
- "I'm getting back into my high school jeans if it kills me."
- "I'll buy these jeans that are two sizes too small and I'll *just have to* lose enough weight to get into them."

It looks silly on paper, but when you are totally motivated, anything seems possible—until all those grandiose ideas backfire.

Remember Oprah on the liquid diet, proudly strutting out in her super-thin dark wash jeans, pulling a red wagon filled with a representation of all the fat she had lost. The next day she confessed that, because of a nighttime binge, she couldn't get comfortably back into the jeans. While we all applauded her success, most of us also identified with what happened, literally, overnight. The rigid diet that rewarded her with the unbelievably svelte figure came crashing down as she broke all the rules and ate through the night.

In other words, goals are tricky. They can be wondrous, magical tools that spur us into achieving healthy accomplishments. But goals can also cruelly set us up for disaster.

"Quick fix" usually means "quick failure." If you've been eating poor quality food in large portions habitually and gaining weight slowly and insidiously over a period of years, do you really expect to undo the damage in four or eight weeks? If you've been a chronic fad dieter, gaining and losing pounds over and over again, do you really expect to break that habitual dieting pattern in a short period of time? If you have raised your children to eat mostly processed foods with extremely sweet, creamy, or salty tastes and you've let them watch TV or play video games with little interference, do you really expect to redirect all their eating and exercising habits in a few short weeks or months?

Whether you are using the HFL plan to lose weight or improve your health, remember: it did not take your family six or eight weeks to get into this situation, so it's not going to take six or eight weeks to dig your way out.

What Really Works

The HFL program walks you through gradual changes in your daily habits with the ultimate goal of sustaining those changes for a lifetime. In reality, small goals, not giant ones, are the most likely to set us up for the best results. Most of my clients who have had long-term success with a lifestyle change have gotten there by achieving small, gradual milestones, one at a time.

WHERE TO BEGIN: TEN STARTING GOALS

Sometimes you need a goal list to get yourself started. Use this as a checklist system and try to hit all these goals in four to six weeks.

1. Step on the scale at the same time every day three or four times a week.
2. Limit TV time.
3. Make more *Yes Foods* a daily priority.
4. Eat breakfast every day.
5. Use a pedometer and shoot for 10,000 steps a day.
6. Keep a daily journal (with food/exercise entries).
7. Keep liquids low calorie or calorie-free.
8. Use visual cues for portion control.
9. Celebrate the small successes.
10. Ask for help when you need it (family as well as professional support).

For example, my client Sandy* decided that if she could lose fifteen pounds and hold at that weight for three months, she would then tackle the next fifteen pounds. She kept right on going once she lost the first fifteen, but I wasn't concerned that she was setting herself up for failure because her initial goal and attitude were so sensible. She did not put unreasonable pressure on herself or set her standards too high.

As a lifestyle coach, part of my job is to temper optimism with a little reality here and there. There's no doubt that some people are able to achieve amazingly difficult goals quickly and stick with them permanently, but they represent a small percentage of the population.

---

*Client name has been changed.

Most of us need to target reasonable goals that mesh with our busy lives, our genetics, physical characteristics, and even our personalities.

Once you begin to follow the HFL program, you will quickly see how individual responses can vary, as some family members shed pounds faster or find some of the guidelines easier to follow. But this is supposed to be a different journey than you typically take when dieting because the plan itself requires the whole family to work together; unlike many fad diets, there is no right or wrong way to apply the program; there is no absolute amount of weight loss that must be achieved; there are no black and white absolutes; there is no time frame for change to occur. The outline is there for you to harness in a time frame that works for the family as a team. The only requirement is that all family members agree to follow certain basic guidelines while at home and avoid sabotaging others as changes are being made. HFL behavior outside the home will hopefully follow in time.

Setting Family Goals

Some goals need to be set up for the sake of the family as a whole. This is especially important for family members who may struggle with individual goals and not feel successful. Family achievements such as, "We nailed four family sit-down meals together this week," or "We all ate five servings of veggies daily for a week," or "We all worked out for thirty minutes daily for a month!" give everyone an opportunity to celebrate as a team. Joy and a sense of accomplishment are a particular boon, even when personal weight or health goals are taking longer to achieve.

As a parent, you may be desperate to see your overweight child lose weight. As a wife, you may be anxious to see your husband reduce his risk for diabetes. Personally, you may want rapid physical changes. However, not everyone will be on the same wavelength, and you don't want to make the mistake of expecting everyone to be moving at the same pace, with the same urgency, toward goals YOU have set. That's a setup for an anguished, frustrating, and very dismal HFL journey.

Yes, you can implement the rules in the kitchen and hang tough on creating an HFL home environment. But you need to set your personal goals and let other family members set theirs. You may feel they are setting the bar too low in terms of initial goals, but remember that these are only the first step. It's okay if family members target simple and easy-to-reach successes. You don't get to harangue or badger someone simply because they aren't trying for what you want or think is appropriate.

However, as household members, everyone has to follow certain basic rules. If certain family members do not want to weigh in on menu planning, that's fine. But if they want to eat, they need to help with food preparation. If they don't like the food being offered, they can eat the back-up choices you have in the fridge—tuna, sliced chicken, salad, fruit, or yogurt—but they don't get to sabotage the process by bringing fast food into the house or derailing your efforts in some other way. And they don't get a special separate dinner cooked for them either.

Your initial objectives have to be to take control of the kitchen, especially the pantry and fridge, and to promote enthusiasm among family members. Your goal has to be to get everyone on board at some level initially, and then encourage more involvement as you continue to implement the four P's of the HFL program. As team captain, your goal is to have patience and pull the team together, while targeting your own personal goals.

One of the most important ways to help your family succeed is to keep your goals positive, with the big picture, lasting lifestyle change, in mind. The whole family needs to know that, unlike most weight loss schemes and plans, this program is not about dieting for a few months or sacrificing taste and fun for a little while before returning to old habits. The natural inclination of many people who have struggled with weight or eating issues is to change their habits for a while, then once goals are met, gently slide back into old habits. The whole point of this program and teamwork is to undo unhealthy habits or habits that are instigating weight gain. The "Yes, No with a Smile, Maybe So" eating plan and the four P's are set up to be adopted as lifelong habits.

HFL goals involve:

- Change that your family can sustain as a new way of life
- Health improvements that last
- Weight loss that remains lost
- Reasonable new habits that can be maintained for a lifetime
- Health-conscious living that is maintained as a true family value

TIPS TO CONTROL HUNGER CRAVINGS AND FEEL FULL

If your goal is to avoid mindless or emotional eating, it can help if you truly feel physically full. In addition to the other ideas throughout this book, here are some quick tips to control cravings and feel full:

1. Eat breakfast every day and make sure it combines protein, healthy carbs, and a small portion of healthy fat so you remain satiated.
2. Add beans to your meal. They add protein and fiber, two very filling components.
3. Double-blend your smoothies to create a frothy, air-filled, and filling beverage.
4. Sniffing scents can help some people control their cravings and impulsive eating: vanilla scent works for me and I use candles in the kitchen and bedroom.
5. Do snack, but snack smart: fruit with a bit of healthy fat, veggies with a healthy dip, a small bowl of warm bean soup, fat-free yogurt with berries. The goal is to fill up on a small calorie investment.
6. Lower your stress with deep breathing, exercise, or meditation, which will reduce or stabilize cortisol levels and its possible impact of appetite stimulation.

Your family goals should reflect an uplifting and enduring approach that is bearable, not overwhelming for your family, and most of all, is attainable. For example, eating more high-fiber foods at meals is a doable, positive goal with lots of delicious and filling options. It's a "Do" rather than a "Don't." This "Do" approach is fundamental to the HFL program. When it comes to kids or even a tough spouse, saying Yes to lots of options improves your likelihood of success.

Examples of Family Goals

Even though my emphasis is on personal goal-setting, as a parent, you will probably have some thoughts on why you want your kids or the family as a whole to follow the HFL program. (You probably have some ideas of goals for your family). For example, you may be thinking:

- "I'd like to help my children lose some weight or at least maintain their current weight while they grow, so they are at lower risk for health problems."
- "I'd like to help my children move with greater ease and feel better about themselves."
- "I'd like to help my children develop healthier habits, more energy, and a more active lifestyle."
- "I'd like everyone in our family to pass a health and physical fitness exam with flying colors."
- "I'd like us to eat less food from fast-food sources."
- "I'd like us to eat less processed foods out of boxes and prepare more meals from scratch."
- "I'd like to feel that, over time, we are in control of our nutrition and activity level, instead of feeling disorganized and out of control."

Your concern and passion for your family's health is the perfect starting point for the HFL program. You can take these initial ideas and turn them into positive, action-oriented family goals. Depending on what stage of health your family is in and the personality types in the family, you can set specific family goals. A mild competitive flavor to these goals is fine, but turn them into "musts" carefully by continuing to explain why this shift in habits is so vital to the health of your family. If you are too pushy, change too many aspects of your household too quickly, or become a rigid taskmaster, forcing many rapid and sudden changes, you may deter a family member from joining the process. You can create a list of "starter" ideas and then meet with your family to create goals on which you can all agree. The most important thing you need to create is an environment of discussion and communication, while stating the obvious reasons why change is needed. Here are some examples of HFL family goals, but you will want to create some that fit your family:

1. "We will have three or four family dinners a week."
2. "We will make one large and organized food shopping excursion and one fill-in every week."
3. "We will eat four fruits and four or five veggie servings at least four days each week."
4. "We will exercise as a family once every weekend."
5. "We will have one or two menu planning nights a week."
6. "We will eat one weekend breakfast together."
7. "We will have only sixty minutes of TV/video viewing time per day (not related to homework)."
8. "We will try one new taste per day."
9. "We will each have a prep job on the designated prep day(s)."
10. "We will not bring personal food items that are not on the family shopping list into the home."
11. "We will choose our 'No with a Smile Foods' before we shop."

Setting Personal Goals

Individual goals are just that—individual. Every family member will have different priorities and approaches. Health goals will be appropriate for some—weight loss or behavior changes for others. Encourage everybody to create personal goals.

Here are some examples of personal goals:

1. "I want to lose some weight so I can fit into a smaller size and feel better about myself."
2. "I want to lose some weight because my doctor has told me it will help prevent (you fill in the blank: heart disease, hypertension, diabetes . . .)."
3. "I want to lose some weight so I can enjoy being active with my kids and set a better health example."
4. "I have some important milestone events coming and I'd like to lose some weight to feel better about myself at these events and then continue to lose weight or maintain this weight loss."
5. "I'd like to meet some personal weight and health goals that my doctor and I have set for myself."
6. "I'd like to stop skipping meals."
7. "I'd like to give up soda and high-calorie coffee drinks."
8. "I'd like to reduce my blood sugar, blood pressure, LDL cholesterol (and raise HDL), and knee joint pain associated with excess weight."
9. "I'd like to increase my walking frequency and distance."
10. "I'd like to ride elevators and use my car less, and climb stairs and walk more."
11. I'd like to eat breakfast every day.

Examples of Reasonable Goals for Kids

Adults in the family should help kids and teens create their personal goals. You may want to share some of the following examples to help them. It's very important to state kids' goals in kids' language. Some kids may feel comfortable with specific weight loss goals, but if they pose too much pressure, other behavior- or results-oriented goals can work just as well. Here are some goal ideas:

1. "I want to fit into clothes more comfortably and shop for regular not plus sizes."
2. "I want to feel better when I look at myself in the mirror."
3. "I want kids to stop making fun of my size."

TRACKING YOUR GOALS

One of the simplest tools you can use for charting progress is journaling. The beauty of a journal is that you can keep an honest record of what is happening. Our memory of eating can be very short or simply unclear. Keeping the journal handy and making quick entries is a good way to track your HFL efforts. You can include food entries, exercise entries, emotional content (especially because it can correlate to eating temptations), goals, and measurements (like weight and inches). When I create a journal with a client, we set up a seven-day cycle of those parameters. We'll usually do a BMI measurement once every four to six weeks, depending on weight loss goals and progress. We also include body measurements and lab profiles every two to three months. The following outline may or may not work for you, but you can use it as a good starting point to create your own.

A daily entry can include these categories (or add your own):

Date:
Day of the Week:
My Goal for the Day (Do this the night before so it's on your mind.):

Breakfast:

Lunch:

Dinner:

Snacks (Include number and food content):
__Servings of fruits:
__Servings of veggies:

TRACKING YOUR GOALS, *continued*

__Servings of dairy:
__Servings of protein:
__Servings of fat:
__Servings of bread-like carbs:
__Dessert or "No with a Smile" food (if applicable):

Exercise:
__Minutes total
__Minutes aerobic
__Minutes weight training

Emotional State:
Weight:

__**Family meal happened (check off)**
__**I met my HFL goals (check off or quantify if you didn't)**

Health Goals:
 BMI:
 Measurements:
 Labs/Health Measurements:

4. "I want to be the one of the first ones chosen when choosing sides for sports."
5. "I want to run faster, jump higher, last longer when I play."
6. "I want to stop feeling bad or guilty when I eat."
7. "I want to stop skipping meals."
8. "I want to stop sneaking snacks."
9. "I want the scale to stay at the same number or move downward."
10. "I want the pediatrician to tell me that my 'numbers' are better."

11. "I want to get really good at a sport."
12. "I want to improve my running times or other athletic parameters."
13. "I want to stop feeling embarrassed, depressed, or anxious about my weight or body image."

As you can see, these goals are phrased to be as positive as possible, without pressure to lose a specific amount of weight, often relating to physical activity or areas that can be important to a child or teen.

Time Frames: How Far, How Fast?

Incorporating high-fiber fruits and vegetables, alternative proteins, whole grains, low-fat and fat-free dairy products, and healthy oils into a family eating program that used to focus on fried chicken, pizza, burgers and fries, spaghetti and meat sauce, macaroni and cheese, ice cream, soda, and lots of treats is a process that requires time. If you're a Stage 3 or Stage 4 family, or if there is a family member who specifically falls into those more urgent health stages, of course, it makes sense to work toward change at a faster pace.

However, a common downfall of an otherwise successful lifestyle change effort is pushing too hard and too fast, even in the name of positive change. I always caution new clients to remember the needs and personalities of each family member and to be patient. Offer new foods and be patient. Discuss the need for change and be patient. And most of all, model the behaviors you want to see from other family members.

You will have to consider health measurements and parameters to assess your lifestyle changes. Health goals such as weight and BMI measurements, blood tests, and other health assessments should be discussed and worked into a schedule. Use the assessment forms I've provided in earlier chapters to gauge how quickly you need to get activity happening or significant amounts of Yes Foods replacing other foods or more control of snacks and entrée choices. A family with serious ongoing weight or health issues may need a more serious discussion when implementing the program to motivate action and change.

If you or family members are in a "pre-stage" of disease, discuss optimal testing times, schedules, and goals (including weight measurements) with your doctor. For example, if you are a diabetic, you are probably doing blood sugar testing and HbA1c testing; if you are hypertensive, you should be doing blood pressure home monitoring; if you have high LDL cholesterol, set up a reasonable testing interval with your doctor. Ongoing evaluations will show the positive impact of your HFL program and may happen independently of weight loss or significant body measure changes.

You may want to check weight once or a couple of times per week, and take body measurements every six weeks. From a health perspective, most professionals agree that one to two pounds/week weight loss after an initial water loss (which sometimes exceeds that amount) is a healthy goal.

When it comes to kids, you really need to determine a reasonable weight loss goal after consulting with the pediatrician and how often you would like to assess weights or measurements. Or, if the child is showing signs of medical problems like insulin resistance, high total cholesterol, or high blood pressure, the doctor can also suggest a schedule of check-ins. It may help kids if the doctor is involved so that both supportive encouragement and reality messages can come directly from a health professional who is not a family member.

Also, discuss with each family member specifically how you all would like to verbalize progress or the lack of progress. Telling your child he "blew it this week" is reverting back to the very techniques that make people unsuccessful dieters. Remember that even if weight loss did not occur, your child ate more healthy foods or was more active or both, and those are important achievements, even in the face of no weight loss.

As adults, we need to apply those same positive reflections on ourselves, as long as honesty is the prevailing policy. If you are in a state of denial, thinking by Week 12 or 14 that eating an extra couple of fruits a week and taking two or three ten-minute walks a week is going to achieve great progress, then you are clearly not ready for the HFL program. That doesn't mean that you're not deriving some benefits from eating more fruit and moving a bit. It's just not enough progress to really dent even a Stage 1 family's health profile significantly.

ACHIEVE YOUR GOALS BY MANAGING HUNGER

You have to work with your daily hunger rhythms (we all get hungry at specific times of the day) and patterns (if you always end dinner with dessert, for example) in order to be successful with nutrition goals. Here are some techniques I recommend:

- Give up the eating until you're stuffed approach. You need to decide that feeling pleasantly full is healthier and will be more likely to help you follow portion control. Finish two-thirds of your main course and agree to have some tastes of dessert and not the whole serving.
- Don't diet. Following an eating program is not about deprivation, which is why if you give into a craving or eat too much on a given day, we suggest starting fresh the next day—not compensating by eating less.
- Exercise should not justify eating though, on occasion, if you feel you are going to overeat (at a party or event) or you've eaten extra food or an extra treat, you should balance it out with extra movement or exercise. The HFL program should be providing enough filling food. Remember to eat an adequate breakfast, lunch, and dinner and time snacks to have a complete and satiating eating experience. You do not want to make a habit of adding exercise to balance out additional calories. It will not work for you in the long term.

Let's take a look at two actual families, and how they created goals to meet their needs.

Real-Life HFL Family Story: Goals from Age Four and Up

The Kay family (their names have been changed) had five members, each with a specific set of personal challenges:

- A hard-working, successful dad, who had developed a borderline high cholesterol problem over the years and had packed on an extra thirty-five pounds (which he carried in his abdominal area)
- A stay-at-home mom who was clearly overweight, probably carrying about fifty to sixty extra pounds
- Three children: a high school senior boy who was slim, an athletic girl in middle school, and a young boy with ADD issues who was gaining weight rapidly

Dad worked long hours and often skipped breakfast, ate fast-food lunches on the go, and came home to dinner (sometimes home-cooked, sometimes fast-food takeout) with non-stop snacking continuing through the evening. He had a variety of goals:

- Lose weight
- Learn how to weight train
- Build a modest home gym so he could do work out at any time that was convenient for his schedule
- Score better on his blood cholesterol panel
- Deal with the issues he was having sexually, which he felt might respond to a less artery-clogging diet

Mom had jumped from diet to diet unsuccessfully in the past. Her extra pounds were a combination of weight that remained after the birth of each child, weight gain due to the start of perimenopause, and the results of what was obviously a poor diet and minimal activity (but did include some doubles tennis playing). She had a family history of Alzheimer's disease and heart disease among her immediate relatives. She had an extensive list of goals:

- Lose forty pounds over six to eight months
- Improve her approach to organization in the kitchen and food prep
- Reduce fast-food meals to once a week
- Clean out the pantry and have only one or two boxed treat choices for each child to choose from once a day
- Begin a three to four times/week workout of cardio/weight training, with one hour duration each time and one family weekend hike or other activity
- Learn to do a large family shopping/prep twice a week

When the kids were interviewed, the eldest son said he wanted "no part" of this family makeover but would obviously eat whatever was available on the home front and he would help with one of the two weekly shopping trips. He also agreed that he would eat fast food only outside of the home; he would not upset the household's "new rules" by bringing in fast food.

The daughter was actually excited about the program because she was concerned that, though she was now slim, she would "become" her mom when she got older. She was also convinced that she would do better in sports if she ate better-quality food (especially home-prepared brown bag lunches and snacks). Together, we outlined a number of goals:

- Help Mom with the shopping once a week
- Participate in the weekend activity with Mom
- Help pack her own lunches and snacks
- Stop drinking so many sugary drinks and switch to flavored waters, except when her coach recommended an electrolyte-replenishing drink

At the age of four, the Kays' youngest child could absorb some of the information we relayed to him, like "helping and choosing new foods," but he didn't like being told there would be no more fast food around the house and that he couldn't just take whatever he wanted from the pantry anymore whenever he wanted it. He also wasn't keen on the reduced TV and video gaming time. He did like the idea of playing more with Mom and Dad and joining a soccer league. He also was a "willing taster" so this would enormously help the shift in food quality and types.

- He agreed to let Mom pack his lunch (instead of eating the higher-fat lunches being served at his private school)
- He asked if he and his mom could bake something once a week. We came up with a fabulous muffin and a brownie recipe chock full of flavor and nutrients, and low in fat
- He also asked for a basketball hoop to start practicing like his favorite member of the Lakers and he willingly started taking a karate class after school

---

SETTING YOUR EXERCISE GOALS: USE THE "ADD-ON" RULE

If you want a simple guide to introducing a workout program into your life, follow this five-step schedule of goals:

1. I will start with a ten-minute walk three times a week.
2. I will add ten minutes to each walk every week until I reach sixty minutes per day, three days a week (this will take six weeks).
3. I will add ten minutes of weight training twice a week during week four.
4. I will add ten more minutes of weight training to each day in week eight.
5. I will add ten more minutes to each of the two days in week twelve.

You will now be walking three days a week for six minutes on each day and weight training twice a week for thirty minutes. Keep this going for six months and then add a class, fun activity, or extra walk day per week, so you will be exercising six days per week.

As you can see, this family was made up of diverse individuals, each having different needs and goals and different levels of initial involvement. Everyone came on board at some point to work together; frankly, everyone ended up really enjoying the menu planning, the food tasting, and the weekly family meals. I was most happy that the youngest child wouldn't require so much habit modification time because the changes were happening while he was young, before his habits became firmly entrenched. Changing

REBOUNDING FROM A RELAPSE

Setbacks happen to anyone who sets goals; it's part of human nature. What steps can you take to deal with those moments when you revert to old habits and eat too much or abandon your exercise commitments?

- Forgive yourself immediately and learn from the experience. Maybe you convinced yourself that you could handle temptation and you couldn't; maybe you allowed a negative emotion to fuel eating or derail exercise.
- Return to normal eating and exercise as soon as possible. Don't skip meals, overexercise, or reduce portions. Just get back on track.
- Try to avoid the same or other temptations for three or four days so you feel in charge and in control of your habits and behaviors again.
- Ask family members to buddy up with you if you feel that it is still a transitional time for you in terms of temptation.
- Really emphasize self-nurturing behaviors like getting enough sleep, practicing relaxation techniques, and making enough "me" time so you don't wallow in negative feelings that put you at risk of temptation again.

ingrained habits can be the hardest part of the HFL program. I was also happy that Dad's health and energy levels improved and that Mom ended up feeling really fulfilled and much more in control of her eating habits and the manner in which her family was engaging in eating and exercising. Frankly, whether families realize this or not, these feelings are also goals to be achieved.

Real-Life HFL Family Story: Progress in Spite of Challenge

The Wilson family* offered me one of my most difficult challenges as a family lifestyle coach and as someone who profoundly believes in the *family connection* as the most vital tool for HFL success. The mom was a computer biller, working out of her home part-time, and suffering from osteopenia, a disease that affects bone density, and a precursor to osteoporosis,. She had fertility issues that were connected to hormonal imbalances. She had also been an on-again, off-again extreme dieter. Both of the fertility and dieting problems may have contributed to her bone density issues. Her workaholic husband was an avid exerciser who would embrace extremely rigid eating plans in pursuit of greater athletic capabilities and stamina. He had some decent food foundations, but he had some rather questionable theories that he used to justify his constant dietary modifications: he would switch from high protein/low carb to high protein/high fat/no carb to high carb/low fat. I never met him directly, but heard about his nutritional views and habits from his wife. He also justified a lot of eating (six to eight mini meals per day) because of his exercise schedule. He had put on about twenty-five pounds over a five-year period (his weight fluctuated tremendously), but he never abandoned his exercise regimen. For the most part, he ate one way and Mom and kids ate another.

Their two children, a ten-year-old and five-year-old, were being raised on restaurant food and highly processed choices like pasta, grilled cheese sandwiches, chicken fingers and fries, pizza, some fruits, and minimal veggies. The kids were slim, but utterly non-engaged

---

*Client name has been changed.

in exercise, and the whole family was disconnected in terms of family meals.

As a whole, the family was not invested in real nutrition and there were no family physical activities. We worked out a plan to address these problem areas:

- Mom's goal was to learn to prepare, shop, and actually cook for a family but we would stick with very simple meals and recipes. She confessed she was "really doing it for the kids," so I was initially concerned about her own needs and goals.
- Dad's goal was to support Mom at home and maybe drop some weight. However, he was really convinced that he fully understood nutrition and was not going to be very receptive to changes in the way he was eating, though he was willing to listen and be supportive.
- The kids were excited that Mom was finally going to let "messes happen in the kitchen." They loved the idea of going

ADULT FIBER GOAL TO TARGET: APPROXIMATELY 35 GRAMS/DAY

Every day, you want to consume enough soluble fiber, which attracts water, slows digestion, and lowers LDL or bad cholesterol. You also want to consume enough insoluble fiber, which adds bulk to stool and lowers cardiovascular risk.

Soluble fiber foods: Oat bran, nuts, seeds, barley, beans, lentils, rice bran, peas (Maybe So Foods). Apples, strawberries, citrus fruits, other fruits and vegetables (Yes Foods).

Insoluble fiber foods: Whole wheat breads, wheat cereals, wheat bran, rye, rice, barley (Maybe So Foods). Cabbage, beets, carrots, brussels sprouts, turnips, cauliflower, apple skins (Yes Foods).

to the market to shop, helping with cooking, and having a say in food choices. They were also going to learn to skate and ride bikes—so the family could do some "moving and grooving" together.

Both nutrition education (me and Mom working one-on-one) and many attempts at planning and preparing menus (on Mom's part) failed miserably. With a lot of humor on my part, some major "count to ten and try again" moments (again on my part), and most importantly, the kids' willingness to see HFL as a fun experiment (and their willingness to beg Mom and Dad to "get with the program"), we were able to establish some very solid HFL habits. Mom would take the girls grocery shopping once a week (often, she made it a special experience by taking one child at a time) and bring home a variety of fruits and veggies.

Fresh-cut veggies were available daily, as were individual cups of low-fat yogurt, healthy cereals, and whole grain muffins and breads. Pre-sized packs of white turkey meat, little cups of hummus and bean dip, and mini apples and tangerines helped make healthy food readily available. Mac and cheese made with lower-fat cheese was served only once a week.

Dad would join the rest of the family for weeknight meals three times a week. Mom began to eat breakfast with the kids as often as possible and this meal incorporated healthier cereals, whole grain waffles, and even wraps with scrambled eggs and salsa. Both girls started dance classes and Dad helped them learn to ride bikes so that they could have a weekend bike ride together. TV viewing time dropped dramatically in lieu of reading time with Mom.

Mom actually took a series of cooking classes and received some easy cookbooks as gifts from the girls and Dad, with the understanding that they all needed to pitch in with prep. Mom started working with weights twice/week and a recent DEXA scan (bone density assessment) showed a small but significant improvement in her bone density.

The shift toward greater activity, more meals together, and lower-fat dairy products yielded distinct health benefits over time. The family came together and definitely benefited from the increased activity and less TV time. Dad lost fifteen pounds, thanks mostly to portioned evening meals and only fruit snacks after dinner. He also got enormous pleasure from teaching the kids to ride bikes and taking them out on weekend rides.

This is an evolving HFL family and they continue to call me in for new "assignments" to further their progress in stabilizing their weight, maintaining their health, and keeping their activity and eating patterns intact.

ADULT DAILY VITAMIN GOAL

One of your goals should be to get your daily vitamin requirements mostly through food, but many of us do need a multivitamin or supplements to meet specific needs like calcium. If you are not eating a number of fortified foods, I find a multivitamin daily is a healthy habit to embrace. These are the amounts adults need each day:

- Vitamin A/beta-carotene: Up to 5,000 IU (retinyl palmitate or acetate and beta-carotene)
- Vitamin D: 400 IU
- Vitamin E: 30 IU (up to 400 IU)
- Vitamin K: 90mcg (mcg=micrograms)
- Folic acid: 400mcg (pregnant women need 600 mcg)
- Vitamin B6: 2mg
- Vitamin B12: 2.4mcg (pregnant women need 2.6mcg)
- Vitamin C: 75mg up to 500mg
- Calcium: 1000mg in divided doses (over age 50: 1200mg)
- Chromium: 25mcg (pregnant women need 30mcg)
- Copper: 2mg
- Iron: 18–25mg
- Magnesium: 400mg
- Omega-3 fatty acids: 1g
- Zinc: Up to 35mg

Don't Let Environment or Economics Stop You

One important consideration for achieving goals is your physical environment—and economics plays a role, too. A Canadian researcher coined the phrase "obesiogenic environment" to describe factors like the lack of access to green space, healthier food, physical activity opportunities, which combine to contribute to obesity. No one can argue that it is far more difficult to find healthier food options in lower socioeconomic neighborhoods and that unsafe neighborhoods can derail outdoor activities.

The solution is to be as creative as you can be. You can do all kinds of exercise for free at home: dancing to music for a set period of time daily, buying a pair or two of free weights or an exercise band (minimal cost), investing in a couple of exercise DVDs if you have access to a TV and DVD player. I have worked with financially challenged families who find used equipment for sale in the local paper, have choreographed at-home dance and movement sessions to radio music, and found other ways to implement better quality food and activity sessions.

It doesn't cost money to refuse to buy fast food. You may have to travel on the weekends to another location for access to healthier food. You may need to form a carpool with a couple of families, buy in bulk, and share the food. You can change what's in your pantry, pre-portion foods, sit down together, ration TV and computer time, and do weekend family activities. Again, this challenge asks for teamwork and communication among family members.

The Realities of Family Dynamics

As a wife and the mother of two children, I do know that you can butt heads with your spouse and your kids on just about everything! Food and exercise are two issues that do seem to encourage conflict.

If you are not yet a parent but are contemplating having kids, getting the HFL plan set up in your home will mean that you raise children who, for the most part, will understand the importance of nutrition and exercise. If you have young children, it's often easy to engage them, especially because the HFL program means more time

AVOIDING RATIONALIZATIONS

It is easy to pledge a goal and then get a bit hazy when it comes to behaviors. If you are meeting daily exercise goals, then you may rationalize larger portions or more frequent meals and snacks. Here are some other "logical" conclusions you may reach:

1. *"It's free, so how can I say no?"* Freebies and samples are everywhere. So is the bread basket every time you go to a restaurant. (I was surprised to find that in Europe you pay for the bread, so it's easy to say no!) When you face a tempting handout, ask yourself, "Would I pay for it if it weren't free?"

2. *"I have to eat it—I'm a guest."* You need to develop a strategy that people will respect without taking offense. Warn them up front, take it home and toss it, or simply take seconds of the least offensive dish and then just take a couple of tastes.

3. *"People are starving everywhere. How can I leave food on my plate?"* Your eating it doesn't help those starving people. Food respect is a private matter and you have to set your own eating guidelines, regardless of world events.

4. *"It's a special occasion."* If you count up birthdays, holidays, anniversaries, graduations, and all the other celebratory events, you'd realize how much "overeating for a cause" goes on. "No with a Smile" has to be your approach. I always bring a fruit dessert and dipping sauce as a rule (and restaurants usually honor my request for this dessert dish).

5. *"Bulk shopping is a bargain."* That's why I suggest dividing up the food in single-serve portions as soon as it comes home—prep your bulk purchases so *you* don't bulk up.

AVOIDING RATIONALIZATIONS, *continued*

6. *"It's no fun without food."* Can't imagine seeing a movie without popcorn? If popcorn is your treat for the week, that's fine. Otherwise, bring cut-up fruit or a low-cal beverage to sip. Gum can also help in this situation.
7. *"I deserve it."* Choose rewards other than food. You need to find new ways to celebrate life.

with Mommy and the whole family, which appeals to young children. You can introduce goal-setting as a game: if you use stickers and other tactile and visual cues and rewards, the process will tend to go more easily. My chapter on kids and teens offers more suggestions and tips.

Don't lose sight of the fact that older kids may embrace the experience wholeheartedly (especially if they are unhappy with their weight, body image, or athletic level of performance) or if they perceive that the whole household will be a lot less negative when it comes to food issues (meaning fewer battles over food). A home-cooked meal with the family gathering around a table can be comforting, and family hikes and picnics may be appealing, so goal-setting may not turn out to be a combative experience with teens either. On the flip side, teens may initially feel like you are just adding more rules and negativity to the home environment. Patience, love, a caring attitude, and admitting your own mistakes (the ones that reflect on why you set the home up in an unhealthful fashion and are now trying to change the environment) will all help to get your kids and teens on board.

One of your best strategies for preventing high levels of conflict is to avoid setting unreasonable goals or enforcing rules too rigidly. Your initial challenge should simply be to get kids to give up fast foods and highly processed foods and to embrace quality foods like fruits and vegetables. They need to want to learn about nutrition, to move more and enjoy physical activity, and to desire change because they connect the dots of "better habits, better health, longer life, more energy, better intellectual capacity" and other benefits.

However, two areas call for firmness and determination. The first is family participation: it's important to have all family members contribute to the food preparation process. This helps everyone understand and appreciate the process, learn by doing, and encourages family responsibility and togetherness. The second is exercise: a little prodding, even a firm hand, is worth the effort when it comes to increasing activity levels and managing TV/computer/videogaming habits. I recommend addressing these issues weekly. Yes, there is likely to be resistance. Replace screen time creatively with more parents-and-kids together time, with new movement activities or even with a reward system that does not involve food.

Setting Your Family Up for Success

Research offers some clues about how to encourage success when you set weight loss or lifestyle change goals. In 2006, *Consumer Reports* did an interesting report on dieters and their thoughts and convictions about losing weight. About 2,000 people weighted in on the poll. Here are some interesting highlights from the report:

- About 75 percent were optimistic that they would reach their target weight goal, 19 percent were unsure, 6 percent were pessimists.
- Roughly 85 percent said their *last effort* to lose weight was successful (meaning they were repeat dieters).
- Roughly 67 percent were trimming down on their own, 16 percent were participating in a free weight loss program, and 8 percent were paying a fee to a group or individual.
- Most said they had been on a diet for about three months and were losing five pounds/month.

Researchers who assessed the data concluded that:

- Dieters probably need to embrace hopefulness in order to fuel their willingness to restrict their eating.
- Most people plateaued after six months of dieting, which set them on a course to "chuck it all" (i.e., eat without bounds and regain weight).

- Most dieters had unrealistic expectations, which set them up for frustration, disappointment, and weight gain.
- If the factors that made you gain weight in the first place were still present, such as high-calorie foods on the home front, a sedentary job, emotional eating issues, or certain food-social interactions, then failure was built into the experience.

The American Medical Association also offers some guidance on weight management strategies. They endorse a number of dietary/exercise programs on the basis that different approaches may be a reasonable fit for different individual needs. They point out that almost any healthy plan of change can work if the patient *adheres* to it.

Lastly, research at the University of California, San Francisco School of Medicine, indicates that "patient adherence is more crucial that diet type." This means that the path that works is the path you *commit to*, regardless of the actual rules and guidelines of the program.

If you want to lose weight and keep it off or shift habits so you achieve a better state of health, you have to commit and feel that you can stick with the commitment long term. That being said, you still need to acknowledge some realities when it comes to changing habits and lifestyle patterns for good:

- You are more likely to follow a program that is organized and appeals to your sensibilities.
- Though daily calorie consumption is important, quality of food is paramount to your health.
- Individuals that work together succeed together.
- A program that has a step-by-step approach will be easier to follow.
- The way the program helps you to deal with a setback is crucial to the long-term success of reaching goals.
- If the program doesn't allow for review, modification, and shifting of goals, then it probably won't serve long-term commitment or success.
- If the program does not address *your needs* specifically, you will probably abandon it.

BE PREPARED WITH A CALENDAR TO HELP AVOID GOAL SABOTAGE

We all think we can defy temptation. We also believe that we can handle any situation. Here is a *calendar alert* you can pencil into your planner to help you decide in advance on seasonal strategies to cope with common food challenges that most of us face:

January 1: Don't let the first brunch of the year be your "last supper" and an out-of-control eating fest. Use portion control and mindfulness to make choices that are satisfying and health conscious.

February 5: This is the time of the Super Bowl bash and other winter parties, so plan choices such as a huge salad bowl, crudités, and bean or hummus dip, fruit salad, and air-popped popcorn to help satisfy munchies without too much of a calorie splurge.

February 14: It's Valentine's Day, so consider healthy ways to treat yourself and your family. For example, a small piece of dark chocolate (full of antioxidants) can be your food dessert splurge.

March: TV and movie awards shows and family celebrations can mean multiple get-togethers. Bring something to the potluck so you'll know there's a healthy HFL dish there for you.

April: It's the season of Easter and Passover, holidays that often revolve around food. Consider food ingredient substitutions (to lower saturated fat and calories) and plan menus carefully.

May: For Mother's Day, give yourself health options to celebrate your healthy new eating habits. You can create a buffet that showcases healthy ingredients.

AVOID GOAL SABOTAGE, *continued*

June: For Father's Day, consider giving Dad (and the whole family) the gift of a hike and picnic.

July 4: Barbecues can showcase veggie shish kabob with white meat chicken, veggie burgers, baked french fries, and lots of watermelon and fruit.

Summer Vacations: Center your summer fun around physical activity you enjoy as a family, not high-calorie drinks and sedentary lounging in the sun.

September: School's starting and this is your chance to start packing HFL lunches for your kids (and for you).

October: Make Halloween about tricks (having fun together), not treats!

November: From white meat turkey to skimming the gravy to salads topped with cranberries to "light" pumpkin pie, your Thanksgiving can be tasty *and* healthy. (This is something you'll get better at with practice every year!)

December: From holiday parties to Christmas and Hanukkah with oodles of "special food" temptations, make sure you keep your exercise schedule going strong, keep portion control habits in place, and maintain your commitment to "No with a Smile" food timing and selections.

Achieving Your Goals

Once everyone in the family member has set his or her personal goals, it's important to remember that goals can change or evolve. Don't expect goals to be permanently carved in stone—this is a learning process.

Also, avoid the natural tendency to be too tough. Depending on your health needs and weight loss needs, it is often better to aim a bit lower than to obsess on impossible, self-defeating goals because even if you do achieve them, they may be too difficult to maintain.

After all, if you ultimately surpass your goals, fabulous! Isn't that a better mindset to have than repeatedly feeling of despair from always falling short of unreasonable goals?

Whether it's weight loss, better health, or a combination of the two, you need to create an environment both at home and away that encourages success. One of the reasons people do well on those TV shows like *The Biggest Loser* is that they are placed in a secluded and controlled environment. Though occasional challenges involve temptation, these overweight individuals are allowed to pursue weight loss goals in a safe and nurturing situation for the most part, supported by a team of professionals and their peers. They do, in a sense, become a family unit or team, guided by the shared goal of wanting a better quality of life. There is no doubt that it is easier to achieve your goals in this very structured and isolated situation.

That's why you need to create a home (and away-from-home) environment that follows the HFL program. Think of it as setting up your own positive reality TV show environment! I know how tough temptation and emotions can be, how hard it is to shift ingrained habits, how discouraging a setback can feel, and how depressing failure can be. That's why you need to embrace habits that will make you feel better—and why you need support to succeed.

A team effort yields a superior outcome. We all need support, cheerleaders, mentors, and those who will force us to get real with our weight and health issues. Your family can be your most powerful tool in the challenge to change habits, get healthy, and/or lose weight.

So stop investing in a series of ridiculous health crazes. Stop accepting short-term success only to realize repeated failures. Stop yo-yo dieting, and stop putting your health and the health of your kids at risk. Genuine health and weight maintenance requires dedication to a set of rules. If you want to use vanity as your starting goal, my hope is that, over time, health becomes your long-term goal. We all know the person who survives a heart attack and is suddenly ready to do anything to live. My hope is that this book has convinced you that you and your family are in a very serious situation, possibly a health disaster waiting to happen. But with the HFL program, you have the power to turn that around—and become a Healthy Family for Life!

Secrets for Changing Kids' and Teens' Habits

....

Creating Healthy Habits
Without Causing Tantrums

....

I suspect that some of you who have purchased this book are jumping right to this chapter for answers. How do I get a five-year-old to eat vegetables—any vegetables? How do I get a hostile fifteen-year-old to want to come on a weekend family hike? What about all the time my kids spend away from home—how can I control those hours?

So let's get right to some answers. There are four invaluable HFL guidelines for parents to adopt in the battle to preserve their kids' health:

1. The Family Is a Team.
2. Mealtime Is Family Time.
3. Let's Negotiate.
4. No Means No.

Now let me explain how each of these four principles plays a role in your efforts to create a Healthy Family for Life.

The Family Is a Team. I continue to emphasize the team concept because when you diet or try to make a major change in habits, solitude can be a stumbling block along the way to long-term success. You and your family need an environment that involves everybody working toward the same goals. Kids and teens especially need this support.

Keeping the family team as your constant mental framework will help you. Kids will be particularly challenging to work with because

THE HEALTH CONSEQUENCES OF CHILDHOOD OBESITY

Through this book, a number of health consequences of childhood obesity have been mentioned repeatedly to highlight how much weight and health issues are interrelated. Here are the health issues by body system:

- *Cardiovascular*: Hypertension, left ventricular hypertrophy, atherosclerosis, high total cholesterol/LDL, low HDL, high blood pressure.
- *Metabolic:* Insulin resistance, dyslipidemia, metabolic syndrome, type 2 diabetes.
- *Pulmonary:* Asthma, obstructive sleep apnea, shortness of breath with exertion.
- *Gastrointestinal:* Gastroesophageal reflux, non-alcoholic fatty liver disease, gallstones.
- *Skeletal:* Blount disease (bowed knees), slipped capital-femoral epiphysis, flat feet.
- *Psychosocial:* Depression.
- *Gynecological:* Early puberty, polycystic ovary syndrome.

HOW MANY CALORIES DO KIDS NEED?

	SEDENTARY		MODERATELY ACTIVE		ACTIVE	
AGES:	GIRL	BOY	GIRL	BOY	GIRL	BOY
2–3	1000	1000	1000–1400	1000–1400	1000–1400	1000–1400
4–8	1200	1400	1400–1600	1400–1600	1400–1800	1600–2000
9–13	1600	1800	1600–2000	1800–2200	1800–2200	2000–2600
14–18	1800	2200	2000	2400–2800	2400	2800–3200

Source: Dietary Guidelines for Americans

even though you may introduce the program as "something the whole family will be doing together," change can be upsetting, threatening, disconcerting—in some cases, frightening to young children and even to older kids or teens. Don't be surprised if kids act up, become defiant, try to play off one parent for sympathy, or "cheat" on the food program. Just don't respond by demanding that every little thing be handled exactly YOUR way. There is no right or wrong way to go about HFL changes. If you are striving for some personal ideal, that's fine as long as you don't set the bar for change too high and don't force your idea of success on your spouse or kids. It's my philosophy to go about making changes at a slow, steady pace because when change happens gradually, it is more palatable.

You are a family, and you approach the HFL program as teammates who support each other—but that doesn't mean everyone will do things exactly the same way and at the same time. Younger kids may want to emulate Mom and Dad who decide to implement their personal changes in a paced and structured way. Teens may have to be wooed a bit. Most commonly, you will find you can change your habits at one pace while the kids get on board on their own terms, at their own pace. Other than my recommendation that you set up the kitchen with many of the *plan and prepare* rules in mind, you have to decide which Family Rules you will enforce in the early weeks of implementing the HFL program. Here are several I recommend:

- No sabotaging of others' efforts.
- Anyone not ready to participate still eats the food being prepared or the back-up foods available on the homefront.
- Food that's not part of the plan should not be brought into the home.
- If kids are old enough, they may still be doing their own thing outside the home in terms of food choices, but once they're on home turf, you, as the parent, have the right to control the environment.

At some point, most kids begin to participate because being part of the family team is ultimately what they desire; they do want Mom and Dad's support, encouragement, and positive feedback—it simply feels good. They also, believe it or not, want Mom and Dad involved. I know this because most families I've worked with over

---

CHOOSE SIX

If I somehow had to choose the "super six" HFL habits for kids to focus on initially when instituting the HFL program, they would be:

- Eating more fruits and vegetables daily
- Reclassifying sweets as "treats" designed to be eaten less often
- Ditching the drive-through
- Instituting controls over TV viewing and video gaming time
- Equipping the house for exercise—putting up a basketball hoop, buying some balls, jump ropes, a Hula-Hoop®, skates
- Getting the family moving on the weekend

the years have an "Aha moment" when the kids say, "I wanted to eat more together—I wanted to share more together—I wanted to hike and play ball and take classes together—I hate being overweight—I wanted to help in the kitchen and weigh in on choices—I wanted to let my mom or dad know that I was unhappy with the way things were—and I couldn't." If you were a disconnected family before, which is a family behavior pattern often associated with weight issues, then this new approach could well encourage togetherness and be very intriguing, even to teens.

Mealtime Is Family Time. Eating meals together allows the family to unite at the end of the day and share with each other—so good for mental health and self-esteem. Kids who eat with their families tend to get better grades, gain less weight, and are less likely to value peer group over family opinion. So when you begin to adopt the habit of eating together as a family on a regular basis, it may even over-shadow poor food choices. The very act of coming together has profound health benefits. Research has shown that:

- The more often families share meals together, the less likely teens are to smoke, drink, get depressed, or have eating disorders, and the more likely they are to get good grades and even delay having sex.
- The more often a family eats together, the better the experience of being together gets, while the less often a family eats together, the worse the experience gets and the less healthy the food is likely to be.
- If families eat more meals together, that often means fewer fried foods and less soda and more fruits and vegetables, according to a report in the *Archives of Family Medicine* in 2006.

The studies also revealed that many of the teens who ate three or fewer meals a week with their families actually wished they would eat together more often—I have found this myself when interviewing families. That's why I came to realize over time that coming together as a family, planning together as a family, and eating together as a family holds such importance when you are dealing with teens and teen eating habits. They may seem to be distant and even downright belligerent and uncommunicative, but internally they are struggling with many issues, and family mealtime can be quite a supportive experience. I have also found that when eating is going on, sometimes communication is truly facilitated. Mealtime can become an opportunity for families to deal with school issues and personal issues even while developing better eating habits and choices.

Miriam Weinstein, author of *The Surprising Power of Family Meals*, suggests that teen children let their parents off the hook a bit too quickly. Because the teen scene going on in households can be fraught with tension and full of arguments and accusations of nagging, parents will often give up on suggesting having meals together with their teens, and teens go along with it. Well, the CASA study found that a recent Arizona State University study of 6,400 teens showed that those who came from families with healthy habits—like eating breakfast in the morning—were 33 percent less likely to be overweight.

Unfortunately, the family dinner today is often lost to the late hours working parents keep, to after-school activities, to time spent in front of the television or computer. Many parents let different people eat dinner at several times and according to their individual needs and tastes, and have given up on any family rules about turning the TV off, gathering together, or eating the same foods.

If you're following the HFL program, you are going to be serving better quality, more nutritious foods, which is a great start. You also want to engage your kids while they are helping to set the table or portion out food: "How was your day? Anything good happen today? Anything special you learned today? Anything you need from me for school tomorrow?" Let them decide which days (I recommend two or three days a week to start) will be *designated* "No with a Smile" treat days, for that special dessert that is supposed to be portion controlled, savored, and enjoyed slowly. Use the time together at meals to let them weigh in on what they do and don't like about the meal so everybody feels like they have a say in the food planning. Give them a sense of ownership or major involvement by letting them pick an "ethnic or buffet night" so there are fun nights where

INSTEAD OF EATING, GET YOUR KIDS TO DO THIS

- Walk the dog.
- Help you to clean out closets (finding old stuff in the back can be fun).
- Select recipes/go buy new recipe books.
- Organize a room (garage, bathroom).
- Plan weekend activities.
- Search out new farmers' markets.
- Map out some new hiking trails.
- Try a new sport or activity together——bowling, belly dancing, yoga.
- Take photos of each family member, date them, and create a scrapbook for charting appearance changes.

they feel they were in charge of the food choices. And again, remember that though you'd like them to choose better-quality "No with a Smile" treats (a low-fat ice cream sandwich instead of a milk chocolate bar), they do get to choose which treats they want—you get to decide frequency and portion size.

Let's Negotiate. Negotiations are important with youngsters and teens because when it comes to food and habits that are already ingrained, you—the parent—will need to look for changes that may not be black and white. You need to pick and choose battles, decide what is really an important behavior change milestone, and what habits or behaviors can be given a pass. You'll need to negotiate new tastes, new meals, and new behaviors creatively—don't just force issues. Be willing to talk it through. "Let's make a deal" may become part of your daily vernacular.

PICKY EATER TRICKS: TURN YUCK INTO YUM

Don't let the picky or unwilling taster or eater defeat you. Here are some tips to help you get over that hurdle:

- Put the "rejected" fruits and veggies out daily on the table; kids need to keep seeing it in order to be willing to try it.
- Let the kids see you eating the suspect foods frequently.
- Display the foods differently—get creative and spear them with toothpicks, cut them up in shapes, use them to make faces (like on an open-face peanut butter sandwich).
- Add purées of them in small amounts to food and then—after they've eaten it a few times—let the kids know they've eaten it and "survived." Down the road, share the actual recipe with them. If they react to the "surprise ingredients," you can let them know it was simply a recipe that they seemed to enjoy and talk about the fact that sometimes using foods they don't like in recipes offers nutritional benefits without making them actually taste the undesired food.
- Make interesting dips for fruits and veggies, but they can only have dip if they actually use the veggies to dip.
- Depending on age, use a reward system and let them amass points for eating a fruit or veggie they have previously rejected. I used a deck of cards and let the child take one card from a particular suit for each new food added to their repertoire. When the kids amassed a full suit—thirteen new foods added to their food repertoire—they would get a small reward. With older kids, give small gifts, movie passes, or even a little time added to curfew.

Here are just a few ways to make compromises and encourage gradual change:

- Start with smaller desserts like mini-size treats if they are used to lots of processed snacks and are really resistant to the changes going on around them.
- Do discuss a "close the kitchen after dinner" policy, with only fruit and zero-calorie beverages allowed after dinner.
- Remember to give individual non-food rewards for small successes, as well as "team family rewards." In order to change habits, you will have to choose rewards selectively (but never hesitate to reward kids with a verbal compliment).
- Let your kids call family meetings whenever they're unhappy about some of the changes being implemented.
- Encourage flexibility. If someone does not like a certain plan or prep job, be willing to shift or defer responsibilities.
- Wean kids off unhealthy snacks with a healthy food with a small amount of "tasty topping." Create and keep small bags of ready-to-grab toppings in the pantry, such as crushed nuts and cereal, dried fruit, and crushed whole grain graham crackers for use on fat-free yogurts or small servings of cottage cheese or just to be eaten with fat-free milk. Or make sprinkles mixes with high-fiber and high-protein cereals, dried fruit and cereal, nuts, Bran Buds®, and mini dark chocolate chips.

No Means No. The "No" word is really hard for most parents, but it is crucial to the HFL program. Ideally, you will want to determine in advance which rules (and there shouldn't be too many) are absolutes and which are up for negotiation. Most parents also don't realize that there are many, many ways of saying No. You silently say No when you don't bring certain foods into your pantry and fridge; you also say No when you are active and *not sitting* in front of the TV; you clearly say No by pushing the bread basket aside in a restaurant—but especially when you hand it back to the waiter to remove the temptation to graze on it mindlessly.

When parents tell me, "I don't want to be the mean parent who always says No," I advise them that the way they set up their home

WHEN TO GO ORGANIC

I think that choosing organic foods has value, especially when you're feeding kids, because many researchers believe that the very young are especially vulnerable to pesticides, dyes and chemicals, preservatives, and hormones. If going totally organic is too pricey, consider buying organic fruits and milk at least.

Here are some foods to consider buying "organic" because of pesticide levels: apples, bell peppers, celery, cherries, grapes, nectarines, peaches, pears, potatoes, red raspberries, spinach, and strawberries (called the *dirty dozen* because of their pesticide content), whole wheat or whole grain crackers, cereals, bread, flour, milk, cheese, yogurt, beef, and lamb (because of possible hormones).

environment can say No in ways that are quite subtle, not adversarial.

Here's an example of saying No and negotiating. When little Dylan says, "I want the sweet cereal I see in the commercial NOW, Mommy," you can easily tell him that you don't buy that cereal on a regular basis because you need to eat mostly Yes Foods like fruits and veggies and Maybe So Foods like whole grain cereals, which are all in the pantry. But you promise the next time you go shopping you'll get Dylan a small box of that cereal, which he can have as a special treat or use as topping on the really yummy, healthy cereal you do keep at home.

Dylan learns patience, which, by the way, is vital to a happy existence. He learns he can have it, but it is now a designated No with a Smile treat. He learns that Mommy really cares about him and wants to give him foods that are good for him and that taste good. He also needs to see you be a role model of the behavior. Otherwise, forget about it. Dylan will get this message: "Mommy says this cereal is bad for me, but she's eating doughnuts, so I guess when I get a little older and I'm big like Mommy, then I can eat like Mommy." That's the ultimate confounding, confusing, very damaging, mixed message that has to stop.

Five Mistakes to Avoid

Mistakes and parenthood seem to go together—we all make them and we hope our kids survive! But let me make the HFL program easier for you by outlining some common mistakes so you can avoid them as you help your kids create better nutrition and activity habits:

1. Being Too Rigid

Diet-obsessed parents, moms in particular, can create a rigid environment that backfires and actually causes their children to hide eating, hoard food, and ultimately gain weight. A mother who constantly berates her child or who condemns her own personal body image is not practicing HFL principles; she is modeling dangerous behaviors that often lead to serious weight and behavior issues in their kids. Studies from the American Dietetic Association and Harvard Medical School

PLAY THE STONE AGE GAME WITH YOUR KIDS

One of the easiest ways for your kids to grasp the HFL program is to play a game with them. Ask them to imagine what people ate in the Stone Age. Their list should include: nuts, berries, veggies, beans, fish, and meat. When just considering those foods, ask them to look at their daily diet and see how many "real foods" they eat (like the food Stone Age people ate) and how many "fake foods" they eat. It's a great way to start the dialogue about the choices you're making about food and how their choices will affect their long-term health and weight.

reveal that girls who observe their mothers dieting frequently are likely to be acutely aware of their weight and may get a disordered message about the need to be thin. These messages can backfire and lead to out-of-control eating, overeating, hoarding, and other behaviors intended to defy the healthy principles their mothers are espousing. Or they can result in the need to constantly strive to lose weight, like Mom is trying to do. Parents, especially mothers, need to understand that even the youngest children receive body image messages from their parents' direct behaviors. Even though we want our kids to be of normal weight and healthy, a mother who is too rigid can actually create an environment that leads to overweight children. Lead by example—sit down with the kids to eat a healthy and balanced breakfast, eat healthy snacks with them, take a walk with them—it can be one of the most important life (and HFL) lessons a parent can model to a child.

2. Using Time as an Excuse

Ask a parent why Dylan has a bag of Cheetos® and a fruit drink in his hand as he goes off in carpool in the afternoon, and you'll hear

OBESE KIDS AND HEART DISEASE

Studies show that kids who are at risk for obesity or who are already seriously overweight or obese show signs of heart disease similar to obese adults with heart disease:[1] a change in the actual motion of the heart muscles as they contract and relax. Researchers normally expect these changes to be present only in adults with long-term obesity. Apparently, these changes can occur in younger people who have been obese for much shorter periods of time. So teenagers with obesity or serious weight issues show decreased myocardial performance, making early intervention with a plan like HFL absolutely vital. You do not want lifestyle choices to lead to these serious consequences.

something like: "I just didn't have time to get anything else on the run and he has to eat something." This isn't a time problem—it's a priority problem. If one of our primary values is not making sure our kids have healthy food most of the time, then we are not meeting one of our core responsibilities as parents: the safety of our children. The consequences of not learning the difference between a red and a green traffic light are easy to grasp—you could cross the road at the wrong time and be struck by a car. The consequences of not learning the difference between Yes (green light) Foods and No (red light) Foods are more subtle because cholesterol accumulation and elevated blood sugar levels are "hidden."

If your children are allowed to eat without boundaries, snack with the TV on, drink sugary fruit and soda beverages, or have fast food regularly, it's causing silent and insidious changes to your children's health and weight. It's well worth the time it takes to teach them healthy habits.

3. Waiting for Your Doctor

It's important to note that one of the important failures of the whole nutrition regulatory picture may be the inaction of your pediatrician or family doctor. Many physicians are still unwilling or unable to engage in discussions with parents about lifestyle choices, excess weight, and the health impact they have, especially if a) the parents themselves are overweight or appear sensitive to these issues being discussed, b) the parents are unwilling to dialogue about their child's weight issues, c) they feel it will cause parents or the child pain or humiliation, or d) they feel the family will leave the practice.

There are other practical issues. A wellness discussion takes time, especially if the doctor needs to tread carefully with a family's response to the discussion, and the physician's schedule just may not accommodate it. Insurance may not cover a referral to a dietician or nutritionist. The whole topic may be uncomfortable. I know very well how hard it is to discuss poor or downright dangerous parenting—no one wants to be told they are a bad parent.

The bottom line is that you can't wait for your doctor to take the lead or solve your problems. Don't get frozen in denial; take an active role in enlisting your physician's help.

4. Ignoring the TV Factor

Your children's TV habits affect them in a variety of ways. If they are watching TV, they're not moving, so they are missing opportunities to burn off calories. If they are watching TV while eating, they are not engaged with their food and may overeat because they are not conscious of how much they are eating and subsequent satiation. Also, advertisements are designed with your child in mind. Your children will clamor to buy fast food that comes with a toy, to buy cereal that has their favorite cartoon figure on it, to buy the luscious high-sugar, high-fat food they can almost taste through the screen. They'll want the foods that come in the pretty packages, the ones that have mail-away offers, the ones their favorite celebrities are touting.

You can have a profound impact on your children's food values and attitudes. The topics you discuss with them, the examples you set, the behaviors you model—particularly when it comes to nutrition—can enhance their health and well-being. An engaged and skillful parent will be the very best educator a child can have. You are the role model to whom they look. If you are drinking meal replacement shakes in their presence, they will take note; if you tell them they cannot sit for hours and play computer games and then you sit for hours with your BlackBerry® personal digital assistant— they will take note. If you tell them the kitchen is closed for the evening and then sit and munch all night—they will take note. Overweight or obese parents tend to underestimate what they eat, overestimate how many calories they burn, ignore the amount of time they spend in front of the TV or in other sedentary pursuits, and then hand off these behaviors to their children. Most health experts are increasingly concerned about the number of sedentary hours children and adults spend in front of the TV. Parents who don't control the TV will be failing in one of the most important lifestyle sectors. The TV should not be turned on during a meal, should not be available in a child's bedroom, should not be used frequently as a babysitter, and should be monitored in terms of total number of viewing hours/day.

COMMENTS THAT CAN ENCOURAGE EATING DISORDERS OR SELF-ESTEEM ISSUES

Even gentle, well-intentioned comments that come out of love or concern may help to trigger an eating disorder. You want your kids motivated by health and positive reasoning; you do not want to increase the likelihood of dangerous dieting or other destructive habits.

Try to avoid comments like:

1. You're big-boned compared to your brother.
2. Maybe this new diet/equipment/supplement will help.
3. I also hated my body when I was your age.
4. You are so clearly talented at this sport—taking off a little weight would really crank it up a notch.
5. You look wonderful—have you lost a lot of weight?

Whether you realize it or not, this is how your teen interprets these comments:

1. You are so much fatter than your brother.
2. You so need help that I'll buy anything to get you to lose weight.
3. You should feel bad because I did when I was a fat child.
4. You need to get better (leaner) so do it at any cost.
5. You looked so awful before so even if you are suffering—keep it up.

FAMILY FITNESS MAKEOVER

Here are some ideas and guidelines for activities by age:

Three months to eighteen months: Consider water workouts playing in the pool gently with the infant, floor playtime, or chasing your baby (crawling or running).

Eighteen months to five years: You can dance with the kids, play ball games, do gymnastics, or even use a small trampoline.

Five to eight years: Create backyard treasure hunts; go for family hikes; spend time at the beach running on the sand and in playtime, have winter snowball fights and build snowmen; use the local park and playground.

Eight to thirteen years: Try biking, jogging, soccer, basketball, or tennis. Remember what activities gave you joy as a kid and do them now with your own child or try something new together. If your child is in an organized sport, run or jog the sidelines while you watch.

Over thirteen: In addition to the suggestions for ages eight to thirteen, find out if your child is willing to prep for a 5K or join a weekend parent-child league. Ask older kids if they'll go to the gym with you and work out or take a class, or work on home projects with you.

5. Letting Weight Be Your Only Guide

Earlier in the book, I mentioned TOFIs—people who are "fat on the inside," meaning their fat deposits are accumulating around vital organs. Kids can certainly fall into this group and appear quite slim to the naked eye. But they may be developing fatty plaque in their arteries, or mild hypertension, or the beginning of insulin resistance.

These problems would typically remain undetected unless your doctor specifically tested for them or there was a catastrophic health event.

We need to stop viewing our kids solely by their weight, BMI, or waist measurements. Different children in the same family can show different physical responses to poor quality food or too much food due to their genetic makeup, particularly their metabolic rates. Although it's obvious when one child is gaining too much weight, for other children, the impact of lifestyle choices can remain hidden.

The autopsies of teen car crash victims are revealing dramatic internal deterioration due to the plaque accumulating in their arteries. Though appearances offer one way to spot poor lifestyle habits, they are not the whole story when you are assessing the true health damage report.

"LATE FOR CARPOOL" BREAKFAST-TO-GO FOR KIDS

1. Use yogurt as your base and add berries or cut-up fruit or dried fruit, nuts, whole grain cereal. Put it in a cup to go.
2. Take a wrap and add peanut butter, cut-up banana, raisins, or apple slices.
3. Make a smoothie with non-fat yogurt, frozen berries, some whey protein powder, and a splash of juice. Use a straw and thermos or portable coffee mug. One great recipe (serves 4): 1 14-ounce can pumpkin, 1 cup fat-free milk, 2 tablespoons maple syrup, 1/4 teaspoon nutmeg, 1/2 teaspoon cinnamon, 1 teaspoon vanilla extract, 1 cup ice. Blend together and top with Redi-Whip® fat-free whipped cream (88 calories/2 grams fat per serving).
4. Top an English muffin with tomato sauce and low-fat shredded cheese and put it in a small plastic container.

Kids Need to Be Active

Getting your kids moving is a big part of creating an HFL lifestyle. Kids need a minimum of ninety minutes of high-energy movement daily. That can mean disciplined exercise plus fun activities plus anything else you can think of to keep them in motion and not sitting: helping with housework, washing the car, mowing the lawn, walking to and from school, choosing the stairs rather than elevators or escalators at the mall. I think every child should be on a sports team or involved in a discipline like karate for the exercise and self-esteem benefits they offer. Teams are a good way to get them used to making exercise part of their lives.

Don't limit yourself or your kids to formal sports activities or indoor gym memberships as ways to get moving. Going to playgrounds and sandy beaches, playing with a Hula-Hoop®, jumping rope, running with the dog, gardening, or building home projects are all ways to get fun activity into your lives. Put up a basketball hoop, get a trampoline—just find ways to get daily activity into your lives. Fitness doesn't have to mean athletics.

In November 2007, the American College of Sports Medicine (ACSM) announced a new campaign aimed at getting doctors to "prescribe exercise" to adult patients at every possible opportunity.

BEVERAGE TIPS FOR KIDS

- If you choose juice, use four ounces as a serving and make sure it is pure or 100% juice.
- Calcium-fortified orange juice is a great way to help your kids meet daily calcium needs. Just watch portion sizes and frequency.
- Make a glass of *supermilk* daily by adding some non-fat powdered milk (up to 1/4 cup of this protein-rich powder) to a cup of non-fat milk.

Pediatricians need to give the same prescription for kids of all ages. That means babies that can crawl should not be sitting in playpens for hours and toddlers should not be sitting in front of the TV—not even educational TV—for hours. Parents need to model active behavior. If you don't do it, your kids will think you're a hypocrite and they'll be right!

For many kids or teens, what motivates them is their personal "Aha" moment—a transformative event that changes their self-image with regard to weight or exercise. It can happen during a serious talk with a pediatrician or other health professional, an athletic moment where they fail due to excess weight or are told their performance could improve if they lose weight. It might be an embarrassing moment like being told they are too fat to date or being called cruel names or being excluded from a clique. The result is usually the start of a change in diet and exercise patterns.

At the 2007 annual meeting of the Eastern Society for Pediatric Medicine, the results of one of the studies presented clearly demonstrated that teenagers who lost weight often had had a transformative event. It was also clear that the kids who experienced this as their motivation to lose weight were more successful than kids "who just thought it was time." The study also noted that the teens who had experienced a transformative event who engaged in lifestyle change often included changes in diet and exercise habits.

Talking to Your Kids

Asking questions is another great technique for engaging with kids, both for parents and physicians. Examples include:

- Are you concerned about your weight or your health?
- Has your weight caused you difficulties?
- Does your weight affect your ability to pursue the things that are important to you (sports, friendships, goals)?

When kids begin to answer those questions, it can then lead to a desire for self-management. Kids will only change when they are ready, which comes from an internal desire to do something about their weight or health. If they are ready for a change, use a series of open-ended questions to spur dialogue:

- What do you want to do about this situation?
- What do you think may be the roadblocks to being success-ful (at weight loss, improved health, more energy)?
- Where do you want to go from here? Shall we make a plan?

Maybe they will ask for a meeting with a dietician or some home exercise equipment, or want to get involved in shopping and plan-ning meals. These kinds of questions can get the discussion moving forward. The next step is an action plan. You can then begin to share the HFL principles and involve them in putting those principles into action.

WHEN TO USE STEALTH

I'm a big fan of being real, so I don't necessarily encourage stealth or deception when it comes to kids and eating. How-ever, I do know that including healthy ingredients that kids may not be aware of is beneficial. I'd call it "Mom's health magic." My kids never knew that the brownies I'd been making for twenty-five years have puréed prunes in them—it makes the chocolate taste even more intense. (They did wonder why after dessert they'd "have to go.") I puréed veggies and added them to turkey loaf and tomato sauces. I've made veggie and fruit muffins, and I'm a big fruit smoothie creator. The value of including these sometimes less-popular foods in recipes is worth the effort involved.

That doesn't mean you shouldn't also put the fruits and veggies on the table. I encourage you always to have a salad and steamed veggies available as well, because kids still need to learn to incorporate these foods into their diet themselves.

You don't want to make it a battle and you do want to avoid making eating a negative experience. React to your kids' negative reaction to the menu plan, entrée, or choices being offered with a calm and patient attitude: A great response is, *"Okay, when you are hungry, there are cut-up carrots in the fridge with hummus dip or apples and peanut butter or yogurt and crackers—you take it when you're ready."* In most cases, they will grab it when they're hungry enough. During the transition period of introducing the HFL program in your home, be prepared for kids refusing to try something new and have some simple alternatives already prepared. Ignore the desire to gush with praise when they finally start eating healthful food, but do acknowledge their good choices.

Talking about true hunger versus other reasons to eat will help your child create better food relationships. When it comes to teens, remember the obvious temptations of dieting to look good or overeating in the name of growth and athletic prowess. Make sure they know that if they are eating and exercising in a healthy manner, they'll be able to lose and maintain weight without damage to their health, and that small increases in healthy protein portions or an extra serving of whole grain carbs supports muscle growth more effectively than eating humongous portions of fast food.

If they had been involved in talking about food since they were little kids, this conversation would be a no-brainer by this point. But reworking ingrained habits in older kids and teens has to be done over time, with as much dialogue and education as possible. The last thing you want to do is try to order them around. While you are setting up a new way to interact with food, be prepared to go slowly.

I can tell you that teens I saw in my practice years ago when I helped their families form new habits have let me know that now, as adults, they are bringing those habits into their homes right from the start. They want their memories of childhood eating to be replaced with memories of teen habits that were newly learned but very special because it involved the family working together, enjoying wonderful meals that everyone had a hand in, and sensing their families coming together. They also don't want their kids to struggle like they did with weight issues and bad habits.

Understanding What They Go Through

You need to understand what your kids face when they leave home every day, especially older teens, who have easy access to outside food. Unless the food program at their school has undergone a dramatic shift, most school lunch programs offer high-fat, processed foods in large portions with high-fat dressings, chips, and juices on the side. Kids are moving less in school, so unless they are on a sports team, they are not burning calories during school hours. They have access to fast food and convenience stores and all the other kids are eating this food, so your kids will be anomalies if they decide to follow HFL guidelines outside the home. They'll be watching their

MANAGING TV TIME

- Make rules—no TV during meals or until homework is done. Require them to do some physical activity before dinnertime.
- Create a TV budget for the week with a certain amount on school nights and a bit more on weekends but have solid viewing numbers pre-established—don't budge on this one.
- Use TV time wisely. For every pure entertainment half-hour, they should watch a half-hour of educational programming—Animal Planet, cooking shows, decorating shows, etc.
- View it together as much as possible so you can monitor commercials that relate to food and discuss them.
- Keep TVs in cabinets that close.
- Avoid using TV as a babysitter.
- Allow no TV time at all for children less than two years old. I know that sounds harsh, but they should be moving constantly at that age.
- Never put a TV in a child's bedroom.

friends downing high-fat/high-sugar blended drinks, sugary sodas, doughnuts, burgers, fries, chips, and other No Foods daily.

If your child is overweight, he or she may also be dealing with ridicule, embarrassment, loss of self-esteem, depression, and other emotions that can complicate the already-difficult teen years. Can you imagine the mortification of having to undress in front of your peers, squeeze into a bathing suit, or try to wedge yourself into a movie theater seat when you are overweight? If you are an overweight parent who was an overweight kid, you know it well. Why would you want your kid to go through that? If a crystal ball could show you some of the prejudice they may experience because the world's cruelty to the seriously overweight and the diseases associated with this condition, how could you want to lead your child down this dangerous, unforgiving path?

Children as young as three report teasing, bullying, rejection, and other negative experiences because of their weight. Studies show there also may be subtle bias among parents and teachers, a kind of ongoing subtle pity and sympathy reaction that puts these children into a situation similar to people with cancer—I compare it to "pity the poor child" syndrome. Overweight kids are two to three times more likely to report suicidal thoughts. Whether you want to face it or not, and whether your child is talking about it or not, it is likely that he or she is being stigmatized, and it is probably an unrelenting assault.[2]

A 1999 study of 115 middle- and high-school teachers found that 20 percent of those teachers said they believed overweight or obese kids were *untidy, less likely to succeed, and more emotional.* This again supports that subtle pitying reaction that teachers will feel for these kids, who they perceive have less ability to succeed. Sylvia Rimm, author of *Rescuing the Emotional Lives of Overweight Children*, surveyed more than 5,000 middle-school kids and found that the overweight kids felt less intelligent, less popular, and really like "a different species." They can actually sense their teachers' pitying behavior; their fellow students tend to be more cruel.

'Tween girls (pre-teens between the ages of nine and twelve) are especially at risk for becoming overweight. A report in the *Journal of Pediatrics* in January 2007 highlighted the serious consequences of this. Chubby 'tweens experience heightened blood pressure and cholesterol levels (early precursors to heart disease), which takes a toll on the health of their arteries because of that cholesterol or plaque that forms. These problems are reversible if you shift their lifestyle habits; otherwise, serious complications like coronary artery disease and diabetes continue to develop. Being overweight at that stage meant a tenfold risk of these girls going on to be overweight adults with all the associated health complications. One explanation for these problems among 'tween girls may be that this is an age where kids are eating out of the home a lot more, so outside eating opportunities and the way their friends eat may have a direct impact on weight. Girls at this age no longer like to "get sweaty," so any exercise or physical activity they might have enjoyed previously may start to disappear as well.

In January 2007, a report in the journal *Pediatrics* revealed that by age nine, 7.4 percent of white girls and 17.4 percent of black girls are already overweight. Between ages nine and twelve, another 2–5 percent of 'tweens who were not already overweight become over-

YOUR KIDS ARE WATCHING YOU

Teens are watching what you do in the kitchen and beyond. They are typically taking mental notes on:

- Exactly what you eat.
- How you cook (or don't).
- What you do (and don't) buy.
- The rules you follow regarding eating and meals.
- Your concerns about nutrition.
- Family meal patterns.
- Whether you eat in front of the TV, on the go, or not at all (miss meals).
- Your relationship to food. Are you an emotional eater, a mindless snacker, a food sneak?

weight. This is an age at which there is extremely high risk for both weight and health issues, and we need to reach these kids them fast. Using the four P's and involving all kids (but especially kids in this age group), talking to them, and emphasizing why you are making these lifestyle changes can be a huge turning point for 'tween girls.

A Word About Babies and Toddlers

Pediatricians know that babies initially *self-regulate* when it comes to appetite and eating. You cannot get them to eat another mouthful if they are full—they will spit out the food. But in their second year of life, toddlers begin to respond to cues other than hunger and fullness. Social cues begin to come in to play. *If Mom is giving me more and it tastes really good, well then, I'll have more. If everyone else is taking seconds, I want to be like them.* Because the huge growth spurts that a child has experienced will slow down a bit at this age, anything that messes with the innate hunger/fullness cues can lead to abnormal weight gain. Toddlers actually need *fewer* calories per kilogram of body weight than infants, but from the way most American parents feed their kids and agonize over so-called picky eaters, it's clear they don't know that.

As they get older, toddlers naturally become pickier about what they eat, so if you decide "I need to get my children to eat at all costs" and bribe them to eat with less healthy foods or foods with higher sugar/fat content, you will create children who prefer processed food quite easily.

An eight-year study at the University of Tennessee determined that most kids develop and establish their food preferences as early as age two. If you consistently offer poor quality foods rather than fruits, vegetables, whole grains, lean meats, and low-fat or fat-free dairy products, don't be surprised if your child is exclusively interested in these processed foods by age four.

If kids are playing at and eating at McDonald's®, Burger King®, Carl's Jr.®, and other fast food haunts frequently, that will be what they want on a regular basis. Early exposure to intensely sweet foods has long-term consequences. If your child becomes accustomed to the sweet and tart tastes of fruits at an early age, that will be their measure of flavor and sweetness. Offer them repeated exposures to concentrated sweets in the form of processed foods and high-sugar drinks, and that's their new measure of satisfaction, and nothing else will quite measure up. Nothing is sweeter than high fructose corn syrup (HFCS), the number one sweetener in many processed foods.

The bottom line is that there is clearly a critical period in a child's development for establishing healthy eating patterns, a window of opportunity between the time when you breast- or bottle-feed a child and the time when school lunches begin. During this time, too many parents choose foods they know kids will like and eat, which typically are high-fat or highly processed foods, instead of relaxing and just letting kids signal which fruits and veggies they do and don't like, preparing baked potatoes, or supplying other finger foods like healthy cereals, beans, and other simple foods.

We also tend not to offer kids foods that we personally dislike. I know parents who shun veggies; therefore, their kids don't get offered a whole lot of them. In my case, I was not a big fan of hard and soft cheeses, and frankly I think most kids can live without those high-fat choices. I'm also not a fan of cottage cheese, but I intentionally gave my kids low-fat cottage cheese as one of their dairy servings so they'd have a chance to decide for themselves.

By the time children are two or three, they are forming a lot of their food preferences. Before that point, they need repeated exposures to lots of flavors in order to expand their repertoire of food choices. And let's also remember there is no particular reason baby food needs to be bland. Parents in many cultures serve their children dishes prepared with many different spices—South Asian parents offer curries, Hispanic parents offer salsas and other ethnic foods, etc.

It's important to note that most overweight toddlers will not shed their baby fat. Scientists at ten universities examined the records of 1,042 students whose height and weight were recorded seven times between the ages of two and twelve. In September 2006, their findings were published in the journal *Pediatrics*.[3] Findings included the fact that 80 percent of kids who were overweight or obese during their early school years were also overweight or obese at age twelve. Forty percent of kids who were at the fiftieth per-

PLAY THE SHOPPING GAME WITH YOUNG CHILDREN

Involve your kids in the food shopping experience:

1. Show them several fruit and veggie pictures and then have them find them at the store.
2. Ask them to find two new fruits and two new veggies they've never tried.
3. Have them describe the shape, color, and size of fruits and veggies.
4. Give them a pad to track all the different types of: mushrooms, potatoes, melons, apples, lettuces, and other fruit and vegetable groupings.
5. Ask them to find a new herb (fresh and/or dried).
6. Help them dissect a cereal label to find the highest fiber or protein cereal or lowest sugar count.

centile of weight or higher by age three were overweight or obese at age twelve; the more times a child reached the "overweight category" during the pre-school and elementary school years, the more likely it was that child would be overweight by age twelve.

By the time a kid is ten or twelve, you are fighting a difficult but not insurmountable problem. It's just much harder to retrain than to train from the beginning. HFL will help you establish a healthy home from inception, if you are new parents or creating a new milieu, such as in the case of a family in need of a makeover.

My older daughter was a ninety-fifth percentile weight (and height) child from the age of about nine months. She was breastfed exclusively until she was six months old, then exposed to many different foods while still being breastfed until she was fourteen months of age. Because I knew my own history with weight and my family profile, I made sure she was extremely active and introduced her to

MIX AND MATCH LUNCHES FOR SCHOOL OR HOME

Start with one of these: whole grain bread, whole wheat tortilla or wrap, whole grain mini bagel, whole grain English muffin or small roll, or a serving of high-protein pasta.

Then add one of these: Lean, low-sodium deli turkey, soy deli slices, tuna, sliced grilled chicken, egg salad, peanut butter and jelly (if your school allows peanut butter based on allergy rules).

Then top with some of these: Chopped broccoli, non-fat cheese, spinach leaves, grated cabbage, cucumber/tomato slices, shredded carrots, roasted peppers.

Then add some: Fat-free mayo, mustard, low-sugar ketchup, balsamic vinegar, non-fat Russian dressing, hummus, relish.

Also add in (one, two, or three snacks depending on age/activity level of child): baby carrots, raw broccoli/cauliflower, raisins, celery, non-fat dip, whole berries, pineapple spears, fat-free popcorn, baked potato, whole wheat pretzels, homemade trail mix, baked crackers, apple slices, small tangerine, fat-free yogurt/pudding, a bag of healthy cereal, soybeans, grapes, dehydrated fruit packs, unsweetened applesauce.

Beverage of choice: water, no-calorie flavored water, fat-free or 1 percent milk, iced tea.

(You can add additional ingredients to this easy outline and keep it handy so kids can make their own choices.)

Create your own lunch scheme and be realistic about portion sizes based on your kid's age and activity level. Older kids may need several small snacks—remember to count the number of Maybe So Foods you are using in snacks. Let your kids choose from these groupings and then add to the choices on the list based on their preferences and your own ideas.

tennis at around age seven. I followed the HFL principles of Yes, No, Maybe So Foods and she ate very little fast food. I am utterly convinced that though my husband is slim, and she may also share some of his gene pool (slim tendencies/faster metabolic rate) as well as mine, it was her commitment to a sport that requires daily practice that kept her slim. It helped motivate her to eat healthy choices, even outside the home, to support her energy and her performance. She found soda made her feel bloated and she felt "awful" the few times she had fast food and then tried to practice or play a match. I can't point to one specific habit but rather to the combination of HFL behaviors at home, lots of physical activity, and the HFL choices she makes outside the home that have helped to defy her genetic predisposition from my side of the family.

No Singling Out

As a parent, you can use the information from this chapter to help you approach the subject directly with your child or to enlist the help of a doctor or health professional. Remember that you, as the parent, want to *help* them out, not *single* them out. If they are not ready, all you can do is continue to try to involve them in the HFL program and model the behaviors you want from them.

Here's one final note about the diversity of kids within a family and how you handle the individual needs versus the needs and goals of the whole family and any rivalries that may occur. The reality is that different family members will have different reasons for needing the HFL program. You may be the family with the one "physically fat" child, but you need to make it clear to the other kids in the family that just because it isn't obvious, it doesn't mean they don't have internal fat or other serious health consequences due to their current eating and exercising habits. Ongoing dialogues are necessary so that one child is not rewarded more, so children don't feel negatively singled out, and so that any rivalries get handled. There's nothing wrong with a competitive family using challenges to get habits changed, but not at the expense of making someone feel that their pace of habit changes is slow, unhealthy, or unacceptable.

We no longer use the word "diabetic" because we don't want the condition to define the patient. By the same reasoning, I'm not sure I'm all for telling a child that they are obese or using the term as a single-word description. However, I am of the opinion that you do need to tell a child if they are "at risk of being overweight" or "already at risk for serious health conditions because of their extra weight," because both descriptions imply hope—"if you change x, y, and z—then you will no longer be at risk." I believe you have to say something, you have to be honest, and you have to offer support, comfort, and a plan they can grasp and implement. If you don't offer them reality, they cannot grasp the importance of changing habits— if you are cruel or too graphic without being hopeful, you risk damaging their self-esteem and creating a bleak picture that may seem too hard to cope with or inescapable.

HABITS OF TEENS WHO LOSE WEIGHT SUCCESSFULLY

- They take initiative.
- They get active.
- They get real about portion sizes and food quality.
- They use a family support system.
- They figure out a personal approach that works for them.
- They get connected with other teens or groups of people who lost weight.
- They do not rush the process.
- They use the scale but also other measures of success: improvements in athletic performance, daily quality of life, relationships, and self-confidence.

ARE YOUR KIDS OFF TO COLLEGE?

You may feel like there's no time to work with young adults on nutrition and exercise recommendations when they're heading off to college. You're too busy with "really serious stuff." Well, it doesn't get more serious than the food choices they're going to be making for the next four years, and whether or not they're planning to exercise something other than their computer fingers!

The beauty of HFL is that the changes can be going on at home while discussions take place anywhere. Here are some quick tips for helping the college-bound develop HFL habits:

- Take time the summer before they leave to get health screenings, weight/BMI/waist assessments.
- Discuss where and how they will approach meals: pre-paid meal plan, cooking in an apartment, a mixture of both?
- Visit the campus and see what food shopping and eating options are available.
- See if there is an on-campus gym, jogging track, or club nearby that they can join and offer to buy them a membership.
- See if there is a nutrition course on campus.
- Invest in a dorm room mini-fridge, toaster oven, blender, and microwave.
- Enroll them in a fruit-basket-a-month delivery service so you know they'll have fresh produce on hand.
- Send them monthly care packages with healthy snacks.
- Make sure they weigh in on menu plans for whenever they come home.

SUFFERING FROM "NATURE DEFICIT DISORDER"?

With shrinking green space and overscheduled lives, are you and your kids suffering from lack of exposure to some of nature's best playgrounds—our forests and parks? According to Richard Louv's book *Last Child in the Woods: Saving Our Children from Nature-Deficit Disorder,* there is a huge disconnect between our children and the great outdoors. How often do you go to the zoo, a park, for a hike in the forest, for a weekend or week in the great outdoors? A number of studies collectively show a positive association between outdoor play and favorable health outcomes. One study showed a 50 percent drop in hiking, walking, and fishing by kids between 1997 and 2003. Not only will kids experience increased activity outdoors (as opposed to in front of the keyboard or TV), but experiencing nature has a variety of other benefits:

- Reduced stress levels.
- The ability to focus on tasks more effectively.
- Enhanced emotional and social well-being as well as self-esteem through unstructured play, self-initiation, and interaction with nature in general.
- Opportunities for a variety of aerobic experiences because kids tend to run, climb, dash, and build things like little beavers outdoors.
- A chance to be physically engaged for an extended period of time: things like building a treehouse or sandcastle, hiking, or going on a scavenger hunt for samples of nature like flowers, plants, or bugs.

Take It from the Kids

I asked you a question at the beginning of the book: are you brave enough to face reality, abandon denial, and embrace the fact that your family is not in a healthy zone?

Maybe we all need a "shock and awe" campaign, like the one high school students suggested at the Young Epidemiology Scholars Competition in 2007, a gathering of talented youth from around the nation who brainstorm ways to deal with ongoing health issues. The students examined the rising rates of obesity and type 2 diabetes in kids and decided a grim campaign akin to those offered on subjects like drunk driving and smoking is needed to have an impact on this epidemic. The kids involved in the competition felt that "a void is filled with food" and everyone needs to look for something else to fill the void (of boredom, anxiety, depression, and other emotional extremes). They also felt participation in sports should be mandatory all through middle school and during the first two years of high school. They did feel that there should be both low- and high-intensity activities, so everyone could participate. Interestingly enough, they also felt that though the idea of a "magic pill to melt fat" would be quite something, the reality is that we need to make changes we can tolerate and do it slowly over time. They did feel exercise was the key to weight loss and better health, especially with kids. They also conjectured with a smile that one day maybe taste buds that prefer healthy food could be engineered. I'm all for that and I appreciate their insights at such a young age.

KNOW YOUR JUNK

With companies offering lighter versions, 100-calorie packs, lower fat/fat free, low-sugar snack options, you do need to really read labels to see just what is in those treats. For example:

	Frito Lay®		Kraft Foods Chips Ahoy!®		General Mills Cheddar	
	Lay's Classic vs. Baked Lay's®		Real chips vs. Thin crisps		Chex Mix® vs. 100 cal	
Amt.:	2.5 ounce	1.0 ounce	1.4 ounce	0.8 ounce	30g	23g
Fat:	2.5g	1.5g	9g	3g	4g	2.5g
Cal.:	380	130	190	100	130	100
Sodium:	480mg	170mg	140mg	140mg	370mg	320mg
Sugar:	0g	2g	13 gm	7g	3g	2g

So when it comes to Chex Mix®, for example, there isn't a whole lot of difference; the sales pitch has to do with *portion control*. You really do need to read labels and make "portion to portion" comparisons, if taste is being sacrificed. Is it worth the "savings" in these highlighted supposedly healthier categories? When dealing with No Foods eaten as treats, taste in the original version often wins out over the supposed better health offering. For me, I know a small portion of deep dark chocolate is the end-all in terms of taste and health benefits whereas milk chocolate may taste good but offers unhealthy saturated milk fat and added refined sugars. (Just remember to control portions and time treats.)

GREAT HEALTH AND NUTRITION WEB SITES FOR KIDS AND TEENS (OR PARENTS)

Teen-Help-Desk.com: http://www.teen-help-desk.com/

The Produce Passport: http://www.producepassport.com/

Cartoon Network's "Get Animated": http://www.getanimated.com/

American Dietetic Association (ADA): http://www.eatright.org/

Batter Up Kids!: http://www.batterupkids.com/

Healthy Kids Challenge (HKC): http://www.healthykidschallenge.com/

National Heart, Lung and Blood Institute's "We Can!": http://wecan.nhlbi.nih.gov/

School Nutrition Association: http://www.schoolnutrition.org/

Share Our Strength: http://www.strength.org/

U.S. Department of Health & Human Services – Report on Obesity: http://www.surgeongeneral.gov/topics/obesity/calltoaction/fact_adolescents.htm/

For Parents:

We Can!: http://www.nhlbi.nih.gov/health/public/heart/obesity/wecan/

iVillage: http://www.ivillage.com/ ("Diet and Fitness" and "Women and Family" centers)

WebMD: http://www.webmd.com/ (Children's Health Center)

Parents.com: http://www.parents.com/ (click on your child's age group and then "Eating and Nutrition")

Aetna IntelHealth®: http://www.intelihealth.com/ (click on "Healthy Lifestyle" and then choose "Fitness/Nutrition/Weight Management")

See Appendix 13A for more great resources.

BEST BETS FOR TREATS

When choosing No with a Smile Foods, they should ultimately be a mix of healthier snacks and portion-controlled general munchies or treats. When you start the HFL program, though, you may choose to allow the kids whatever snacks they like. Your kids may crave or want snacks that are not necessarily the best choices in terms of HFL guidelines, but they can fit into the program with portion control. Some examples of satisfying, single-serve options include:

1. Pepperidge Farm® chocolate chunk dark chocolate 100-calorie cookie pouches
2. Back to Nature® banana walnut bakery squares
3. Figamajigs®—one serving has 150 calories/4g fat
4. Mott's® Healthy Harvest blueberry delight
5. Hungry Sultan® hummus snack pack
6. Special K® honey nut bar
7. Pacific Natural Foods® organic light sodium creamy tomato soup
8. Julie's Organic Ice Cream® mandarin sorbet bars
9. VitaMuffin® VitaTops
10. Any 100-calorie pack that does not contain any trans fats

For some heartier homemade snack or mini-meal recipes, choose from these ideas:

• For a veggie baked potato, scoop out the inside of the potato after baking and mix with mashed, cooked broccoli, some cottage cheese (1 percent) and spices. Stuff filling back in.
• Mix cubed sweet potatoes with steamed green beans and a dressing of honey mustard and olive oil. Top with slivered almonds.

BEST BETS FOR TREATS, *continued*

- A serving of Barilla® high-protein pasta with veggies and a bit of marinara sauce.
- Create strips of carrots and sweet potatoes, brush with olive oil and a bit of kosher salt, and bake at 450 degrees. Serve with bean dip (2 tablespoons).
- Use hollowed-out pepper halves as "containers" for tuna or cottage cheese.
- Whenever you make plain brown rice, jazz up a serving with cooked veggies and add some cubed tofu marinated in teriyaki sauce.
- Whole grain bite-size crackers topped with nut butter and a raisin.
- A half-cup serving of cooked high-fiber pasta like Amish Naturals® or high-protein pasta like Barilla® spaghetti with steamed veggies and 1/8 cup tomato sauce.
- Large berries with a bit of dark chocolate dipping sauce and a sprinkle of crushed nuts.
- Vanilla non-fat yogurt topped with crushed cereal, nuts, and cubed fruit.

PARENT REALITY CHECK

You are going to integrate the HFL program into your household as the team leader. That means that you have some tough choices to make as you navigate the program and decide the pace you will use to implement the plan (based mostly on your family's health status, how receptive they are, and other evaluations you make). Consider these concepts:

- Parents, especially moms, are the "nutrition gatekeepers" who set the home lifestyle tone.
- Eating together as a family is a huge step toward improving your family health profile.
- Eating too much sugary and high-fat foods, and not moving enough, contribute significantly to the obesity epidemic.
- Mom's health before and during pregnancy is a huge determining factor in a child's weight and health.
- Mom and Dad are both models of behavior kids can observe and learn from.
- Every small change is a step toward better health and little changes have considerable impact.
- You are working this program into your family life because the health, weight, and future of your family's quality of life worry you.
- Each *sustained* habit change you make puts you and your family members in a better health zone.
- Integrating the four P's into your family's day-to-day life over time will make you a Healthy Family for Life.

Yes, No, Maybe So Food Choices

....

An At-A-Glance List

....

Yes Foods

Fruits

Serving size: as listed, sixty to eighty calories
  Apple: one whole
  Banana: one small (6-inch)
  Peach: one whole
  Pear: one small
  Orange: one small
  Grapefruit: one half
  Melon (medium size): one quarter
  Strawberries: five large or seven medium
  Blackberries: one-half cup
  Blueberries: one-half cup
  Raspberries: one-half cup

Nectarine: one medium
Cherries: eleven large
Grapes: twelve
Plum: one medium
Mango: one half
Papaya: one half
Pineapple: two to three rings (one-quarter-inch thick)
Watermelon: one slice (one-inch thick)
Kiwi: one large
Prunes: five

Vegetables

Serving size: one-half to one cup of cooked or chopped raw vegetables will usually fall between twenty-five and sixty calories; most lettuces can be measured as several cups.

Asparagus: twelve spears
Broccoli: four to five florets
Brussels sprouts: six to eight medium
Cabbage: several cups
Onion: one medium
Artichoke: one
Cauliflower: several cups
Celery: several cups
Chicory: two to three cups
Cucumbers: unlimited
Eggplant: two cups, cubed
Carrots: two medium or ten baby
Escarole: several cups
Green beans: one and one-quarter cups or forty four-inch beans
Greens (collards, kale, mustard, turnips): one and one-half to
    two cups
Lettuces: several cups
Mushrooms: depends on type (see expanded list)
Okra: one and one-half to two cups
Peppers: up to several cups, cubed
Radishes: unlimited

Sprouts: several cups
Summer squash: up to several cups, cubed
Tomatoes: one medium or ten cherry

No Foods (Treats Only!)

Cookies
Cakes
Candy
Chips
Granola bars and cereals (refined)
Milk chocolate products
Many bakery goods
Crackers (fried)
Regular cut meats (any that aren't less than 20 percent lean-cut)
Dark meat poultry with skin
White meat poultry with skin
White rice
White pasta
Cereal (sweetened, with low fiber content or minimal whole grain)
Soda
Juices (refined, not fresh-squeezed, with pulp and rind)
High-fat or high-sugar condiments
Dressings
Mayonnaise
Gravies
Canned soups
Alcoholic beverages
High-fat, high-sodium frozen foods
Whole-fat dairy products (unless child is less than two years old)

Maybe So Foods

Dairy

Low-fat or preferably fat-free.

Serving size: approximately eighty calories per serving.

Cottage cheese

Milk

Yogurt

Hard and soft cheese

Non-fat dry milk

Ricotta cheese

Low-fat soymilk and buttermilk

Meats/Poultry/Fish

Serving size: two to three ounces, children; three to four ounces, women; six ounces, men. Most of these have approximately fifty calories/ounce.

White meat skinless breast of chicken or turkey

Extra-lean (17 percent fat) meat

Low-sodium white deli meats

Fresh fish (steer clear of tilefish, shark, swordfish, king mackerel, and other high mercury fishes)

Water-packed tuna/salmon (chunk light tuna has less mercury)

Veal

Pork

Lamb without the bone

Eggs: two

Egg whites: several

"High-protein" pastas: one cup

Grains

Serving size: Since grains are served in a variety of forms use the calorie count of sixty to eighty calories per serving. For breakfast, if cereal is your main meal, you may choose a two-serving portion.

Whole grain breads (includes sourdough)

Whole grain crackers

Air-popped popcorn

Whole grain English muffin, tortilla, roll

Whole grain cereals

Brown rice/wild rice
Whole grain pasta

Beans and legumes

Serving size: one-quarter cup, rinsed, which equals one ounce of lean animal protein or about fifty calories.
> All beans (red, black, kidney, broad, lima, fava, great Northern, navy, pinto, soybean)
> Tofu

Nuts and seeds

Serving Size: one-quarter cup (warning: high fat content). For most varieties, a serving of ten to twenty-five nuts will equal four ounces of protein or about 160–200 calories.
> Dry roasted peanuts: thirty nuts, 170 calories
> Almonds: twenty-four nuts, 160 calories
> Cashews: twenty nuts, 170 calories
> Walnuts: fourteen nuts, 180 calories
> Pecans: twenty halves, 190 calories
> Macadamia nuts: eleven nuts, 200 calories
> Brazil nuts: seven nuts, 170 calories
> Pistachios (not jumbo): forty-seven shelled nuts, 170 calories
> Seeds (includes pumpkin or sunflower): one and one-half ounces
> Peanut butter (choose trans-fat-free): two level tablespoons

Starchy Vegetables

Serving size: sixty to eighty calories—these correlate to bread-like servings.
> Potatoes (including sweet potatoes, though they have higher fiber content): one-half to two-thirds cup or one small
> Peas: one-half cup
> Corn: one small ear or one-half cup
> Beets: one and one-half cups

Yucca: one-quarter cup

Pumpkin: two-thirds cup, canned, unsweetened

Rutabaga: two-thirds cup

Taro: one-half cup

Turnips: one and one-half cups

Winter squash: one cup, mashed

Yams: one-half cup, cubed

Oils

Serving size: varies, but in general one tablespoon has 120 calories, so I recommend trying to use it by the teaspoonful in individual servings of salad dressing or for cooking. Cooking sprays are another option, which you can use to coat cooking surfaces with far fewer calories.

Olive oil, nut oils, canola oil: one tablespoon equals 120 calories

Cholesterol-lowering margarines: three servings/daily are needed to achieve a health benefit, so be sure to factor in the calories. For example: Benecol® Light Spread has fifty calories/tablespoon.

Nuts, seeds and peanut butter: see the "Nuts and seeds" list

Avocado: three ounces

HFL Recipes

The following recipes are favorites of mine (and my family) and include entrées, side dishes, soups, smoothies, and baked goods. Some have calorie counts and breakdowns while others simply offer a healthier twist on traditional recipes.

Root of the Earth Veggie Soup

1 onion, chopped
3 cloves garlic, minced
4 celery ribs, chopped
1 tablespoon vegetable oil
1 zucchini, sliced
3 carrots, sliced
1 parsnip, peeled and sliced
1 rutabaga, peeled and chopped
1/2 pound green beans, chopped
1 turnip, peeled and diced
1 cup fresh corn kernels
1 bay leaf
6 cups low-sodium vegetable broth
Salt and pepper

Preparation: Sauté onion, garlic, and celery in the oil over medium heat till softened. Add remaining ingredients, cover, and reduce heat. Simmer, stirring occasionally, for 30–40 minutes (until vegetables are tender).

Nutrition information: Makes 12 servings, 86 calories per serving.

Orange Creamsicle Milkshake

1 cup skim milk
1 (6-ounce) container fat-free vanilla yogurt
1/2 cup calcium-fortified orange juice concentrate
1/4 teaspoon vanilla extract
5 ice cubes

Preparation: Blend the first 4 ingredients. Add ice cubes and blend again.

Nutrition information: 198 calories, 1.5g fat, 10g protein, 38g carbohydrate, 1.5g fiber, 128g sodium.

Berry Berry Oatmeal

Cook 1/2 cup of dry oatmeal (regular or instant)

Top with:
1 tablespoon brown sugar (or Splenda® artificial sweetener)
3/4 cup berries
2 teaspoons chopped pecans
1/2 cup warm skim milk

Banana-Strawberry Shake Up

Blend:
1/2 cup skim milk or low-fat soymilk
1/2 cup fat-free plain yogurt
1 (medium) ripe banana
1-1/2 cups sliced strawberries

1 tablespoon honey
2 tablespoons wheat germ

Waffle and Topping Breakfast

2 Kashi® GOLEAN waffles

Top with:
3/4 cup non-fat yogurt
1 tablespoon low-sugar maple syrup
1/2 cup berries
1 tablespoon chopped nuts

Chive and Egg Scramble Up

Scramble 1 egg plus 2 egg whites, 2 teaspoons of chopped chives in a pan prepared with cooking spray. Stuff into half of a whole grain pita pocket. Serve with skim latte.

Crunchy Curry Chicken Salad

2/3 cup cooked, cubed white meat chicken breast
1 tablespoon non-fat mayo
1 teaspoon curry powder
2 tablespoons diced celery
1 tablespoon raisins
1 tablespoon cashews or almonds

Place on top of spinach leaves tossed with:
1 tablespoon olive oil
Dash balsamic vinegar

Serve with 4 whole grain crackers.

Southwestern Salad with Salsa

3/4 cup drained and rinsed black beans
3/4 cup low-sodium canned corn
1 chopped red pepper
3 tablespoons salsa
1/4 cup shredded low-fat cheese

Place on bed of mixed greens.

Chicken, Garbanzo, and Couscous Salad

Cook 1/4 cup of whole grain couscous.

Toss with:
2 ounces cubed fat-free chicken
1/4 cup drained and rinsed garbanzo beans
1 cup steamed broccoli florets
1 tablespoon lime juice
1 teaspoon olive oil
2 tablespoons chopped cilantro

Plate and surround with thin tomato slices.

Radish, Tomato, and Onion Salsa

2 large ripe plum tomatoes
1/2 cup trimmed and grated radishes
1/2 cup minced sweet red onion
1 minced jalapeno
2 tablespoons minced cilantro

Preparation: Stir ingredients and add a pinch of coarse salt. Let sit at room temperature before serving.

Nutrition information: 4 servings, 19 calories per serving.

Sweet Potato Air Fries

4 (8-ounce) sweet potatoes, scrubbed
1 teaspoon olive oil
1/2 teaspoon cayenne pepper (or other seasoning)
Salt to taste
Nonstick cooking spray

Preparation: Pre-heat oven to 450 degrees. Cut unpeeled sweet potatoes lengthwise into 1/2-inch slices. Cut slices into sticks. Toss sweet potatoes in olive oil/seasoning mixture. Transfer potatoes to baking sheet prepared with cooking spray. Bake 15 minutes, turning once, then bake for an additional 15–20 minutes, and cook till golden. Sprinkle with salt before serving.

Nutrition information: 250 calories, 2g fat, 4g protein, 50g carbohydrate per serving. Serves 4.

Butternut Squash and Garlic Purée

1–2 pound butternut squash, halved and seeded
2 cloves garlic, unpeeled
2 teaspoons olive oil
1/2 teaspoon chopped sage leaves
1/4 teaspoon cayenne pepper
1/4 teaspoon grated nutmeg
Optional: salt to taste

Preparation: Pre-heat oven to 375 degrees. Put squash cut-side down in a shallow baking dish sprayed with a bit of cooking spray. Bake until tender, approximately 50 minutes. After the first 25 minutes, wrap garlic cloves loosely in foil and place them next to the squash for the final 25 minutes of baking. Remove squash pulp from peel and squeeze garlic to separate it from the skins. Purée garlic and squash with a food mill into a bowl. Add olive oil, cayenne, nutmeg, and salt and stir well.

Nutrition information: 106 calories, 2g fat, 20g carbohydrate, 2g protein per serving. Serves 4.

Halloween (Pumpkin) Oat Muffins

1-1/4 cups unbleached white flour
1 tablespoon baking powder
1/2 teaspoon salt
1/4 teaspoon ground cinnamon
1 cup rolled oats
1 egg or 2 egg whites or comparable Egg Beaters®
1 additional egg white
1/4 cup pumpkin purée
3/4 cup evaporated skim milk
1/2 cup unsweetened pineapple juice
2 tablespoons canola oil
1/8 cup brown sugar and 2 single-serving packets of Splenda® (less brown sugar can be used or sweet taste can come from 1/4 cup apple butter)
4–5 tablespoons All-Fruit® apricot preserves

Preparation: Preheat oven to 400 degrees. Prepare standard muffin tin with liners or use silicone muffin pan. Into a large bowl, sift flour, baking powder, salt, and cinnamon. Whirl oats in blender until they are the consistency of cornmeal, then add to dry mixture. In a separate bowl, beat 1 egg and 1 egg white. Add in purée, evaporated milk, oil, brown sugar (or apple butter). Fold wet ingredients into dry ingredients and mix well. Spoon into muffin pans. Create a small well in the batter in each cup and top with apricot jam. Bake 20–25 minutes (until a toothpick inserted in a muffin comes out clean). Cool.

Nutrition information: 162 calories, 3.4g fat, 5g protein, 24g carbohydrate per serving.

Tangy Split Pea Soup

3 cups chopped onions
1 tablespoon vegetable oil
1-1/2 teaspoons ground cumin
1/2 tablespoon turmeric
1 tablespoon ground coriander
1 teaspoon grated fresh ginger
1 cup dried yellow split peas

6-1/2 cups water
1 (3-inch) cinnamon stick
2 cups peeled and cubed sweet potatoes
1 (3-inch) cinnamon stick
1 cup peeled, cored, cubed green apples
2 tablespoons chili powder
3/4 cup chopped tomatoes
1-1/2 tablespoons fresh lime juice
1 tablespoon low sodium soy sauce
1/2 cup non-fat yogurt
1/4 cup minced cilantro (optional)

Preparation: In a soup pot, sauté onions in oil for 8 minutes, stirring frequently till golden. Add cumin, turmeric, coriander, and ginger and cook 1 additional minute. Add split peas, water, sweet potatoes, apples, cinnamon stick, chili powder. Cover and bring to boil. Lower heat and simmer for 40-45 minutes (until split peas are tender). In a separate medium bowl, combine tomatoes, lime juice, and soy sauce. Add this mixture to soup pot when peas are tender. Purée soup in blender in batches, with additional water when needed to thin it down a bit. Return soup to pot and heat slowly. Divide into 8 bowls (or save extra servings) and top with a bit of non-fat yogurt and a sprinkle of cilantro.

Nutrition information: 187 calories, 1.4g fat, 6g protein, 38g carbohydrate per serving.

"Wake Up" Breakfast Burrito

2 (7-inch) fat-free tortillas
1 container Egg Beaters® egg substitute or 3 egg whites
1/4 cup fat-free shredded cheese (I recommend cheddar)
1 small can fat-free refried beans
Salsa

Preparation: Scramble Egg Beaters® or egg whites. Spread 3 tablespoons of refried beans on each tortilla. Top with egg, sprinkle with cheese, and then microwave until the cheese melts.

Nutrition information: 285 calories, 26g protein, 39g carbohydrates, 0.7g fat, 900mg cholesterol, 5g sodium per serving. Serves 2.

Squash Purée Elegante

3–4 winter squash
1/2 cup warmed low-fat soymilk
1–2 tablespoons low-sugar maple syrup
1/4 teaspoon nutmeg
1/4 teaspoon white pepper

Preparation: Pre-heat oven to 400 degrees. Cut squash lengthwise and scoop out seeds and stringy fibers. Place squash cut-side down on sheet pan filled with 1/4 inch of water. Bake 25–35 minutes (until tender). Remove, flip over, and allow the mixture to cool down. Scoop out pulp, transfer to bowl, and add milk, syrup, and seasonings and mash the mixture. Place mixture in serving bowl and serve immediately.

Nutrition information: 62 calories, 2.8g fiber, 7mg sodium, 2.3g protein per serving. Serves 4.

Cornmeal Crusted Mahi-Mahi with Corn Relish

1-3/4 cup chopped tomatoes
1/2 cup fresh corn kernels
1/4 cup finely chopped green bell peppers
1/4 cup finely chopped onions
2 tablespoons red wine vinegar
1 tablespoon minced fresh cilantro
1 clove garlic, minced
1-1/2 teaspoons yellow cornmeal
1/4 teaspoon salt
1/4 teaspoon pepper
4 (6-ounce) mahi-mahi filets
Cooking spray

Preparation: Combine first 7 ingredients in bowl. Cover and chill. Sprinkle cornmeal, salt, and pepper over filets and place filets on a grill rack that's been well sprayed with cooking spray. Grill about 6 minutes on each side. Top filets with refrigerated mixture and serve.

Nutrition information: 288 calories, 9g fat, 2g saturated fat, 41g protein, 9g fiber, 9g carb, 2g fiber, 222mg sodium per serving. Serves 4.

No-Fail Low-Fat Mushroom Gravy

1/2 cup sliced celery
1/2 cup chopped carrots
1/2 cup chopped onion
3 cloves garlic, peeled
Pinch each of dried sage and thyme
2 cans reduced-fat, low-sodium chicken broth (or vegetable broth for a meat-free option)
1 package (about 10g) dried mushrooms
1/4 cup all-purpose flour
1/4 teaspoon hot pepper sauce
Extra broth in case mixture thickens too much during cooking
Cooking spray

Preparation: Coat nonstick pan with cooking spray. Add first 5 ingredients. Spray a bit more cooking spray, cover, and cook for about 10 minutes, stirring occasionally. Add broth, mushrooms, and simmer for 30 minutes. Remove mushrooms with slotted spoon and chop fine. Pour gravy mixture plus flour into blender and purée. Return to the pan, add hot sauce and mushrooms. Reheat to a boil and thin with extra broth if necessary.

Nutrition information: 33.5 calories, 0.1 fat, 0 saturated fat, 2.1g protein, 6.3g carbohydrate, 216mg sodium per serving. Makes 8 servings

Bran and Cherry Muffins

1-1/2 cups dried tart cherries
1 cup wheat bran
1 cup evaporated skim milk
Splenda® to equal the sweetness of 1/4 cup of sugar
1/2 cup unsweetened applesauce
1/4 cup low-sugar molasses
1 cup all-purpose flour
1/2 cup whole wheat flour
1 teaspoon baking soda
2 large egg whites

Preparation: Pre-heat the oven to 375 degrees. Use a 12-cup silicone muffin pan. In a large bowl, mix cherries, bran, milk, sugar, applesauce, molasses, eggs. Let stand 10 minutes. In a separate bowl, mix flour and baking soda. Add flour mixture to bran mixture and stir just past moistening. Batter should remain quite lumpy. In a clean dry bowl, beat egg whites till soft peaks form. Gently fold the egg whites into batter. Spoon into muffin tins and bake 20–25 minutes (until muffins are lightly brown on top). Test with a toothpick for doneness.

Nutrition information: 190 calories, 5g fat, 1g saturated fat, 32g carbohydrate, 107mg sodium per serving. Makes 12 muffins.

Oven-Poached Salmon with Scallions

1/4 cup white wine
1/4 cup fish stock (now available in supermarkets)
3/4 cup low-sodium soy sauce
1 1/2 inch piece of ginger root, thinly sliced
2 scallions, chopped
Fresh black pepper to taste
1 pound salmon filet, tail end

Preparation: Mix ingredients in shallow pan (except fish) for 1 minute. Lay fish in it, cover. Bake at 350 degrees for 10 minutes. Serve fish on bed of fresh steamed spinach and brown rice. Sprinkle with lemon juice.

Nutrition information: 345 calories, 49g protein, 13g carbohydrate, 8g fat, 114mg cholesterol, 1g fiber per serving. Serves 2.

Herb-Seasoned Crusted Haddock

1 tablespoon each: oregano, thyme, basil, garlic, chives, chopped parsley
1/4 cup dried bread crumbs
3/4 pound haddock
1 egg white
1/4 cup white wine
Kosher salt to taste

Preparation: Mix herbs and bread crumbs. Dip haddock in egg white and cover with bread crumb mixture. Place gently in pan with white wine. Bake in an oven pre-heated to 350 degrees for 10–12 minutes. Sprinkle with salt and serve with steamed zucchini, red pepper, and asparagus.

Nutrition information: 395 calories, 55g protein, 24g carbohydrate, 9g fat, 150mg cholesterol, 3g fiber per serving. Serves 2.

Golden Tomato and Wine Vinaigrette

Non-stick cooking spray
1 shallot, diced
1/2 cup white wine
1 lemon
1 large golden tomato, cored and seeded
Salt and fresh pepper to taste

Preparation: Coat a small saucepan with cooking spray, then sauté shallot over medium heat until translucent. Add white wine and grated lemon zest, and cook to reduce the sauce by half in volume and transfer to blender. Add tomato and juice of lemon to blender and purée. Store in fridge.

Easy Chocolate Blended Shake

1 cup skim milk
1 cup sugar-free chocolate soda
1/4 tablespoon cinnamon
Ice cubes

Preparation: Blend in blender for 1 minute. To make a thicker version, add a scoop of fat-free frozen yogurt and use only a half-cup of skim milk.

Nutrition information: 86 calories, 8g protein, 12g carbohydrate, 0.4g fat, 126mg sodium (without additional scoop of frozen yogurt) per serving. Makes 2 cups.

Black Bean Hummus

1 (15-ounce) can black beans, drained and rinsed
1/4 cup low-sodium vegetable stock
2–3 tablespoons tahini (sesame seed paste)
2 to 2-1/2 tablespoons lemon juice
1-1/2 tablespoons of low-sodium soy sauce
Salt and cayenne pepper to taste
Whole grain pita bread cut into wedges

Preparation: Process first 5 ingredients in food processor until smooth. Season to taste with salt and cayenne. Refrigerate 1–2 hours, then spoon into a serving bowl and serve with pita. Makes 4 servings.

Grilled Tuna with Mango-Carrot Salsa

1/4 cup diced and peeled mango
1 cup grated carrot
3 tablespoons fresh lime juice
1 tablespoon minced fresh chives
1/4 teaspoon crushed red pepper
1/4 teaspoon salt
1/8 teaspoon coriander

1/8 teaspoon ground cumin
1/4 teaspoon Mrs. Dash® salt-free seasoning
1/4 teaspoon black pepper
4 (6-ounce) tuna steaks (about 1 inch thick)
Cooking spray

Preparation: Combine first 8 ingredients in a bowl, stir well and set aside. Season fish with salt/pepper and grill on each side. Top with salsa.

Nutrition information: 296 calories, 9g fat, 40g protein, 2g fiber, 13g carbohydrate, 298mg sodium per serving. Makes 4 servings.

Antioxidant-Rich Carrot Ginger Soup

3 tablespoons olive oil
2 medium onions, chopped
1 tablespoon each of minced garlic and fresh ginger root
4 cups vegetable stock
2 pounds carrots, peeled and chopped
1 tablespoon grated orange zest
1-1/2 cups low-sugar orange juice
Salt, white pepper

Preparation: Add onions and 1 tablespoon of garlic and 1 tablespoon of ginger to heated oil and sauté till golden. Add stock and carrots, then reduce heat and cook until tender (about 40 minutes). Add in orange zest and stir. Strain soup through a fine strainer and transfer solids to a food processor or blender. Add 1 cup of orange juice liquid and purée till smooth. Return to pot along with remaining orange juice liquid. Cook over low heat. Add salt and pepper to taste.

Three-Apple Chunky Chicken Salad

2 (4-ounce) skinless chicken breasts
3/4 cup diced Gala apples
3/4 cup diced Red Delicious apples
1/2 cup diced Granny Smith apples
1/2 cup thinly sliced celery
3 tablespoons chopped pecans
1/4 cup fat-free mayo
2 tablespoons fat-free sour cream
1-1/2 teaspoons stone-ground mustard
1/2 teaspoon dried tarragon
1/4 teaspoon salt
1/8 teaspoon fresh pepper

Preparation: Boil chicken and cool. Cube chicken and combine with apples, celery, nuts and toss. Whisk mayo, sour cream, mustard and spices. Mix in chicken and toss gently. Chill for 30 minutes.

Nutrition information: 246 calories, 12g fat, 24g protein, 8g sugar, 13g carbohydrate, 2g fiber, 287 mg sodium per serving. Makes 4 servings.

Light 'n' Easy Monte Cristo

4 slices toasted whole grain bread
1 ounce low-sodium low-fat ham
1 ounce low-sodium low-fat turkey
2 slices fat-free Swiss cheese
2 pinches nutmeg
2 egg whites
1/4 teaspoon confectioner's sugar

Preparation: Layer cheese and ham and turkey between bread (making 2 sandwiches). In a separate shallow pan, beat egg whites and nutmeg. Lay sandwich bread into egg mixture on one side, and then flip to coat other side. Coat skillet with cooking spray and heat. Place sandwich and cook about 3 minutes on each side, medium heat. Before serving, sprinkle with sugar and slice diagonally.

Nutrition information: 319 calories, 18g protein, 40g carbohydrate, 10g fat, 4.5g saturated fat, 6g fiber, 706mg sodium per sandwich. Makes 2 sandwiches.

Banana Peach Smoothie

Blend:

1 medium banana
1 cup frozen peaches
6 ounces fat-free vanilla yogurt
2 tablespoons orange juice concentrate
1 tablespoon toasted wheat germ
Dash almond extract

Turkey Southwestern Breakfast Burgers

1 pound ground white meat turkey
1/2 cup drained low-sodium corn
1/4 cup minced onions, sautéed
1/4 cup diced sweet red peppers
1/2 cup fresh cilantro
2 cloves garlic, minced
1 teaspoon salt
1/2 teaspoon crushed red pepper flakes
1/2 teaspoon ground cumin
1 cup fresh whole wheat bread crumbs
1 large egg white
1 teaspoon canola oil (for sautéing patties)

Preparation: Mix meat and all ingredients and shape into 4–5 patties. Sauté patties for 2 minutes on each side, then lower heat and brown.

Mega-Citrus Rush Smoothie

Blend:

1-1/2 cups diced pineapple
1-1/2 cups diced cantaloupe
1/2 cup fresh-squeezed orange juice
1/2 cup carrot juice
Pinch nutmeg
3 ice cubes

Nutrition information: 152 calories, 3g protein, 1g fat, 37g carbohydrate, 30 mg sodium.

Vitamin C Blended Sipper

Blend:

1 medium banana, cut up
1 ripe peach, peeled, pitted, and cubed
1 cup raspberries
1-1/2 cups fresh-squeezed orange juice
3 ice cubes

Nutrition information: 185 calories, 3g protein, 1 gram fat, 7g fiber, 2 mg sodium.

Piña Colada Smoothie

Blend:

1 frozen banana
1/2 cup crushed pineapple (in its own juice)
1 cup plain non-fat yogurt
Dash coconut extract
1/2 cup skim milk

Nutrition information: 348 calories, 1.3g fat (you can share to make a snack).

Fresh Fruit Parfait Delight

Cut up a variety of fresh fruit: melons, pineapple, kiwi, blueberries, strawberries, and bananas. Layer non-fat vanilla yogurt, a bit of marmalade, and fruit and repeat pattern until parfait glasses are full. Top with fat-free whipped cream or Soyatoo!® Soy Whip™.

Nutrition information: Approximately 240 calories, 3g fat (based on standard parfait glass).

Red Lentil Soup with Bulgur

6 teaspoons olive oil
2 onions, chopped (1-1/2 cups)
3 cloves garlic, finely chopped
2 teaspoons ground cumin
8 cups low-sodium, fat-free chicken broth or vegetable broth
1-1/2 cups red lentils, rinsed
1/3 cup bulgur
2 tablespoons tomato paste
1 bay leaf
3 tablespoons fresh lemon juice
Salt and pepper
1 teaspoon paprika
1 teaspoon cayenne pepper

Preparation: Heat 2 teaspoons of oil in saucepan. Add onions and soften for 3 minutes. Add garlic and cumin and cook for 1 minute. Add broth, lentils, tomato paste, bay leaf, and bulgur and simmer, stirring occasionally. Cook 20–30 minutes until lentils soften. Take 4 cups of mixture and purée in food processor and then return to cooking mixture. Stir in lemon juice, salt, and pepper to taste. Heat the rest of the oil in a separate pan, adding paprika and cayenne pepper. Serve soup and drizzle seasoning over top just before serving.

Nutrition information: 220 calories, 5g fat, 12g fiber, 190mg sodium (if no salt added), 1g saturated fat per serving. Makes 8 servings.

Untraditional Peanut Butter Sandwich

1 slice whole grain bread
1 tablespoon peanut butter
1/3 cup fresh pineapple chunks

Nutrition information: 199 calories, 7g protein, 23g carbohydrate, 2g saturated fat, 9g total fat, 5g fiber, 250mg sodium.

Chili and Bean Stuffed Sweet Potato

1 medium sweet potato, baked

Mix together:
1/2 cup rinsed black beans
1/4 cup chopped onions
1/2 teaspoon minced garlic
1 tablespoon canned diced green chilies

Preparation: Top potato halves with mixture, sprinkle on 1 ounce of grated fat-free cheddar cheese, then top generously with cubed tomatoes.

Unfried Fried Chicken

Dip skinless chicken breasts into egg whites and coat with whole grain bread crumbs seasoned with your choice of dried herbs. Pre-heat oven to 450 degrees, coat a shallow pan with cooking spray, and bake chicken for 30 minutes.

Spicy 'n' Hot Skillet Potatoes

1 tablespoon olive oil
1 tablespoon peeled and diced mustard seeds
1-1/2 cups fat-free chicken broth

2 teaspoons cumin seeds
2 teaspoons coriander
2 pounds small potatoes, finely diced (about 12 cups)
1 medium onion, peeled and chopped fine
Salt to taste

Preparation: Cook spices in oil over medium heat for 30 seconds. Add potatoes and onion and sauté for 10 minutes. Lower heat, add broth. Cook 10 more minutes. Drain and season with a minimum of salt.

Nutrition information: 93 calories, 1.8g of fat, 136mg sodium, 16.4g carbohydrate, 2.4g protein per serving. Makes 12 servings.

Super Light "Parfait" Cheesecake

In a parfait glass, alternate layers of non-fat cream cheese with Splenda®-sweetened non-fat ricotta cheese. Add fresh or frozen raspberries combined with All-Fruit® jam. Top with fat-free whipped cream and vanilla wafer crumble.

Nutrition information: Approximately 244 calories per 8-ounce parfait glass, 6g of fat.

Appendices

APPENDIX 2A

Family Health Tree

Gt. Grandparents
___ diabetes
___ stroke
___ high BP
___ early heart attack

Grandma
___ diabetes
___ stroke
___ high BP
___ early heart attack
___ obesity

Gt. Grandparents
___ diabetes
___ stroke
___ high BP
___ early heart attack

Grandpa
___ diabetes
___ stroke
___ high BP
___ early heart attack
___ obesity

MOM
___ breast cancer
___ obesity/overweight

Gt. Grandparents
___ diabetes
___ stroke
___ high BP
___ early heart attack

Grandma
___ diabetes
___ stroke
___ high BP
___ early heart attack
___ obesity

Gt. Grandparents
___ diabetes
___ stroke
___ high BP
___ early heart attack

Grandpa
___ diabetes
___ stroke
___ high BP
___ early heart attack
___ obesity

DAD
___ cancers
___ obesity/overweight

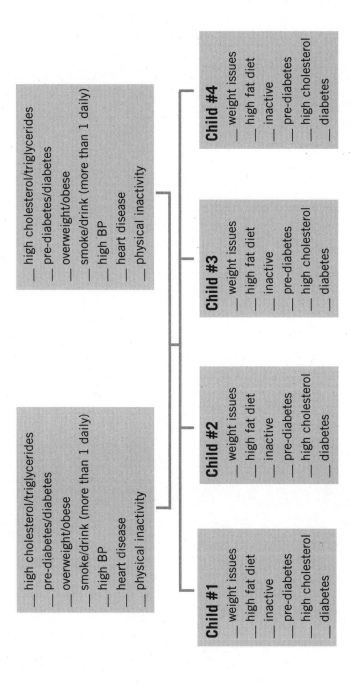

— high cholesterol/triglycerides
— pre-diabetes/diabetes
— overweight/obese
— smoke/drink (more than 1 daily)
— high BP
— heart disease
— physical inactivity

Child #1
— weight issues
— high fat diet
— inactive
— pre-diabetes
— high cholesterol
— diabetes

Child #2
— weight issues
— high fat diet
— inactive
— pre-diabetes
— high cholesterol
— diabetes

Child #3
— weight issues
— high fat diet
— inactive
— pre-diabetes
— high cholesterol
— diabetes

Child #4
— weight issues
— high fat diet
— inactive
— pre-diabetes
— high cholesterol
— diabetes

Name each relative (from great-grandparents if possible, or at minimum, grandparents and aunts/uncles) and identify any diseases that contributed to poor health, or are identified as a lifestyle-related disease. Include heart disease, hypertension, diabetes, thyroid disease, cancers, arthritis, and gum disease (which is associated with inflammation and is a risk factor to other chronic diseases).

APPENDIX 2B

Health Profiles

Adult Health Profile

Height _____
Weight_____
BMI _____
Waist measurement_____
Right bicep measurement _____
Hips_____
Right thigh (six inches above knee) _____

Blood pressure_____
Pulse_____

Blood panel:
    Total cholesterol_____
    HDL_____
    LDL_____
    Triglycerides_____
    Fasting blood sugar_____

HbA1c (if applicable—diabetes)_____

___Smoker ___Non-smoker

Surgeries:

Hospitalizations:

Diagnoses:

Current Medications:

Vitamins/Supplements:

Allergies:

Current Daily Diet:
Chart at least one week's worth of meals per family member, with approximate serving sizes when possible, so you can see food patterns emerge. Areas to assess after you have one week's worth of

entries include: glaringly missing food groups like fruits or veggies, total disregard of portion sizes, a lot of creamy high-fat dishes or fried greasy food, a lot of red meat or high-fat dairy, inadequate low-fat or fat-free dairy servings, or a lot of high-calorie beverages like soda or juices. You need to see clearly what's wrong and right with your diet before you can implement changes.

Breakfast:

Lunch:

Dinner:

Snacks:

Number of coffees daily:
Number of smoothies/blended drinks daily:
Number of sodas/juice beverages daily:
Number of fast food meals weekly:

Teen Health Profile

Height _____

Weight_____

BMI _____

Waist measurement_____

Right bicep measurement _____

Hips_____

Right thigh (six inches above knee)_____

Blood pressure_____

Pulse_____

Blood panel:

    Total cholesterol_____

    HDL_____

    LDL_____

    Triglycerides_____

    Fasting blood sugar_____

    HBA1C (if applicable—diabetes)_____

___Smoker ___Non-smoker

Surgeries:

Hospitalizations:

Diagnoses:

Current medications:

Vitamins/supplements:

Allergies:

Current daily diet:
Breakfast:

Lunch:

Dinner:

Snacks:

Number of regular sodas daily:
Number of juices daily:
Number of fast food meals weekly:

Child Health Profile

Blood pressure_____
Pulse_____

Blood panel highlights (any results that are red flags):
Total cholesterol_____
     HDL_____
     LDL_____
     Triglycerides_____
     Fasting blood sugar_____
     HBA1C (if applicable—diabetes)_____

Surgeries:

Hospitalizations:

Diagnoses:

Current medications:

Vitamins/supplements:

Allergies:

Current daily diet:
Breakfast:

Lunch:

Dinner:

Snacks:

Current exercise/activity/sports:

Number of regular sodas daily:_____

Number of juices/high cal beverages daily:_____

Number of cups of full fat milk daily:_____

Number of fast food meals weekly:_____

Number of daily treats:_____

APPENDIX 2C

Determining Your Body Mass Index (BMI) and Weight Measurement

Body mass index, or BMI, is a new term to most people. However, it is the measurement of choice for many physicians and researchers studying obesity. BMI uses a mathematical formula that takes into account both a person's height and weight. BMI equals a person's weight in kilograms divided by height in meters squared. ($BMI=kg/m^2$).

Risk of Associated Disease According to BMI and Waist Size			
BMI		Waist less than or equal to 40 in. (men) or 35 in. (women)	Waist greater than 40 in. (men) or 35 in. (women)
18.5 or less	Underweight	—	N/A
18.5–24.9	Normal	—	N/A
25.0–29.9	Overweight	Increased	High
30.0–34.9	Obese	High	Very High
35.0–39.9	Obese	Very High	Very High
40 or greater	Extremely Obese	Extremely High	Extremely High

Source: Partnership for Healthy Weight Management (http://www.consumer.gov/weightloss/bmi.htm)

Determining Your BMI

The following table has the math and metric conversions already done. To use the table, find the appropriate height in the left-hand column. Move across the row to the given weight. The number at the top of the column is the BMI for that height and weight. Or, use the BMI calculator at http://www.consumer.gov/weightloss/bmi.htm#BMI.

Body Weight in Pounds According to Height and Body Mass Index

BMI (kg/m²)	19	20	21	22	23	24	25	26	27	28	29	30	35	40
Height (in.)							Weight (lb.)							
58	91	96	100	105	110	115	119	124	129	134	138	143	167	191
59	94	99	104	109	114	119	124	128	133	138	143	148	173	198
60	97	102	107	112	118	123	128	133	138	143	148	153	179	204
61	100	106	111	116	122	127	132	137	143	148	153	158	185	211
62	104	109	115	120	126	131	136	142	147	153	158	164	191	218
63	107	113	118	124	130	135	141	146	152	158	163	169	197	225
64	110	116	122	128	134	140	145	151	157	163	169	174	204	232
65	114	120	126	132	138	144	150	156	162	168	174	180	210	240
66	118	124	130	136	142	148	155	161	167	173	179	186	216	247
67	121	127	134	140	146	153	159	166	172	178	185	191	223	255
68	125	131	138	144	151	158	164	171	177	184	190	197	230	262
69	128	135	142	149	155	162	169	176	182	189	196	203	236	270
70	132	139	146	153	160	167	174	181	188	195	202	207	243	278
71	136	143	150	157	165	172	179	186	193	200	208	215	250	286
72	140	147	154	162	169	177	184	191	199	206	213	221	258	294
73	144	151	159	166	174	182	189	197	204	212	219	227	265	302
74	148	155	163	171	179	186	194	202	210	218	225	233	272	311
75	152	160	168	176	184	192	200	208	216	224	232	240	279	319
76	156	164	172	180	189	197	205	213	221	230	238	246	287	328

Adapted with permission from Bray, G.A., Gray, D.S., Obesity, Part I, Pathogenesis, West J. Med. 1988: 149: 429–41.

Determining Your Waist Measurement

Women with a waist measurement of more than thirty-five inches or men with a waist measurement of more than forty inches may have a higher disease risk than people with smaller waist measurements because of where their fat lies. To measure your waist circumference, place a tape measure around your bare abdomen just above your hip bone. Be sure that the tape is snug, but does not compress your skin, and is parallel to the floor. Relax, exhale, and measure your waist.

APPENDIX 2D

Individual Activity Profile

Have each family member fill this form out. Help little ones by making the questions as child-friendly as possible. I think self-evaluation through these kinds of questionnaires is very helpful. It's unnecessary for me to give you "right and wrong answers." The truth lies in your own reality check. We all think we move more than we really do. When you see how much or, more likely, how little you move on a daily basis, how you personally view exercise, how long TV and computers keep you motionless, you'll be more open to change. The same will hold true for your kids. You'll probably get some eye-opening dialogue going, which is another positive outcome.

Adult Activity Profile

1. I do some form of exercise daily. ( ) Yes ( ) No
2. I take the opportunity to walk and climb stairs whenever possible. ( ) Yes ( ) No
3. I take lunchtime walks at work. ( ) Yes ( ) No
4. After I exercise, I always snack or eat. ( ) Yes ( ) No
5. I like sports. ( ) Yes ( ) No
6. I belong to a gym or have fitness facilities at work and use them. ( ) Yes ( ) No

7. I do a lot (more than two hours/day) of computer work without a break. ( )Yes ( ) No
8. I watch more than two hours of TV daily. ( ) Yes ( ) No
9. I look for ways to be active. ( ) Yes ( ) No
10. I do a lot of home housework, gardening, home mainte-nance. ( ) Yes ( ) No
11. I would enjoy an active vacation. ( ) Yes ( ) No
12. My current home gym equipment gets used frequently. ( ) Yes ( ) No
13. I watch TV and don't move during commercials. ( ) Yes ( ) No
14. I feel like exercise is just work. ( ) Yes ( ) No
15. I've never liked any kind of exercise. ( ) Yes ( ) No

Children's Activity Profile

1. I play ball at school, move at recess time and lunchtime. ( ) Yes ( ) No
2. I walk or bike to and from school. ( ) Yes ( ) No
3. I do after-school sports. ( ) Yes ( ) No
4. I do team sports at school. ( ) Yes ( ) No
5. I play outdoors at home after school. ( ) Yes ( ) No
6. I watch more than two hours of TV daily. ( ) Yes ( ) No
7. I would play more if my parents played with me. ( ) Yes ( ) No
8. I am very active on the weekend. ( ) Yes ( ) No
9. I play a lot of computer games and do a lot of computer work daily. ( ) Yes ( ) No
10. I like all kinds of physical activity—running, playing ball, jumping rope. ( ) Yes ( ) No

We need to move daily as often as possible, with some form of pulse-raising cardiovascular activity (at least thirty minutes/day). Adults should also engage in a regular weight-training program. Kids need to play, run around and bike outdoors, and have set parameters on how much time is spent watching TV and on the computer. There is no doubt that too much sedentary time is a major contributor to obesity.

APPENDIX 2E

Family Activity Profile

The purpose of this assessment is to increase your awareness of your family's activity level. Ideally, fill this out with some or all members of your family present, and encourage discussion, along with ideas for change.

1. We all do physical chores in the house. ( ) Yes ( ) No
2. Weekends are very active for all family members.
   ( ) Yes ( ) No
3. We do a family hike, bike, or other activity at least once on the weekend. ( ) Yes ( ) No
4. We monitor TV watching time. ( ) Yes ( ) No
5. We monitor video gaming time. ( ) Yes ( ) No
6. We monitor computer time (other than homework).
   ( ) Yes ( ) No
7. Our vacations involve walking and other physical activities.
   ( ) Yes ( ) No
8. We have exercise equipment in the home. ( ) Yes ( ) No
9. We belong to a gym or community center. ( ) Yes ( ) No
10. We play outside the home at least three times/week.
    ( ) Yes ( ) No

11. Our children are in after-school/weekend sports team.
( ) Yes ( ) No

12. We actively garden, maintain our outdoor property as a family. ( ) Yes ( ) No

13. We do family winter sports together like skiing; we do summer activities like swimming/surfing/boating/water skiing. ( ) Yes ( ) No

14. We plan physical activities together as a family on a regular basis. ( ) Yes ( ) No

APPENDIX 4A

Our Family's No Food Strategies Plan

Create this plan with your whole family, and be creative in coming up with strategies!

Our Family's No (or Treat) Foods Are:

Our Strategies for Keeping These Goods to Treats, Rather Than Overeating Them Are (see page 96 for examples):

APPENDIX 4B

My Yes, No, Maybe So Favorite Foods and Strategies Plan

Create your own "At-a-Glance" Yes, No, Maybe So list of foods that you eat frequently. It's helpful for every family member to do this. Talking about your choices and working together helps foster understanding and cooperation.

My Favorite Yes Foods (list all the fruits and veggies you commonly eat):

My Strategies for Eating More Yes Foods Will Be:

My Favorite NO Foods:
This list should include variety: some desserts, some snack foods, some higher fat or higher calorie proteins. My personal list would include: pizza, muffins, chocolate, chocolate chip cookies, rice pudding, licorice, frozen yogurt, Pirate's Booty snacks, lite cheese puffs, and french toast.

My Strategies This Week for Keeping No Foods as Treats, Rather than Overeating Them, Will Be (see page 99 for examples):

Week #1:
I plan on having _____ on _____
and then_____

I plan on having _____ on _____
and then_____

I plan on having _____ on _____
and then_____

I plan on having _____ on _____
and then_____

My Favorite Maybe So Foods:

My Strategies for Portion Control Will Be:

APPENDIX 4C

My HFL Food and Activity Journal

Every member of the family who is old enough can track his or her food consumption for a week or two—some may want to track it longer. Copy enough of these pages, or use the format to create your own and fill out one page per day. Make sure that all family members realize they can be creative, and encourage everyone to share their experiences. Your HFL Journal is your window into your "food soul." Tally up the number of servings of fruits, vegetables, dairy foods, grains, proteins, and fats you eat daily so you evaluate "missing food groups" and those that appear too often in a day. Remember that it is also fun to compare your initial assessment journals with journal entries during your transition so you can applaud progress and see continuing food patterns that need to be addressed. See more information on Food Journals on page 100.

Name:

Date (week of):

Goals:

Feelings About My Food and Exercise Today:

	FOOD GROUP	**AMOUNT** (be as specific as you can)
Breakfast		
Snack		
Lunch		
Snack		
Dinner		
Snack		
Extras		
Exercise (Minutes/Type)		

Note: To clarify which food groups you are eating enough of, not enough of, or too much of, you can add these categories as headings at the top of the page: Dairy, Fruits, Veggies, Fats, Protein, and Breads (any grain food).

APPENDIX 8A

MY PYRAMID FOOD INTAKE PATTERN CALORIE LEVELS
U.S. DEPARTMENT OF AGRICULTURE

MALE Activity level AGE	Sedentary	Mod. active	Active	FEMALE Activity level AGE	Sedentary	Mod. active	Active
2	1000	1000	1000	2	1000	1000	1000 (cal)
3	1000	1400	1400	3	1000	1200	1400
4	1200	1400	1600	4	1200	1400	1400
5	1200	1400	1600	5	1200	1400	1600
6	1400	1600	1800	6	1200	1400	1600
7	1400	1600	1800	7	1200	1600	1800
8	1400	1600	2000	8	1400	1600	1800
9	1600	1800	2000	9	1400	1600	1800
10	1600	1800	2200	10	1400	1800	2000
11	1800	2000	2200	11	1600	1800	2000
12	1800	2200	2400	12	1600	2000	2200
13	2000	2200	2600	13	1600	2000	2200
14	2000	2400	2800	14	1800	2000	2400
15	2200	2600	3000	15	1800	2000	2400
16	2400	2800	3200	16	1800	2000	2400
17	2400	2800	3200	17	1800	2000	2400

18	2400	2800	3200	**18**	1800	2000	2400
19–20	2600	2800	3000	**19–20**	2000	2200	2400
21–25	2400	2800	3000	**21–25**	2000	2200	2400
26–30	2400	2600	3000	**26–30**	1800	2000	2400
31–35	2400	2600	3000	**31–35**	1800	2000	2200
36–40	2400	2600	2800	**36–40**	1800	2000	2200
41–45	2200	2600	2800	**41–45**	1800	2000	2200
46–50	2200	2400	2800	**46–50**	1800	2000	2200
51–55	2200	2400	2800	**51–55**	1600	1800	2200
56–60	2200	2400	2600	**56–60**	1600	1800	2200
61–65	2000	2400	2600	**61–65**	1600	1800	2000
66–70	2000	2200	2600	**66–70**	1600	1800	2000
71–75	2000	2200	2600	**71–75**	1600	1800	2000
76 and up	2000	2200	2400	**76 and up**	1600	1800	2000

APPENDIX 8B

The Food Exchange Program Flow Sheet

One of the most helpful tools I've created for clients is this flow sheet, which you can copy and tack onto your fridge, carry with you, or post in your workplace kitchen. This is a great quick reference for understanding portion sizes for popular, healthy food choices in each food group; it offers the measured amounts that correspond to a serving size. You can pick and choose your Maybe So Foods easily from this sheet, particularly your protein and fat choices, as well as your bread and grain choices. From there, follow the basic guidelines for setting up your meal plan and all you've got to do is prep the food. I've used it myself for years and continue to use it.

The Exchange Program

One serving of any food on the following list can be exchanged for one serving of any other food in the same group, as long as it's the same portion size. Each food has approximately the same calorie count and the same number of carbohydrate, fat and protein grams. For example, a small baked potato substitutes for a serving of lentils.

Protein/Lean Meat 55 calories per ounce, or as otherwise listed	Starch/Bread 80 calories per serving	Fruit 60 calories per serving
Chicken breast, skin removed	1/2 cup cooked green peas, corn or lima beans	1/2 cup fruit juice
Fish or shellfish (35 calories per ounce)	1/2 cup cooked pasta	1/2 medium grapefruit
Luncheon meats: turkey breast, lean ham or other "light" cold cuts with 3 g of fat per ounce of less	2 slices "light" pumpernickel or whole grain bread	1/2 cup fresh fruit salad
	2 rice cakes	1/2 small banana
Beef: flank, eye, round or tips	6-in. ear of corn	2 tangerines
Lamb: roast, leg or loin cuts	1/3 cup cooked rice	1 cup berries
Lean red meats (no more than once or twice a week)	1/3 cup cooked legumes (dried beans, lentils)	1 cup melon
	1 slice pumpernickel or whole grain bread	1 medium apple, orange, pear or peach
Pork: tenderloin	1/2 cup bran flakes or shredded wheat	
1 medium egg (75 calories)	1/4 cup yam or sweet potato	
Veal: chops or roast	4 slices melba toast	
	3/4 cup unsweetened flaked cereal	
	1 small baked potato (3 oz.)	

Vegetable 25 calories per serving	Dairy/Milk 90 to 110 calories per serving	Fat 45 calories per serving
1 cup salad greens (including endive, romaine lettuce and spinach)	1 cup skim or 1% fat milk	1 tsp. oil (preferably olive or canola)
1/2 cup cooked vegetables	1/2 cup nonfat 1% fat cottage cheese	1 tbsp. light mayonnaise
1/2 cup vegetable juice	1/2 cup evaporated skim milk	1 tbsp. regular salad dressing
1 cup raw vegetables	1 cup plain or artificially sweetened nonfat yogurt	1/8 medium avocado
		1 tsp. regular butter or margarine
		1 tbsp. cream cheese
		10 small olives
		1 tbsp. diet butter or margarine (made from nonhydrogenated oil)

APPENDIX 9A

Our Family HFL Activity Plan Contract

Month:

Activities Planned:

Date, Location:

What We Need to Do to Make This Happen:

Excuses We Will Ignore:

We commit to being more active as a family for the month of:
_____

Signed (all family members):

_____

_____

_____

_____

APPENDIX 9B

Individual HFL Activity Plan

Month:

Activities Planned:

Date, Location:

What I Need to Do to Make This Happen:

Excuses I Will Ignore:

I commit to being more active, and doing thirty minutes of activity most days of the week for the month of:_____

Signed:

APPENDIX 13A

Useful Web Sites

Health Web Sites

Revolution Health: http://www.revolutionhealth.com/

WebMD: http://www.webmd.com/

KidsHealth: http://www.kidshealth.org/

National Institutes of Health: http://www.nih.gov/

National Cancer Institute: http://www.cancer.gov/

Centers for Disease Control and Prevention (CDC): http://www.cdc.gov/

American Academy of Family Physicians: http://www.familydoctor.org/

U.S. Department of Health & Human Services: http://www.healthfinder.gov/

Mayo Clinic: http://www.mayoclinic.com/

MedlinePlus: http://www.medlineplus.gov/

iVillage: http://health.ivillage.com/

Prevention: http://www.prevention.com/

American Diabetes Association: http://www.diabetes.org/

American Heart Association: http://www.americanheart.org/

HealthCentral.com: http://www.healthcentral.com/

American Dietetic Association: www.eatright.org

Diet and Fitness Web Sites

CalorieKing: http://www.calorieking.com/

FitDay: http://www.fitday.com/

5 A Day: http://www.cdc.gov/5aday/

MyDietExercise.com: http://www.mydietexercise.com/

MyPyramid.gov: http://www.mypyramid.gov/

Ace Fitness: http://www.acefitness.org/

The President's Council on Physical Fitness and Sports: http://www.fitness.gov/

Smallstep Adult and Teen: http://www.smallstep.gov/

Center for Science in the Public Interest—Nutrition, Health, and Diet: http://www.cspinet.org/nutrition/

Nutrition Data: www.nutritiondata.com

Light Cooking Web Sites

FabulousFoods.com: http://www.fabulousfoods.com/

HealthyCookingRecipes.com: http://www.healthycookingrecipes.com/

NutriStrategy—Low Calorie Cooking Tips and Low Fat Recipe Ideas: http://www.nutristrategy.com/lowcal.htm

Cooking Light: http://www.cookinglight.com/

REFERENCES

Chapter 1 References

[1] Revill, Jo. "Are you a Tofi? (That's thin on the outside, fat inside)." *Guardian Unlimited.* 10 Dec. 2006. <http://www.guardian.co.uk/science/2006/dec/10/medicineandhealth.health>

[2] Trust for America's Health. "F as in Fat—How Obesity Policies are Failing in America 2007." *Issue Report.* August 2007. <http://healthyamericans.org/reports/obesity2007/Obesity2007Report.pdf>

[3] "Study: Diabetes drug use spikes in girls." *USA Today,* 16 May 2007. <http://www.usatoday.com/news/health/2007-05-16-diabetes-drug_N.htm>

[4] Mayo Clinic Staff. "Obesity." *Mayo Clinic Web site.* 9 May 2007. <http://www.mayoclinic.com/health/obesity/DS00314>

[5] Gaziano, J. Michael, JoAnn E. Manson, and Paul M. Ridker. "Primary and Secondary Prevention of Coronary Heart Disease." *Heart Disease: A Textbook of Cardiovascular Medicine.* 6th edition. 2001.

[6] Committee on Prevention of Obesity in Children and Youth, Jeffrey P. Koplan, Catharyn T. Liverman, Vivica I. Kraak, editors. *Preventing Childhood Obesity: Health in the Balance.* Washington, DC: The National Academies Press, 2005.

[7] Fletcher, Anthony. "France heading for US obesity levels says study." *Food Navigator.com | Europe.* 2 Jan. 2006. <http://www.foodnavigator.com/news/ng.asp?id=65515-obesity-wholegrains-france>

[8] Manning, Anita. "Pregnant Women with High Blood Sugar More Likely to Have Overweight Kids." *USA Today,* 29 Aug. 2007. <http://www.ksdk.com/news/health/health_article.aspx?storyid=128075>

[9] American Heart Association (news release). "High numbers of men and women are overweight, obese and have abdominal fat, worldwide." *AHA News.* 22 Oct. 2007. <http://www.heart.org/presenter.jhtml?identifier=3051347>

[10] "Increases in Morbid Obesity in the USA: 2000–2005," *Public Health*, 2007. <http://www.ncbi.nlm.nih.gov/pubmed/17399752>

[11] R. C. Whitaker and W. H. Dietz. "Role of the prenatal environment in the development of obesity," *Journal of Pediatrics* 132.5 (1998): 768–776.

[12] J. J. Reilly, J. Armstrong, A. R. Dorosty, P. M. Emmett, A. Ness, I. Rogers, C. Steer, A. Sherriff. "Early life risk factors for obesity in childhood: cohort study," *BMJ* (formerly *British Medical Journal*) 0330 (2005): 1357.

[13] "Bill Clinton in drive to tackle childhood obesity." *Medical News Today.* 4 May 2005. <http://www.medicalnewstoday.com/articles/23813.php>

[14] R. C. Whitaker, J. A. Wright, M. S. Pepe, K. D. Seidel, W. H. Dietz. "Predicting obesity in young adulthood from childhood and parental obesity," *New England Journal of Medicine* 337.13 (1997): 869–873.

[15] Leonard H. Epstein, Jennifer L. Temple, Brad J. Neaderhiser, Robbert J. Salis, Richard W. Erbe, and John J. Leddy. "Food Reinforcement, the Dopamine D2 Receptor Genotype, and Energy Intake in Obese and Nonobese Humans," *Behavioral Neuroscience* 121.5 (2007): 877–886.

[16] Henig, Robin Marantz. "Fat Factors." *New York Times,* 13 Aug. 2006. <http://www.nytimes.com/2006/08/13/magazine/13obesity.html?_r=1&oref=slogin>

[17] T. A. Wadden, K. D. Brownell, and G. D. Foster. "Obesity: Responding to the Global Epidemic," presentation on 8 January 2004. From an article originally published in *Journal of Consulting and Clinical Psychology* 70.3 (2002): 510–525.

[18] M. K. Fox, S. Pac, B. Devaney, L. Jankowski. "Feeding infants and toddlers study: What foods are infants and toddlers eating?" *Journal of the American Dietetic Association* 104.1 Suppl1 (2004): S22–S30.

[19] S. L. Johnson, L. McPhee, L. L. Birch. "Conditioned preferences: Young children prefer flavors associated with high dietary fat." *Physiological Behavior* 50.6 (1991): 1245–1251.

[20] Rachel Tolbert Kimbro, Jeanne Brooks-Gunn, and Sara McLanahan. "Racial and Ethnic Differentials in Overweight and Obesity Among 3-Year-Old Children," *American Journal of Public Health* 97, 2 (2007): 298–305.

[21] Szakacs, Gergely. "TV ads double obese children's food intake: UK study," *Reuters,* 24 April 2007. <http://www.reuters.com/article/idUKL24575 54220070424>

[22] Hitti, Miranda. "Eat as a Family, Lose Weight: Family Dinners Have Many Benefits, but Teens May Need Extra Effort." *WebMD Medical News.* 25 May 2005. <http://www.webmd.com/diet/news/20050525/eat-as-family-lose-weight>

[23] S. A. Lederman, S. Akabas, B. J. Moore, M. E. Bentley, B. Devaney, and M. Gillman. "Preventing childhood obesity: A national conference to address

pregnancy, infancy and very early childhood factors." *Pediatrics* 114 (2004): 1146–1173.

[24] B. J. Rolls, D. Engell, and L. L. Birch. "Serving portion size influences 5-year-old but not 3-year-old children's food intakes." *Journal of the American Dietetic Association* 100.2 (2000): 232–234.

[25] J.O. Fisher and L.L. Birch. "Restricting access to foods and children's eating." *Appetite* 32.3 (1999): 405–419.

Note: References 8, 11, 12, 14, 15, and 17–25 are from a report published by California WIC Association. "Starting Earlier: What We Know about Preventing Overweight in Children from Birth to Five Years Old." Feb. 2006. Available at: http://healthyeatingactivecommunities.org/downloads/Diabetes_and_Obesity-General/Starting_Earlier_02_2006.pdf.

Chapter 2 References

[1] "Global Initiative in Nutritional Genomics." *UC Davis News & Information.* 24 Feb. 2006. <http://www/news.ucdavis.edu/search/news_detail.lasso?id=7640>

[2] Adler, J. and A. Underwood. "Diet and Genes." *Newsweek,* 17 Jan. 2005.

[3] Underwood, Anne and Jerry Adler. "Health For Life: Diet & Genes." *Newsweek.* 17 January 2005.

[4] Lye, B. "Diet Science Chews DNA." *Chicago Tribune,* 24 July 2005.

Chapter 3 References

[1] D. Gie Liem, A. Westerbeek, S. Wolterink, "Sour Taste Preferences of Children Relate to Preference for Novel and Intense Stimuli," *Chemical Senses* 29.8 (2004): 713–720.

[2] S. Yanovski, "Sugar and Fat: Cravings and Aversions 1," *American Society of Nutrition Symposium*, 133 (March 2003): 835S–837S.

[3] S. L. Teegarden and S. L. Bale, "Decreases in dietary preference produce increased emotionality and risk for dietary relapse," *Biological Psychiatry* 61 (2007): 1021–1029.

[4] C. Colantuoni, P. Rada, and J. McCarthy, "Evidence that intermittent, excessive sugar intake causes endogenous opioid dependence," *Obesity Research* 10 (2002): 478–488.

[5] C. Colantuoni, J. Schwenker, and J. McCarthy, "Excessive sugar intake alters binding to dopamine and mu-opioid receptors in the brain," *NeuroReport* 12 (2001): 3549–3552.

[6] B. Spring, J. Chiodo, M. Harden, M. J. Bourgeois, J. D. Mason, and L. Lutherer, "Psychobiological effects of carbohydrates," *Journal of Clinical Psychiatry* 50 Suppl (1989): 27–33.

[7] Cheng, M., "Thin people may be fat inside, some doctors say," *USATODAY .com*, 11 May 2007. < http://www.usatoday.com/news/health/2007-05-10-thin -fat-people_n.htm>

[8] R. Ley, F. Bäckhed, P. Turnbaugh, "Obesity alters gut microbial ecology," *Proceedings of National Academy of Science,* August 2005. <http://www.pnas .org/cgi/content/abstract/102/31/11070>

Chapter 4 References

[1] "A new proposed guidance system." See 3.

[2] Gavin, M., "Carbohydrates, Sugar, and Your Child," *KidsHealth,* December 2007. <http://www.kidshealth.org/parent/nutrition_fit/nutrition/sugar.html>

[3] Warner, J., "Artificial Sweeteners May Damage Diet Efforts—Sugar Substitutes May Distort Body's Natural Calorie Counter," *WebMD Medical News*, 30 June 2004. <http://www.webmd.com/diet/news/20040630/artificial-sweeteners -damage-diet-efforts>

[4] B. Popkin, L. Armstrong, G. Bray, and B. Caballero, "A new proposed guidance system for beverage consumption in the United States," *American Journal of Clinical Nutrition*, 83.3 (2006): 529–542.

[5] LeWine, H., "News Review from Harvard Medical School—AHA Updates Diet Guidelines," *Intelihealth,* 20 June 2006, <http://intelihealth.com/IH/ihtIH?d =dmtContent&c=467071&p=~br,IHW|~st,8059|~r,WSIHW000|~b,*|>

[6] N. Napoli, J. Thompson, and R. Civitelli, "Effects of dietary calcium compared with calcium supplements on estrogen metabolism and bone mineral density," *American Journal of Clinical Nutrition* 85 (2007): 1428–1433.

[7] C. Elwood, J. E. Pickering, and A. M. Fehily. "Milk and dairy consumption, diabetes and the metabolic syndrome: the Caerphilly prospective study," *Journal of Epidemiology and Community Health* 61: 695–698.

Chapter 5 References

[1] Pizzorno, J. E. and M. T. Murray. *Textbook of Natural Medicine,* Third Edition, Volumes 1 and 2. St. Louis: Churchill Livingstone, 2006, 1085–1087.

[2] Hingdon, J. "Glycemic Index." Linus Pauling Institute at Oregon State University. 19 Dec. 2005. <http://lpi.oregonstate.edu/infocenter/foods/grains/ gigl.html>

[3] J. K. Ransley and D. C. Greenwood, "Does the Fruit and Vegetable Scheme Improve Children's Diet? A Non-Randomized Control Study," *Epidemial Community Health* 61 (2007): 699–703.

[4] Prior, R., Cao, J. and Shukitt-Hale B, "Can Foods Forestall Aging?" *Agricultural Research*, February 1999, 15–17.

Chapter 8 References

[1] B. T. Hunter, "America's Eating Habits," *Consumer Research* 83.20 (2000): 10–15.

[2] David A. Levitsky and Trisha Youn, "The More Food Young Adults Are Served, the More They Overeat," *Journal of Nutrition* 134 (2004): 2546–2549.

[3] S. J. Nielson and B. M. Popkin, "Patterns and Trends in Food Portion Sizes, 1977–1978," *Journal of the American Medical Association* 289.4 (2003): 450–453.

[4] M. B. Schultz, J. E. Manson, D. S. Ludwig, et al. "Sugar sweetened beverages, weight gain, and incidence of diabetes Type II in young and middle aged women," *Journal of the American Medical Association* 292.8 (2004): 927–934.

[5] Brian Wansink and Jeffery Sobal, "Mindless Eating: The 200 Daily Food Decisions We Overlook," *Environment and Behavior* 39.1 (2007): 106–123.

[6] John S. A. Edwards, Katja Engström, and Heather J. Hartwell, "Overweight, obesity and the food service industry," *Food Service Technology* 5.2-4 (2005): 85–94.

[7] Eric Turkheimer, Andreana Haley, Mary Waldron, Brian D'Onofrio, and Irving I. Gottesman, "Socioeconomic status modifies heritability of IQ in young children," *Psychological Science* 14.6 (2003): 623–628.

[8] Denis Lairon, "Dietary fiber and control of body weight," *Journal of Nutrition, Metabolism and Cardiovascular Disease* 17.1 (2007): 1–5.

[9] Douglas A. Raynor, Suzanne Phelan, James O. Hill, and Rena R. Wing, "Television Viewing and Long-Term Weight Maintenance: Results from the National Weight Control Registry," *Obesity* 14.10 (2006): 1816–1824.

Chapter 9 References

[1] Hellmich, Nanci. "Research Fleshes Out the Benefits of Exercise." *USA Today.* 24 April 2007. <http://www.usatoday.com/news/health/2007-10-23-exercise-maintenance_n.htm>

[2] Mayo Clinic Staff. "Exercise: 7 benefits of regular physical activity." *Mayo Clinic.com.* 26 July 2007. <http://www.mayoclinic.com/health/exercise/HQ01676>

[3] Centers for Disease Control and Prevention. "The Link Between Physical Activity and Mortality and Morbidity." *Physical Activity and Health.* 17 Nov. 1999. <http://www.cdc.gov/nccdphp/sgr/mm.htm>

[4] Doyle, J. Andrew, "The Benefits of Exercise," The Exercise and Physical Fitness Page. 6 Nov. 1997. <http://www2.gsu.edu/~wwwfit/benefits.html>

[5] Centers for Disease Control and Prevention. "Why should I be active?" Physical Activity for Everyone. 22 May 2007. <http://www.cdc.gov/nccdphp/dnpa/physical/importance/why.htm>

[6] Gerald F. Fletcher, Gary Balady, Steven N. Blair, et al. "Statement on Exercise: Benefits and Recommendations for Physical Activity Programs for All Americans." *Circulation* 94 (1996): 857–862.

[7] NutriStrategy. "Health Benefits of Exercise." *NutriStrategy.com*. 2005. <http://www.nutristrategy.com/health.htm>

[8] Eloi F. Rosa, Antonio C. Silva, Silvia S. M. Ihara, et al. "Habitual exercise program protects murine intestinal, skeletal, and cardiac muscles against aging." *Journal of Applied Physiology* 99 (2005): 1569–1575.

[9] Mayo Clinic Staff. "Strength training: OK for kids when done correctly." *MayoClinic.com*. 11 Jan 2008. <http://www.mayoclinic.com/health/strength-training/HQ01010>

[10] Mendosa, David. "New Exercise Guidelines." MyDiabetesCentral.com. 2 Aug. 2007. <http://www.healthcentral.com/diabetes/c/17/11958/exercise-guidelines>

[11] W. L. Haskell. "Physical Activity and Public Health: Updated Recommendation for Adults from the American College of Sports Medicine and the American Heart Association." *Medicine & Science in Sports & Exercise* 39 (2007): 1423–1434.

[12] Antronette K. Yancey, Paul A. Simon, William J. McCarthy, et al. "Ethnic and Sex Variations in Overweight Self-perception: Relationship to Sedentariness." *Obesity* 14 (2006): 980–988.

[13] Mayo Clinic Staff. "Aerobic exercise: What 30 minutes a day can do." *MayoClinic.com*. 16 Feb. 2007. <http://www.mayoclinic.com/health/aerobic-exercise/EP00002>

[14] Centers for Disease Control and Prevention. "Fact Sheets." *Physical Activity and Health: A Report of the Surgeon General*. 17 Nov. 1999. <http://www.cdc.gov/nccdphp/sgr/fact.htm>

[15] James O. Hill. "Walking and Type 2 Diabetes." *Diabetes Care* 28. (2005): 1524–1525. Also: E.S. Horton. "Role and management of exercise in diabetes mellitus." *Diabetes Care* 11.2 (1988): 201–211.

[16] America on the Move Foundation. "Help us turn September into Steptember." *Planning Guide and Sample Presentation*. September 2007. <http://www.americaonthemove.org/steptember/2007PDF/Planning_Guide_and_Sample_Proclamation.pdf>

[17] Jason L. Talanian, Stuart D. R. Galloway, George J. F. Heigenhauser, Arend Bonen, and Lawrence L. Spriet, "Two Weeks of High-Intensity Aerobic Interval Training Increases the Capacity for Fat Oxidation During Exercise in Women," Journal of Applied Psychology 102: 1439–1447, 2007.

[18] National Diabetes Education Program. "Overview of Diabetes in Children and Adolescents." *Fact Sheet from the National Diabetes Education Program*. <http://www.ndep.nih.gov/diabetes/youth/youth_FS.htm#Exercise>

[20] Weight Control Information Network. "Waist circumference." *Weight and Waist Measurements: Tools for Adults*. June 2007. <http://win.niddk.nih.gov/publications/tools.htm#circumf>

Chapter 10 References

[1] N. A. Christakis and James H. Fowler. "The Spread of Obesity in a Large Social Network Over 32 Years." *New England Journal of Medicine* 357 (2007): 370–379.

Chapter 11 References

[1] Mary F. Dallman, Norman Pecoraro, Susanne E. la Fleur, et al. "Chapter 4: Glucocorticoids, Chronic Stress, and Obesity." *Hypothalamic Integration of Energy Metabolism*, Vol. 153 of *Progress in Brain Research*. Amsterdam: Elsevier, 2006.

[2] Mary F. Dallman, Norman Pecoraro, Susan F. Akana, et al. "Chronic stress and obesity: A new view of 'comfort food.'" *Proceedings of the National Academy of Sciences* 100.20 (2003): 11696–701.

[3] Mayo Clinic Staff. "Weight-loss help: How to stop emotional eating." *MayoClinic.com.* 1 Dec. 2007. <http://www.mayoclinic.com/health/weight-loss/MH00025>

[4] Crawford-Clark, Brenda. "Stress and Eating." *WebMD.* 20 Oct. 2005. <http://www.webmd.com/content/chat_transcripts/2/111279.htm?pagenumber=2>

[5] Elissa Epel, Sherlyn Jimenez, Kelly Brownell, Laura Stroud, Catherine Stoney, Ray Niaura. "Are Stress Eaters at Risk for the Metabolic Syndrome?" *Annals of the New York Academy of Sciences* 1032 (2004): 208–210.

[6] American Heart Association. "What is the metabolic syndrome?" *Metabolic Syndrome.* 2008. <http://www.americanheart.org/presenter.jhtml?identifier=4756>

Chapter 13 References

[1] "Obese Children Show Early Signs Of Heart Disease." *ScienceDaily.* 20 Oct. 2007. <http://www.sciencedaily.com/releases/2007/10/071017131917.htm>

[2] Woodrow Wilson School of Public and International Affairs: Princeton University–Brookings Institution. "*The Future of Children: Obesity* 16.1 (2006). <http://www.futureofchildren.org/usr_doc/Obesity_Volume_16,_Number_1_Spring_2006.pdf>

[3] Philip R. Nader. "Identifying Risk for Obesity in Early Childhood." *Pediatrics* 118.3 (2006): e594–e601.

ABOUT THE AUTHOR

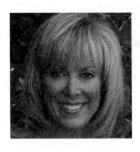 **Amy Hendel, R-PA, IDEA, ASCM**, is a popular and recognizable medical and lifestyle reporter, expert, columnist, and health host. In addition to her Master's Level R-PA (Registered Physician Assistant), Hendel is also certified in nutrition and exercise physiology and has combined her PA degree with this background in nutrition/exercise physiology to create a private family lifestyle therapy, physician-referred practice that has been helping individuals and families for more than twenty years. As a Wellness Coach, Ms. Hendel trains and councils patients with her own unique blend of nutrition, fitness, and psychology for the whole family.

Hendel began her media career as a recurring contributor/lifestyle reporter for KCBS on *Women 2 Women* as well as on their afternoon news. There, she completed more than 100 live segments between 1999 and 2002. In all, Hendel has completed more than 1,000 live and taped segments covering medical and health topics, nutrition, exercise, and lifestyle issues. Other noted appearances include: *Today*, *The Early Show*, *Discovery Health*, *The 700 Club*, Fox News, KNBC Morning and Noon News, KABC local news affiliates, *EXTRA!*, *HouseSmarts*, and *Good Day LA*. She is also a print journalist and her work has appeared in the *Los Angeles Times* and the *Los Angeles Daily News*. She has been a quoted guest expert in *Family Circle*, *InStyle* magazine, and *Fit Pregnancy*.

Hendel's book *Fat Families, Thin Families* (BenBella Books, June 2008) was re-released in paperback in June 2010 as *The 4 Habits of Healthy Families*.